DRUGS: APPROVAL AND EVALUATION, DELIVERY AND CONTROL

DRUGS: APPROVAL AND EVALUATION, DELIVERY AND CONTROL

ANNA O. HARTMANN AND LEA K. NEUMANN
EDITORS

Nova Science Publishers, Inc.
New York

For permission to use material from this book please contact us:
Telephone 631-231-7269; Fax 631-231-8175
Web Site: http://www.novapublishers.com

LIBRARY OF CONGRESS CATALOGING-IN-PUBLICATION DATA

Drug approval and evaluation, delivery, and control/Anna O. Hartmann and Lea K. Neumann,(editors).
P.; cm.
Includes bibliographical references and index
ISBN 978-1-60456-533-1(hardcover)
1. Drugs—Testing.2.Drugs—Safety regulations. I. Hartmann,Anna O. II. Neumann,Lea K..[DNLM: 1. Drug Approval.2.Drug Evaluation.3.Drug and Narcotic Control.4.Pharmaceutical Preparations—supply & distribution.QV771 D7934 2008]
RM301.27.D78 2008
615'.1—dc22 2008016253

Published by Nova Science Publishers, Inc. ≃ New York

CONTENTS

PREFACE

This book provides a wide range of research in both illegal and legal drug substances from around the globe such as examinations of FDA approved pharmaceuticals, different methods of drug delivery, and the investigation of illegal distribution of drug products and its effects on substance abuse.

Chapter 1 - Biomagnetism involves the measurement and analysis of weak magnetic fields detected from physiological activity or magnetic sources within the human body. The implementation of biomagnetic methods in pharmaceutical studies as a non-invasive monitoring of drug delivery is currently an alternative to nuclear medicine. This chapter will present a short review of biomagnetic techniques, particularly AC Biosusceptometry (ACB) as an innovative method in pharmaceutical research.

ACB uses induction coils for recording the magnetic flux variation obtained from the response of a magnetic material ingested. This material has a high magnetic susceptibility that produces a strong response when an alternating magnetic field is applied in a biological system containing small amounts of magnetic material

As this technique has been continuously improved, novel instrumental arrangements became a suitable tool not only for gastrointestinal (GI) motility studies but also as an alternative method for pharmaceutical purposes.

A multisensor system was initially implemented to characterize the disintegration process of tablets *in vitro* in the human stomach. Disintegration process was quantified by the transition of a magnetic marker (non-disintegrated dosage form) to a magnetic tracer (disintegrated dosage form). Moreover, ACB was employed to monitor magnetic tablets and hypromellose capsules in human GI tract showing the disintegration in colonic region and intestinal transit.

Imaging techniques provide valuable information on the *in vivo* performance for any dosage forms. ACB was able to characterize the disintegration process through magnetic images introducing a novel concept in imaging of biological systems.

Several pharmaceutical approaches which have been used for targeting drugs to the proximal GI tract are based on gastroretentive drug delivery systems. In addition, colon-specific delivery has renewed interest in the development of therapeutic agents for treating colonic diseases providing systemic absorption of drugs susceptible to enzymatic digestion in upper GI tract.

Recently, ACB has been used in the monitoring of multiparticulate gastroretentive and colonic delivery systems in human GI tract, since multiparticulate systems are ideal for controlled drug delivery and have advantages over single unit formulations.

This magnetic method will be associated with pharmacokinetic parameters ("magnetopharmacokinetics") to predict the drug absorption for optimized pharmacotherapy, deserving the same importance as conventional techniques in pharmaceutical research. Biomagnetic techniques are harmless and have added new insights in the evaluation of solid dosage forms in human GI tract.

Chapter 2 - Innovation in pharmacology can be achieved designing polymer nanoparticles to rationalize drug delivery by enhancing the oral bioavailability of peptides and proteins. New types of formulations were designed during the last couple of years promoting interactions with the mucus for bioadhesion, with the gastro-intestinal fluids for decreasing antiprotease activity and possibly with cells constituting the epithelium to enhance permeability. As they will be presented in the present chapter, they result from the formation of core-shell poly(alkylcyanoacrylate) nanoparticles coated with chitosan and thiolated chitosan. The design and characterization of such core-shell polymer nanoparticles will be described in this chapter. Their evaluation as a tool to improve the bioavailability of peptides and proteins by the oral route will be discussed thanks to data obtained from different *in vitro* models and set ups. The more advanced research will then be presented on the last part of this chapter opening the conclusion and the discussion for future developments.

Chapter 3 - Over the past years the awareness of the importance of intestinal drug transporters for the bioavailability of certain drugs has grown steadily. More and more drugs are being identified as substrates or inhibitors of one or another transporter. Aside from drugs, however, numerous excipients have been found to modulate the functioning of drug transporters, too. Thus, they might also interfere with the absorption of drugs on a physiological level either enhancing or decreasing their absorption.

For developing rational drug formulations it is important to take into account such effects when conceiving a new formulation or redesigning existing formulations. In the first case, choosing the right excipient might result in higher bioavailability or even allow for absorption in the first place. In the second case unwanted changes of the performance of the redesigned dosage form might be prevented. The knowledge of such excipients is also important from a drug regulatory point of view in order to evaluate post-approval changes in the formulation.

This chapter will review the current findings on excipients with modulatory potential on intestinal transporters. With respect to excipients the article will mainly discuss Cremophor EL, Tocopheryl Polyethylenglycol Succinate (TPGS), Polysorbate 80, Pluronic P85, Polyethyleneglycol (PEG), Solutol HS15 and Labrasol. In addition, a comprehensive table of excipients with modulatory effects on drug transporters will be included. With respect to intestinal drug transporters the article will concentrate on interactions between excipients and two important members of the ABC-transporter family (P-glycoprotein and MRP) as well as two members of the solute carrier family (PEPT1 and the monocarboxylate transporter).

The article shall serve both as an introduction and reference for those active in the field of drug formulation or drug regulatory affairs.

Chapter 4 - Vitamin B_6 includes a series of compounds containing the pyridoxal structure, such as pyridoxol, pyridoxamine, pyridoxaldehyde and their derivatives. The pyridoxal structure, the catalytically active form of vitamin B_6, possesses specific hepatocyte uptake by the pyridoxine transporter at the sinusoidal pole because the pyridoxine transporters that exist in hepatocytes can selectively recognize and bind to the pyridoxal structure, and transport it into the cells via a member transport system. Thus pyridoxine can be adopted as a liver-targeting group and be incorporated into the low molecular weight compounds and macromolecules for the use as magnetic resonance imaging (MRI) contrast agents and anticancer conjugates. The research progress of liver-targeting drug delivery system is discussed briefly. Previous researches have demonstrated that the incorporation of pyridoxine into these molecules can increase their uptake by the liver, and that these molecules containing pyridoxine groups exhibit liver-targeting properties.

Chapter 5 - Biomedical research is the largest scientific enterprise; the twentieth century was its golden age. In that period, almost all therapeutic and preventive substances that participated in the doubling of life expectancy of humans were either discovered or synthesized. As natural consequence, the pharmaceutical industry grew immensely to become among the most successful of all economical investments. Human pathology moved from the acute infectious diseases, which were the principal causes of disease along the history, to the chronic degenerative and proliferative disorders, which have become nowadays the most frequent. The therapeutics of human disorders have also changed, from the preventive or curative, brief intervention (vaccines, antibiotics, vitamins, etc.), to the need for chronic, long-lasting ingestion of palliative remedies (antidepressants, antirheumatics, antihypertensives, lipid-lowering drugs, antiepileptics, etc.). This shift has produced an enormous and adverse impact on the economy of patients and medical institutions, together with a huge proliferation of innovative substances that attempt to participate in this lucrative market.

Evaluation by cost-benefit on the pertinence of new (generally expensive) vs. traditional (generally unexpensive) drugs, as well as fairness of new prices and propaganda strategies used by the pharmaceutical industry have become issues of paramount importance for the medical profession, as doctors are the necessary link between patients and drug-producers [1,2]. Nonetheless the ancestral codes of medical practice state undoubtedly that the moral and professional compromises of physicians are only with the patient [3]. Several peculiarities of research, testing and marketing of pharmaceutical substances indicate that novel and imaginative mechanisms of access to new substances must be found in the benefit of patients, particularly those with limited economical means, which are the great majority of humans, whether living in rich or in poor countries.

Chapter 6 - The number of new molecular entities (NMEs) approved in 2006 was 20 in Japan, 24 in US and 25 in EU, respectively. Among 70 NMEs approved in both Japan and US and/or EU during 2002 to 2006, 69 NMEs had been approved in US and 35 in EU by 2006, and there was only one common approval solely between Japan and EU. On the other hand, 39 NMEs were solely approved in US and EU during this period. Among 109 NMEs approved in either two or three regions, the number of preceding NMEs was 3 in Japan, 85 in US and 21 in EU.

Chapter 7 - The public health strategy to conquer tuberculosis is focused on primary prevention. Normally with an infectious disease, this would entail the use of a vaccine but, in the case of tuberculosis, the vaccine currently available acts as secondary prevention: it does not prevent infection but rather, prevents progress from infection to disease during the phase of dissemination following primary infection. Consequently, the approach to primary prevention differs for tuberculosis as compared with other infectious diseases; focus on the 'control' of the patients who are the most potent sources of transmission of the contagion. In order to understand this focus, and its difference from other infectious diseases, it would be important to understand the sequence of events that leads to disease with tuberculosis and to transmission of its causative organism, *Mycobacterium tuberculosis* and the role of various interventions in cutting this 'chain of transmission'.

Chapter 8 - For more than 160 years anesthetic techniques are being carried out, in order to facilitate surgical procedures without pain sensation. Sufficient, reliable and reproducible control of anesthetic depth is of essential importance in modern anesthetic practice. Unnecessary deep anesthesia may lead to hemodynamic deterioration or prolonged emergence in case of high dose administration of anesthetic agents. Inadequate low anesthetic depth may lead to intraoperative awareness and recall, a frightening event for patients. Some of them may develop a posttraumatic stress disorder (PTSD) and need psychotherapeutic support for several years.

Chapter 9 - More than three decades have passed since Richard Nixon became the first U.S. president to declare "war" on drugs, and despite the investment of billions toward eradicating the abuse of substances such as cocaine and heroin, public officials continue to witness sustained use of the very drugs Nixon, followed by Ronald Reagan and George H. W. Bush, sought to curtail. To keep up the fight, as it were, and to keep at least part of the U.S. population in support of it, political actors who support the "war" on drugs have had to ensure that new threats continually emerge, thus allowing officials to call for intensified efforts and "new" approaches to the problem. Examining heroin reports in the *New York Times* and the *Los Angeles Times* from 1988 to 2003, this article identifies several enemies in the U.S. drug war, including the "Golden Triangle" (i.e., Laos, Thailand and Myanmar), the "Indian Connection," the "Nigerian Connection" and the "Notorious Bekaa Valley" in Lebanon. "Russian drug gangs" and "porous European borders" were also to blame for heroin problems during the last decade of the 20th century.

Chapter 10 - The existence of deterministic processes behind the beat-to-beat fluctuations of heart rate has been postulated since the 1970´s. As autonomic balance is believed to be one major driving force behind this phenomenon heart rate variability (HRV) and its measurement have attracted significant attention from several medical disciplines including neurology, cardiology, somnology, anaesthesiology and intensive care. The large number of methods that have been developed to analyse HRV not only reflects the wide range of information that can be gained from this parameter but also the fact, that there is no single algorithm that can be considered generally suitable for this task.

A short overview of the two basic classes of HRV algorithms (time domain and frequency domain methods) and their application will be given. The mathematical validity of Fourier Transform (FT), the most prevailing algorithm for frequency domain analysis, will be critically discussed. Wavelet Transform (WT) will be proposed as a possible alternative that does not share FT's theoretical limitations for this application.

Chapter 11 - Efforts to significantly reduce the flow of illicit drugs from abroad into the United States have so far not succeeded. Moreover, over the past decade, worldwide production of illicit drugs has risen dramatically: opium and marijuana production has roughly doubled and coca production tripled. Street prices of cocaine and heroin have fallen significantly in the past 20 years, reflecting increased availability. The effectiveness of international narcotics control programs in reducing consumption is a matter of ongoing concern. Despite apparent national political resolve to deal with the drug problem, inherent contradictions regularly appear between U.S. anti-drug policy and other national policy goals and concerns. Pursuit of drug control policies can sometimes affect foreign policy interests and bring political instability and economic dislocation to countries where narcotics production has become entrenched economically and socially. Drug supply interdiction programs and U.S. systems to facilitate the international movement of goods, people, and wealth are often at odds. U.S. international narcotics policy requires cooperative efforts by many nations which may have domestic and foreign policy goals that compete with the requirements of drug control. The mix of competing domestic and international pressures and priorities has produced an ongoing series of disputes within and between the legislative and executive branches concerning U.S. international drug policy. One contentious issue has been the Congressionally-mandated certification process, an instrument designed to induce specified drug-exporting countries to prioritize or pay more attention to the fight against narcotics businesses. Current law requires the President, with certain exceptions, to designate and withhold assistance from countries that have failed demonstrably to meet their counternarcotics obligations. P.L. 106-246, "Plan Colombia," a $1.3 billion military assistance-focused initiative to provide emergency supplemental narcotics assistance to Colombia, was signed into law July 13, 2000. Recently, U.S. policy toward Colombia has focused increasingly on containing the terror- ist threat to that country's security. The Bush Administration's FY2005 budget request continues a policy, begun in FY2002, to request authority for the State and Defense Departments to supply assistance to Colombia for counterterrorism purposes. For instance, U.S.-supplied helicopters and intelligence could be used to support military operations against guerrillas financed by drugs as well as against drug traffickers themselves.

An issue likely to achieve increased attention in the 109th Congress is that of sky-rocketing opium poppy cultivation in Afghanistan and whether to press for aerial crop eradication against the wishes of the local Afghan leadership. Drug control approaches addressed in this chapter brief include:

- Expansion of efforts to reduce foreign production at the source.
- Expansion of interdiction and enforcement activities to disrupt supply lines.
- Expansion of efforts to reduce worldwide demand.
- Expansion of economic disincentives for international drug trafficking.

In: Drugs: Approval and Evaluation, Delivery and Control ISBN: 978-1-60456-533-1
Editors: A.O. Hartmann, L.K. Neumann

Chapter 1

BIOMAGNETIC APPROACHES APPLIED TO DRUG DELIVERY STUDIES

L. A. Corá[1], J. R. A. Miranda[1], M. F. Américo[2], R. B. Oliveira[2] and O. Baffa[3]

[1]Dep. Física e Biofísica – IBB, UNESP, Botucatu, São Paulo, Brazil
[2]Dep. Clínica Médica – FMRP, USP, Ribeirão Preto, São Paulo, Brazil
[3]Dep. Física e Matemática – FFCLRP, USP, Ribeirão Preto, São Paulo, Brazil

ABSTRACT

Biomagnetism involves the measurement and analysis of weak magnetic fields detected from physiological activity or magnetic sources within the human body. The implementation of biomagnetic methods in pharmaceutical studies as a non-invasive monitoring of drug delivery is currently an alternative to nuclear medicine. This chapter will present a short review of biomagnetic techniques, particularly AC Biosusceptometry (ACB) as an innovative method in pharmaceutical research.

ACB uses induction coils for recording the magnetic flux variation obtained from the response of a magnetic material ingested. This material has a high magnetic susceptibility that produces a strong response when an alternating magnetic field is applied in a biological system containing small amounts of magnetic material

As this technique has been continuously improved, novel instrumental arrangements became a suitable tool not only for gastrointestinal (GI) motility studies but also as an alternative method for pharmaceutical purposes.

A multisensor system was initially implemented to characterize the disintegration process of tablets *in vitro* in the human stomach. Disintegration process was quantified by the transition of a magnetic marker (non-disintegrated dosage form) to a magnetic tracer (disintegrated dosage form). Moreover, ACB was employed to monitor magnetic tablets and hypromellose capsules in human GI tract showing the disintegration in colonic region and intestinal transit.

Imaging techniques provide valuable information on the *in vivo* performance for any dosage forms. ACB was able to characterize the disintegration process through magnetic images introducing a novel concept in imaging of biological systems.

Several pharmaceutical approaches which have been used for targeting drugs to the proximal GI tract are based on gastroretentive drug delivery systems. In addition, colon-specific delivery has renewed interest in the development of therapeutic agents for treating colonic diseases providing systemic absorption of drugs susceptible to enzymatic digestion in upper GI tract.

Recently, ACB has been used in the monitoring of multiparticulate gastroretentive and colonic delivery systems in human GI tract, since multiparticulate systems are ideal for controlled drug delivery and have advantages over single unit formulations.

This magnetic method will be associated with pharmacokinetic parameters ("magnetopharmacokinetics") to predict the drug absorption for optimized pharmacotherapy, deserving the same importance as conventional techniques in pharmaceutical research. Biomagnetic techniques are harmless and have added new insights in the evaluation of solid dosage forms in human GI tract.

INTRODUCTION

Nowadays, biomagnetic techniques are capable to evaluate conventional dosage forms and also the most sophisticated drug delivery systems in the human gastrointestinal tract. A primary difference of this is the non-invasivity and radiation-free characteristics which are potential advantages over classical methods.

In order to understand how these methods may be employed for pharmaceutical investigation, it is essential to know the complex interactions among the drug, the dosage form and the human gastrointestinal tract. Consequently, it allows optimizing the drug delivery systems to increase the effectiveness of drugs orally administered.

In this chapter, we will discuss a basic knowledge of the Superconducting Quantum Interference Devices (SQUIDs), Magnetoresistive Sensors, Hall-Effect Sensors, and Induction Coils and how these techniques can be applied in the pharmaceutical research.

HUMAN GASTROINTESTINAL TRACT – THE TARGET

Despite some disadvantages oral administration remains the most common route for drug delivery. Moreover, the gastrointestinal (GI) tract is an appropriate site for drug absorption. Absorption of an orally administered drug from the gastrointestinal tract can be regarded as a part of a serial process that includes the drug release by the disintegration of the dosage form, the dissolution of the drug, the solubility and physicochemical properties and its effective permeability coefficient.

Additionally, physiological properties of the GI tract such as the diameter, length and surface area, pH profile, the gastric emptying, the intestinal transit times and the GI motility are the major determining factors in bioavailability of the drug and can limit the absorbed fraction dose.

Gastrointestinal tract is a complex environment and presents regional differences that must be fully investigated to provide more reliable information when a local or systemic effect is desirable.

Absorption from Stomach, Small Intestine and Colon

The primary function of the stomach is the digestion, to perform this function this organ is subdivided into two compartments performing different functions. The proximal region acts as a reservoir whereas the distal stomach has a grinding and mixing capacity. The coordinated actions of these regions allow the gastric emptying to the duodenum at a required rate. The thick mucus layer with a small surface area and high electrical resistance limits the absorption process in the stomach.

In contrast, the small intestine has an extremely large surface area with low electrical resistance which facilitates the absorption of nutrients and, consequently, most of the drugs. The absorption process in the small intestine is modulated by motor activity including aboral movement of its content and by chemical digestive process.

The colon is a suitable site for the slow absorption of drugs which are targeted at the large intestine or designed to act systemically. Colonic physiology is complex and influenced by many factors including diet, bacterial metabolism, and also colonic mixing and transit time. Compared with the small intestine, the colon has a lower surface area that is compensated by the slow transit rate, which provides a significant opportunity for the absorption of drugs and other materials.

Gastrointestinal Variables

The dynamic interaction between the gastrointestinal tract variables and the orally administered dosage form determine the rate and extent of drug absorption. The major physiological variables are gastrointestinal motility, gastric emptying time, intestinal transit time and pH. Moreover, the physicochemical properties of a drug such as solubility and particle size, beyond the formulation parameters including controlled-release mechanism, pH sensitivity, size, shape and density can also affect the absorption. An understanding of the factors involved in drug absorption and how the gastrointestinal variables can interfere with this process is important to develop more reliable drug delivery system.

Gastrointestinal Motility

The gastrointestinal tract is structurally complex and its functions depend on coordinating actions. The gastrointestinal smooth muscle has the ability to produce coordinated motion which is called motility. Hence, the knowledge of the motility aspects is fundamental to understand the gastrointestinal physiological functions and how the interactions between these parameters and the orally administered solid dosage forms can interfere with drug release.

Spatial and temporal patterns of contractions or relaxation of smooth muscle cells and their integration are modulated by a complex neuro-hormonal regulatory system control. Basically, gastrointestinal motility is organized into two motor patterns according to the prandial state.

After cessation of the digestive processes a cyclic motility pattern, called interdigestive migrating motor complex (MMC) initiates. This pattern is organized into alternating cycles of activity and quiescence, as illustrated in Figure 1. Phase I is characterized by a period of motor quiescence; phase II consists of an irregular phasic contractile activity; and phase III presents a short period of intense and rhythmic contractions, termed *housekeeper waves* (Quigley, 1996). During the phase III occurs the emptying of indigestible particles, including solid dosage forms, retained in the stomach. Contractile waves of the MMC propagate distally from the stomach to the terminal ileum and are interrupted by food ingestion. Phase IV is the transition period between phases III and I.

With the ingestion of food the MMC is replaced by the fed pattern characterized by contractions of variable amplitude and frequency according to gastrointestinal segment (Hasler, 1995). This pattern persists as long as the bulk of food remains in the stomach and depends on multiple factors including energy content, volume, and the nature of nutrients.

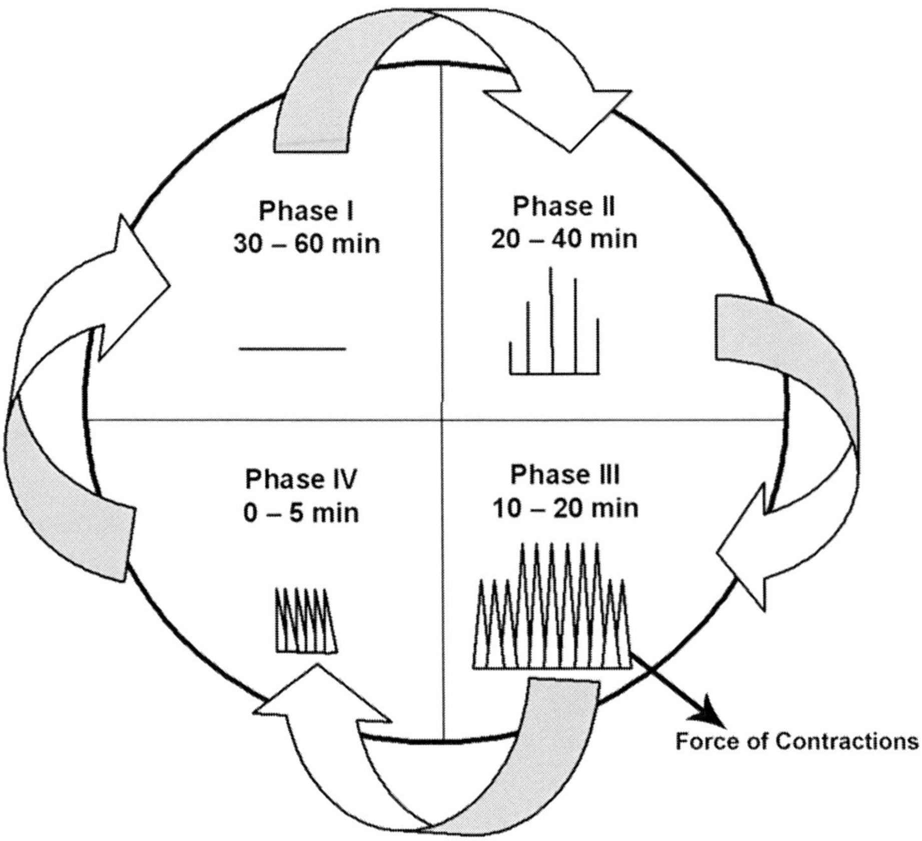

Figure 1. Interdigestive gastrointestinal motility pattern (Modified from Chawla et al, 2003).

Contractions are based on electrophysiological properties of smooth muscle and triggered by a non-neural pacemaker system in the wall of the gut known as interstitial cells of Cajal. Electrical activity propagates through the gut because every region of phasic muscle has intrinsic pacemaker capability (Camilleri, 2006). However, the necessary discontinuity in the pacemaker cell network between segments of the gastrointestinal tract generates a pacemaker frequency gradient. The frequency registered in the stomach is approximately 3 contractions per minute (cpm), reaching 11-12 cpm in the duodenum with decreasing gradient to distal ileum. In the colon two rhythms appears to occur: a frequency of 5-6 cpm and another around 3 cpm (Rao & Schulze-Delrieu, 1993; Frexinos & Delvaux, 1993). Moreover, the human colon presents a duality of the motility pattern: phasic contractions ensure the mixing and the aboral progression of colonic contents while the tonic activity acts as a brake. Thus, complexity of the electrical motor activity, differences in recording techniques and methods of data analysis might explain the discrepancies observed until now in this frequency gradient.

Motility patterns determine the rate of transit and residence time for pharmaceutical dosage forms in the human gastrointestinal tract, and hence the drug release.

Gastric Emptying

Gastric emptying of solid and liquids are controlled by coordinated actions promoting changes in gastric tone and the propagating gastric peristalsis. Gastric emptying depends mainly on nutrient content, viscosity and volume of the meals.

Ingested non-caloric liquids are rapidly distributed throughout the entire stomach and the emptying begins immediately in a first-order exponential process directly proportional to the volume. On the other hand, solid particles empty from the stomach by fundamentally zero-order kinetics that is independent of gastric volume. Hence, the gastric emptying of solids shows a *lag phase*, where the solids are redistributed and broken down to smaller particles able to pass through the pylorus during the *linear phase*(Siegel et al, 1988). Figure 2 gives an overview of the biphasic characteristic of the gastric emptying of solids.

Gastric emptying rate plays an important role in determining the gastric retention time of oral dosage forms. Density, size and shape of the dosage form, concomitant ingestion of food, simultaneous administration of drugs affecting gastrointestinal motility and biological factors, such as gender, posture, age, sleep, body mass index, physical activity and disease states are the most important parameters influencing gastric emptying rate.

The relationship between the tablet size and its gastric emptying varies significantly among the subjects. Indigestible solids including non-disintegrating dosage forms larger than the pyloric opening remains retained in the stomach for as long as the digestive phase is maintained and are emptied during the passage of the housekeeper wave.

Multiple-unit systems containing pellets pass through the constricted pylorus with a gradual emptying profile. Pellets administered with a light meal follow an initial short lag phase and a linear emptying pattern. A delay gastric emptying occurs when pellets are administered with a heavy meal. Therefore, the prandial state is the primary consideration for modulating gastric residence time in relation to drug administration. While feeding substantially delays the gastric emptying of large single-unit preparations, little effect is observed on the emptying of multi-unit preparations which leave the stomach at rates similar to fasting.

On the other hand, prolonged gastric retention of the dosage form provides an excellent opportunity for drug absorption, especially for drugs with an absorption window in the upper gastrointestinal tract.

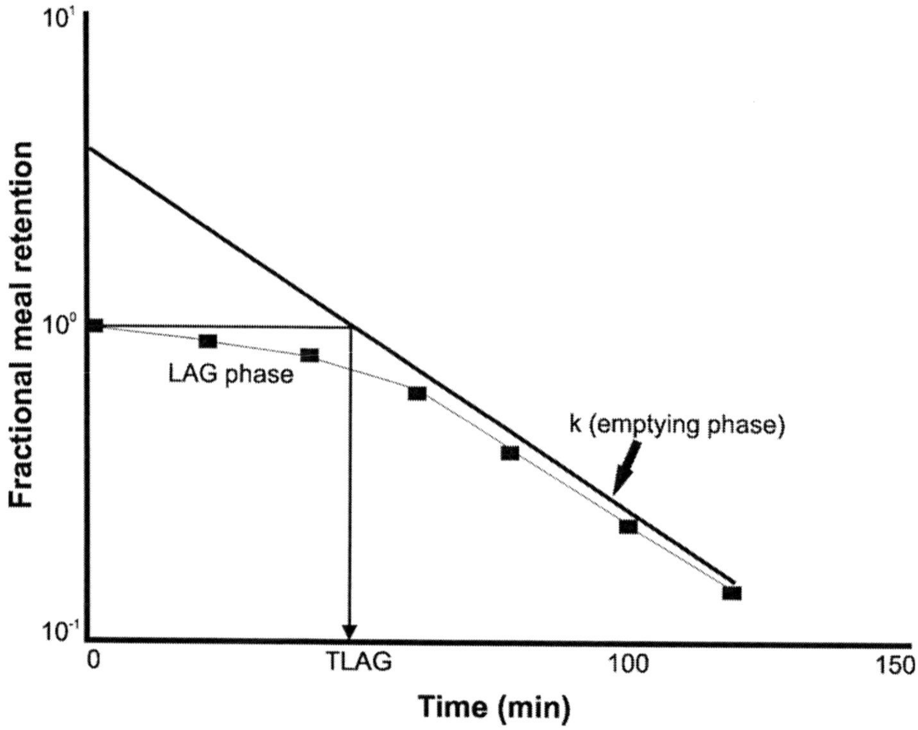

Figure 2. Solid emptying curve fitted of the function $y = 1-(1-e^{-kt})^{\beta}$. The *lag phase* is indicated by *TLAG* and *k* is the emptying rate. (From Siegel et al, 1988).

Gastrointestinal Transit

Propulsion of the contents of the small bowel is dependent on the lumen, intestinal wall tone, and the amplitude of intestinal phasic contractions. Age and gender have no effect; however, intersubject variability is expressive.

Similar to the gastric emptying, intestinal transit is influenced by the MMC activity. After a meal, the distribution of small intestinal contents is more uniform and the transit is faster than during the interdigestive period.

For pharmaceutical purposes, the transit of a dosage form through the gastrointestinal tract determines how long a compound remains in contact with its absorptive site. The bioavailability of a drug can be affected by factors that change gastrointestinal transit.

As demonstrated by Davis et al (1986) small intestinal transit time of pharmaceutical dosage forms in humans is relatively constant at around three to four hours and appears to be independent of both the type of dosage form and prandial state.

Compared with the stomach and small intestine, the colon moves its contents slowly. The slow rate of colonic transit is an excellent opportunity to drug delivery since the drug remains in contact with the mucosa for a longer period than in the small intestine. The residence time in any particular segment of the colon determines the absorption at that site.

Total colonic transit tends to be highly variable and is influenced by factors such as diet, mainly dietary fiber content; stress, disease, drugs and type of pharmaceutical form. When the dosage forms reach the colon, the transit depends on its size since the colonic transit of small units is slower than large ones. Hence, there may be advantages in formulating multi-unit dosage forms for colonic drug delivery to ensure that the entire drug will be released during the transit time.

Gastrointestinal fluids and pH

Drug absorption and clinical response from an orally administered dosage form depends on drug solubility in the gastrointestinal contents and the surface area. Aqueous solubility, crystalline form, drug lipophilicity and pK in relation to the gastrointestinal pH profile determine the solubility of a drug. The dissolution rate of a drug is a function of the surface area and diffusion coefficient of the compound in the dissolution media. Variability in the constituents of the gastrointestinal fluids such as electrolytes, enzymes, bile acids will affect the dissolution and consequently the absorption and bioavailability of drugs.

The pH gradient in the human gastrointestinal tract is one of the most important influences on the solubility of ionizable drugs. The gastrointestinal pH is not constant; rather it is influenced by factors such as diet, disease, gases, fatty acids, and other fermentation products exhibiting intra- and inter-subject variation. This variation in pH may significantly influence the performance of orally administered drugs.

The mean value of gastric pH in fasted healthy subjects is 1.10 ± 0.15. In addition, the mean gastric pH in fed state in healthy subjects arises to 3.60 ± 0.4 and returns to basal level in about 2 to 4 hours.

Evans et al (1988) reported that the mean pH in the proximal small intestine and terminal ileum is 6.6 ± 0.5 and $7.5 + 0.4$, respectively. There is a decrease in pH to a mean of 6.4 ± 0.4 in the caecum, apparently due to the presence of short-chain fatty acids produced by bacterial fermentation of dietary fiber. The pH then rises progressively from the right to the left colon, with a final value of 7.0 ± 0.7. The variation in the pH profile is exploited as an alternative to deliver drugs in a controlled manner.

ORAL DRUG DELIVERY

Oral administration is a widely accepted route for drug delivery, mainly due to patient's acceptance. For this reason, solid dosage forms are often chosen since it affords of advantages such as stability, ease to ingestion, and convenience of dosing.

When a solid dosage form is administered, the active substance has to be released first so that it can be absorbed. If this process is slow or incomplete the bioavailability of a drug will be inadequate. Therefore, the appropriate choice of excipients and its consistency of performance have critical importance to the formulation development.

The pharmaceutical development of solid dosage forms is a key focus to assure the product quality. The challenge is to use a therapeutic agent whose clinical response can be predicted among individuals or to establish the in vitro drug release information to in vivo drug profiles.

Drug Release from Tablets and Capsules

Tablets and capsules are still the most popular solid dosage forms due to ease of manufacture, convenience of dosing and stability. Active substances are available for absorption after release from solid dosage form by the disintegration process. The disintegration is a time-dependent process that promotes a fast fragmentation of the dosage form under the action of disintegrants (Melia & Davis, 1989). Appropriate choice of disintegrant and its consistency of performance have critical importance to the formulation development.

Proposed mechanisms for the action of disintegrants include water uptake through wicking, swelling, deformation or particle repulsion. However, the swelling of disintegrant particles is perhaps the most widely accepted mechanism for tablet disintegration since almost all disintegrants swell to some extent. A detailed revision about the mechanism of action of disintegrants was reported by Lowenthal, 1972.

The most important quality parameter of drug formulations is bioavailability, which is limited by the extent and rate of drug release. The bioavailability is strongly influenced by the type of dosage form, the properties of its components, and the production methods. Because of its influence on the bioavailability of drugs administrated on conventional tablets, Caramela et al (1988) described a mathematical approach to analyze the disintegration process. According to this model, the disintegration force as a function of time is dependent of compression force. Hence, an increase in the compression force causes a reduction of tablet porosity and, as a consequence, a linear increase of the disintegration time.

Differences in the qualities of excipients as particle size distributions, surface properties and impurities can alter the chemical, physical, and biopharmaceutical properties of solid dosage forms.

In vitro – In vivo Correlation

A good understanding and application of the concept of the *in-vitro* and *in-vivo* correlation (IVIVC) is essential for pharmaceutical development of solid dosage forms. The concept of IVIVC refers to a mathematical model describing the relationship between *in vitro* drug dissolution characteristics and *in vivo* bioavailability parameters. Five correlation levels based on the suitable correlation reflecting the complete plasma drug profile following the dosage form administration is defined (Demírtürk et al, 2003; Emami, 2006).

Level A is the highest category of correlation and represents the point-to-point relationship between *in vitro* dissolution profile and *in vivo* absorption rate. In this correlation level, percent of drug absorbed can be calculated by methods such as Wagner-Nelson, Loo-Riegelman or numerical deconvolution. The objective of a Level A correlation is to achieve a direct measurement of *in vitro* dissolution profile able to predict the *in vivo* performance.

Level B correlation utilizes statistical moment analysis to compare the *in vitro* mean dissolution time (MDT_{vitro}) to *in vivo* mean dissolution time (MDT_{vivo}) or mean residence time (MRT_{vivo}). MDT_{vitro} is the mean time for the drug to dissolve under *in vitro* dissolution medium. MDT_{vivo} is defined as the mean time for *in vivo* drug dissolution from a dosage form and the MRT_{vivo} is the time that the drug remains in the body. This level does not reflect a point-to-point correlation and cannot alone predict a reliable *in vivo* bioavailability data.

In the Level C correlation, one dissolution time point ($t_{50\%}$ or $t_{90\%}$) is compared to one mean pharmacokinetics parameters such as the traditional area under the plasma concentration time curve (AUC), t_{max} or C_{max} as a single point correlation. The doses not represent the complete plasma drug concentration curve which is fundamental for an ideal indicative of the dosage form performance. Therefore, this level represents a partial relationship between dissolution and absorption limiting to predict *in vivo* data.

Multiple-level C relates one or several pharmacokinetics suitable parameters to the amount of drug dissolved at several points of the dissolution profile. In this level, a relationship between *in vivo* performance and *in vitro* data can be demonstrated by providing a correlation over the entire dissolution profile and one or more pharmacokinetics parameters.

Level D is a qualitative analysis, not a formal correlation, but helpful in the development of formulation or processing.

An IVIVC is developed concerning formulating parameters, dissolution conditions and pharmacokinetics/pharmacodynamics models. Based on Biopharmaceutical Classification Systems (BCS), the permeability of a drug is a key factor in establishing the feasibility of a formulation and the interpretation of the observed *in vivo* absorption profile of a dosage form (Amidon et al, 1995). Thus, BCS allows estimating the contribution of dissolution, solubility and intestinal permeability in the rate and extending of drug absorption from solid oral dosage forms.

According to knowledge of the solubility and permeability characteristics of specific drugs, it is possible to predict which variables can alter the drug absorption from orally administered dosage forms. In the BCS, pharmaceutical compounds are classified based solely on its solubility and intestinal permeability.

Class I drugs exhibit a high solubility and high permeability and are well absorbed. IVIVC is expected if dissolution rate is slower than gastric emptying. Class II compounds presents low solubility, high permeability and exhibit dissolution-rate limited absorption. IVIVC is expected if *in vitro* and *in vivo* dissolution rate are similar. Class III groups drugs that presents high solubility and low permeability, with high variability in rate and extent of absorption. This variation can be attributed to gastrointestinal transit, luminal contents and membrane permeation rather than dosage form characteristics. As absorption rate is controlled by permeability, limited or no IVIVC is expected. Class IV are low solubility and low permeability compounds with poor oral bioavailability.

Following this classification, IVIVC is generally expected for highly permeable drugs or drugs under dissolution rate-limiting conditions. The AC Biosusceptometry may be useful as a tool to correlate *in vitro* drug release information to the *in vivo* profile considering the lack of techniques able to provide this kind of analysis. The effectiveness of IVIV correlation from theory to practice has been recognized to minimize the need for additional bioavailability studies in the formulation design.

Formulation Strategies for Delivery Systems

Strategies to designing oral solid dosage forms and delivery systems to release drugs at optimal rate to improve the therapeutic effectiveness and to minimize adverse effects are desirable.

The enhancement of therapeutic efficacy of a drug depends on the clinical condition of the patient, its mechanism of action, including side effects, the dose–response relationship, its biopharmaceutical and physicochemical properties, and its route of administration. Modern pharmaceutical approaches for delivering drugs in a controlled manner include gastroretentive and colonic systems.

Gastroretentive Systems

A variety of drugs are characterized by a narrow absorption window in the upper gastrointestinal tract. An absorption window exists due to physiological or physicochemical factors, including the pH profile, and the presence of certain enzymes in a specific gastrointestinal region.

Pharmaceutical dosage forms with gastroretentive properties are able to delivery drugs with narrow absorption window in a controlled manner by releasing the drug for a prolonged period of time, supplying continuously its absorption site. This approach has applications for local drug delivery to the stomach and proximal small intestine ensuring optimal bioavailability (Davis, 2005). Furthermore, gastric retention provides better availability and therapeutic effectiveness of drugs with substantial benefits for patients.

Figure 3 illustrates the possibilities to achieve gastric retention based on swelling, mucoadhesive, hydrogel, floating or high-density systems. Floating dosage forms are low-density single or multi-unit systems that have sufficient buoyancy to float over the gastric contents providing continuously drug release at the desired rate. Floating systems improve the absorption of various drugs in the upper gastrointestinal tract, however cannot provide for a long gastroretentive effect. In addition, the effect is dependent on the amount of food and liquid within the stomach, which makes these systems relatively unstable.

High-density systems are based on the assumption that the dosage forms might be positioned in the lower part of the antrum and generally are made of heavy materials. Initially these systems appeared as greatly promising, but the main disadvantages are the dependence on the prandial state and the need to use relatively large and heavy structures for obtaining the desired effect.

Mucoadhesive systems are intended to extend the gastric retention by adhering them to the gastric mucous membrane by hydration, bonding, or receptor mediated. Several natural or synthetic polymers have been exploited to control as well as to prolong the gastric retention. The main drawback of these systems is the susceptibility to adhere to diverse particles in the stomach. In addition, the pH-dependent behavior of bioadhesive materials can reduce acidity of the gastric juice decreasing the adhesive properties and, hence, the gastroretentive effect.

Swelling systems are constituted by polymers promoting the swelling to a size that prevents their passage through pyloric sphincter resulting in prolonged gastric retention. However, a balance between the rate and extent of swelling and the rate of erosion of the polymer is the key to achieve optimum benefits and to avoid side effects.

Indeed, the challenge to the development of successful gastroretentive system is to overcome differences in gastric physiology as well as inter-subject variability influencing substantially on the retention time and drug release.

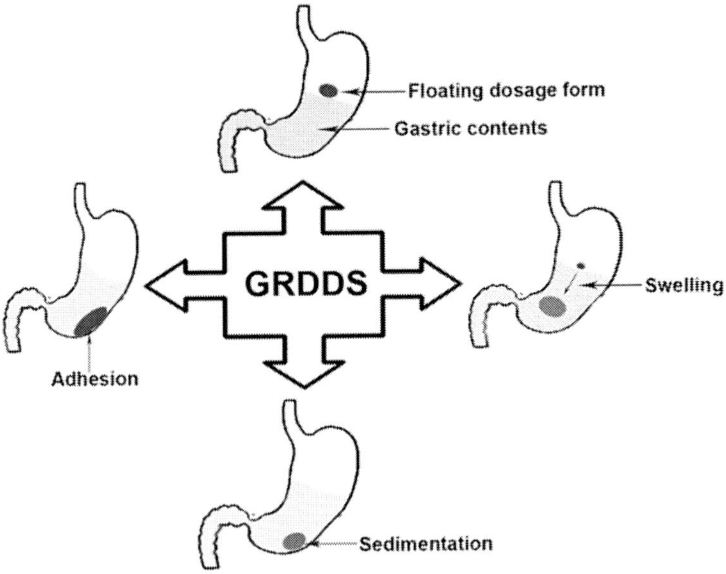

Figure 3. Gastroretentive techniques based on floating, swelling, high-density and mucoadhesive delivery systems. (Modified from Chawla et al, 2003).

Colonic Drug Delivery

Specific targeting of drugs to the colon is potentially useful not just for the topical treatment of intestinal diseases but also for the delivery of therapeutic peptides and proteins. Pharmaceutical approaches include the development of colonic delivery systems to maximize the effectiveness of these drugs.

Therapeutic strategies proposed for colonic targeting rely on the gastrointestinal features for their functionality such as pH, transit time, pressure or microflora. Concerning these characteristics, orally administered colonic drug delivery is based on four main mechanisms including bacterially triggered, pressure-controlled, pH-dependent, time-dependent; or CODES™ systems (Chourasia & Jain, 2003; Schareef et al, 2003).

Colonic microflora is constituted by complex microorganisms whose physiological functions playing vital roles in health and disease. Microbially degradable polymers and certain plant polysaccharides are used for colon target drug delivery systems. The linkage between the drug and the polymer is susceptible to enzymatic degradation in the colon and the drug is released. These systems appear to be promising because of their practicality and exploitation of abundant colonic microflora.

A wide range of suitable polymers are available for the use as enteric coating for tablets, capsules or multi-unit dosage forms. In the development of colonic delivery systems, the major progress was made with the introduction of semi-synthetic cellulose derivatives as well as synthetic polymethacrylates with specific solubility properties according to the pH conditions of the gastrointestinal tract. Despite of inherent limitations, pH controlled delivery systems are widely accepted due to its functionality and effectiveness ensuring excellent performance for the product.

Timed release systems are based on the delaying of the drug release until it reaches into the colon. Pulsincap® was developed using this principle; it is similar to a conventional hard gelatin capsule, however, the body is water insoluble. The drug is enclosed within the body by a hydrogel plug that is covered by a water-soluble cap. The whole unit is coated with an enteric polymer to avoid the drug release in an undesirable site. Once the cap is dissolved, the hydrogel swells and the drug is released. Time Clock® is another system proposed and it is composed of a solid core coated with hydrophobic material, surfactant, and water soluble polymer. After a predetermined time interval, the polymer is dissolved and the drug is slowly released.

Pressure controlled delivery systems are based on relatively strong colonic contraction waves that leads to luminal pressure. These systems are constituted by capsules coated with water-soluble polymers (cellulose derivatives). Colonic peristalsis causes the rupture of the system and release the drug.

CODES™ technology was developed as a colonic specific drug delivery to avoid the limitations associated with pH- or time-dependent systems. CODES™ systems use polysaccharides that are degraded by colonic microflora in combination with three layers of pH-dependent polymers: the inner layer is an acid-soluble polymer, the outer layer is an enteric coated barrier and the core contains the drug, as shown in Figure 4.

Significant benefits were achieved with the development of technologies for colonic target of drugs. Colon-specific delivery systems based on the mechanisms exploited above are sufficiently reliable for most applications and also, in some cases, they are relatively inexpensive and easy to manufacture.

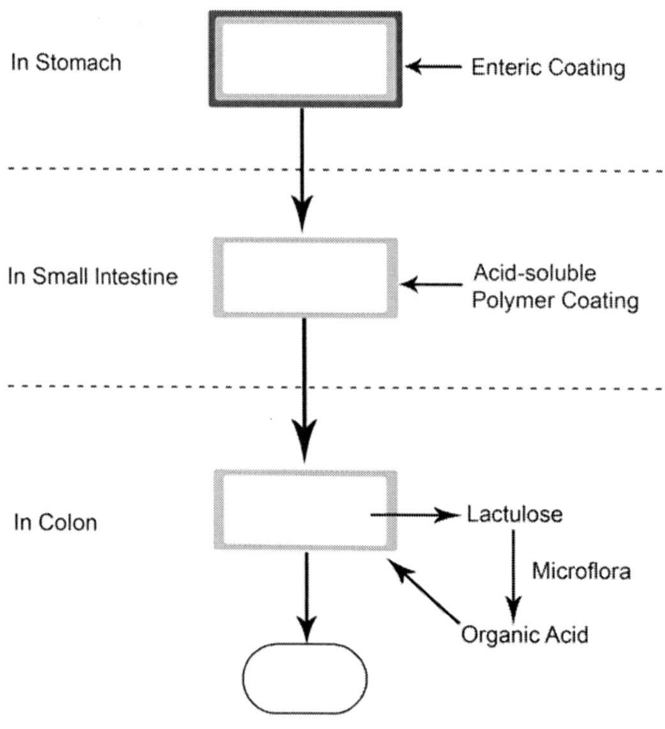

Figure 4. Schematic representation of CODES™ drug delivery system in the human gastrointestinal tract. (Modified from Yang et al., 2003).

EVALUATING DRUG DELIVERY IN MAN

The variation of absorption profiles along the human gastrointestinal tract and the ability to target drugs by adequate dosage forms to distinct sites is the challenge in the pharmaceutical development of solid dosage forms.

Experimental determination of drug release may be assessed by well-established in vitro methodologies. However, these tests are often not predictive of the more complex in vivo behavior of drug products.

Biomagnetic methods has gained increasing acceptance in pharmaceutical applications due to its ability to evaluate non-invasively solid dosage forms in the human gastrointestinal tract.

Biomagnetism embraces the measurement, analysis, interpretation and application of extremely weak magnetic fields, which are spontaneously generated by physiological electric currents that flow in excitable tissues or as a result of ferromagnetic particles. This property can be exploited for quantifying physiological iron storage, for detecting ferromagnetic impurities or the behavior of magnetically marked dosage forms.

Biomagnetic Fields

For more than 200 years, biomagnetic fields have been associated with the normal functioning of biological tissues. Briefly, Galvani discovered that muscles are activated by electric currents produced by nerve cells and later Örstedt demonstrated that when an electric current flows in a conductor, it generates a magnetic field around it. In the early 19th century, Biot and Savart calculated the magnetic field generated by a current carrying wire. Maxwell unified the theory of electromagnetism describing the behavior of the electric and magnetic fields, as well as their interactions with the matter. Maxwell's equations are the most elegant and concise methods to demonstrate the fundamentals of electricity and magnetism (Hobbie, 2001).

Nowadays, it is well known that all excitable cells base their functioning on the exchange of ions. The displacement of these electrically charged particles produces biomagnetic fields that are several orders of magnitude smaller than the Earth's magnetic field.

This section focuses mainly on the biomagnetic fields generated by the gastrointestinal activity. Smooth muscle layers of the gastrointestinal tract exhibit a periodic cyclic electrical activity also called electrical control activity or slow waves, originated by rhythmic depolarization and repolarization of the cell membrane (Irimia & Bradshaw, 2004). This electrical activity shows specific frequencies according to the gastrointestinal regions and can be detected by mucosal, serosal, or surface electrodes.

The source of the externally recorded magnetic field is the intracellular current associated with the membrane potential, since the extracellular current flows over the body cavity which could be consider a homogeneous volume conductor. Bioelectric fields depend on tissue conductivity and are therefore attenuated by the abdominal wall. On the other hand, magnetic fields depend basically on the permeability of biological tissues instead of the abdominal wall.

Biomagnetic fields in the human gastrointestinal tract can be measured as a result of electrical currents associated to the ions movement, magnet or by ferromagnetic sources in response to an applied external magnetic field. The magnetic field due to the distribution of electric currents in the abdomen, can determine the location, orientation, and time evolution of electric current dipoles.

The precise location of the magnetic marker is useful in studies measuring frequency of gastrointestinal motility. In transit studies, the position of the marker is tracked along the gastrointestinal tract.

Detection of magnetic fields generated by magnetically marked dosage forms provides an opportunity for pharmaceutical research involving functional analysis of drug delivery mechanisms.

Biomagnetic Instrumentation – Fundamentals and Applications

Biomagnetic fields may be generated as a result of the electric activity of the excitable tissues or due to magnetic markers and they are extremely weak. Thus, potential applications of biomagnetism in pharmaceutical research require sensitive magnetic sensors.

Currently, the most important sensors for biomagnetic measurements are Superconducting Quantum Interference Devices (SQUIDs), Magnetoresistive Sensors, Hall-Effect Sensors, and Induction Coils.

SQUID System

SQUIDs are a class of the most sensitive detector of magnetic flux and consist basically of a superconducting loop interrupted by one or two weak links. These weak links are Josephson Junctions (JJ) that can be formed between two superconductors as a single or multiple point contacts, microbridges, and tunnel junctions. The components of the detection system must be maintained at a low temperature that generally is achieved by immersion in liquid helium (4.2 K) contained in a special insulated vessel known as a Dewar. Figure 5 summarizes a simple single channel SQUID.

The physical phenomena of flux quantization and Josephson effect are the basis of the SQUIDs. Magnetic flux quantization is the state that the magnetic flux through a superconducting loop is always quantized in units of the flux quantum. While Josephson effect involves the coherent tunneling of a pair of electrons (Cooper pair) through a thin barrier separating two superconductors.

The SQUID can be used to detect a magnetic field directly, but this is not the most practical arrangement for biomagnetic studies due to the need to minimize the detection of ambient noise. It is advantageous to sense the field with a detection coil magnetically coupled to the SQUID which forms a closed circuit that is known as a flux transformer. As with an induction coil, the application of a magnetic field induces a current; but because the flux transformer is a superconducting circuit, the current is proportional to the magnetic flux applied to the coil. As this current passes through the input coil it imposes a field on the SQUID and it is the field to which the SQUID responds.

An electronic circuit outside the Dewar monitors the response of the SQUID, and it includes a sensitive preamplifier as close as possible to the SQUID to enhance its signal. The preamplifier and control unit constitute the active portion of the circuit, and its output voltage is proportional to the magnetic flux which is applied to the detection coil. A complete review of the principles of SQUIDs was reported by Williamson & Kaufman, 1981; Romani et al 1982 and Pizella et al, 2001.

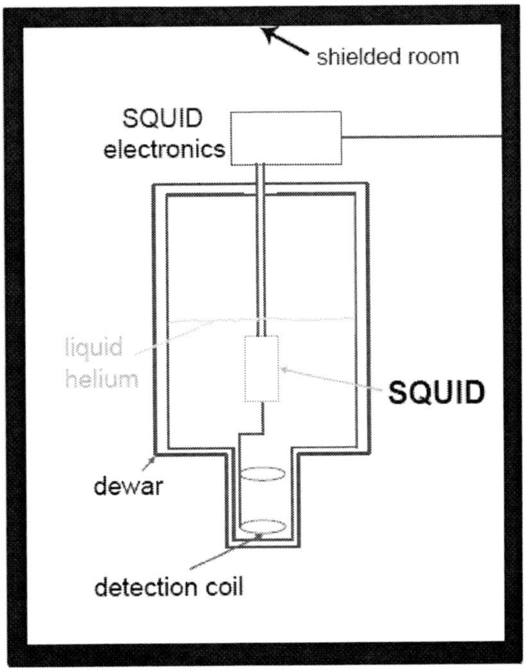

Figure 5. Schematic diagram of a single channel SQUID system. (Modified from Pizzella et al., 2001).

The high sensitivity of SQUIDs devices makes these sensors suitable for a wide range of applications. These include magnetocardiography, magnetoencephalography and magnetogastrography for the study of ionic currents generated by nervous and muscular tissue of the human body (Sternickel & Braginski, 2006).

In the pharmaceutical research, SQUIDs systems have been applied as an alternative to investigate the behavior of solid dosage forms in the human gastrointestinal tract. For this purpose, the technique called Magnetic Marker Monitoring (MMM) uses the dosage forms marked as a permanent magnetic dipole by incorporating small amounts of ferromagnetic material and subsequent magnetization (Weitschies et al, 2005).

For magnetic monitoring of a dosage form, it is essential labeling the dosage form as a permanent magnetic dipole. The ferromagnetic iron oxides are nontoxic and insoluble color pigments for food and drugs often used.

The dosage form magnetically marked is magnetized in a homogenous magnetic field in order to align all magnetic particles in the direction of the magnetization field. This alignment produces a net magnetic moment generating a measured dipolar magnetic field. Hence, any process that can disturb the alignment of the particles reduces its net magnetic moment.

This property is the basis for investigating the disintegration process of the magnetically marked dosage forms. During the disintegration the magnetic material is released in the fluid medium. Consequently, the particles lose their orientation resulting in a decrease of the net magnetic moment over time, as illustrated in Figure 6.

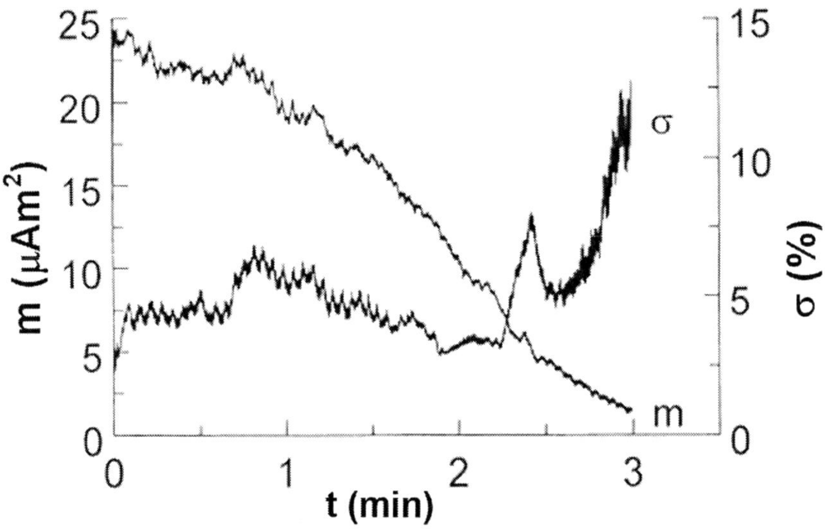

Figure 6. Magnetic signals of the disintegration of capsules *in vivo*. Magnetic moment (m) and the standard deviation (σ) are represented. (From Weitschies et al, 2001).

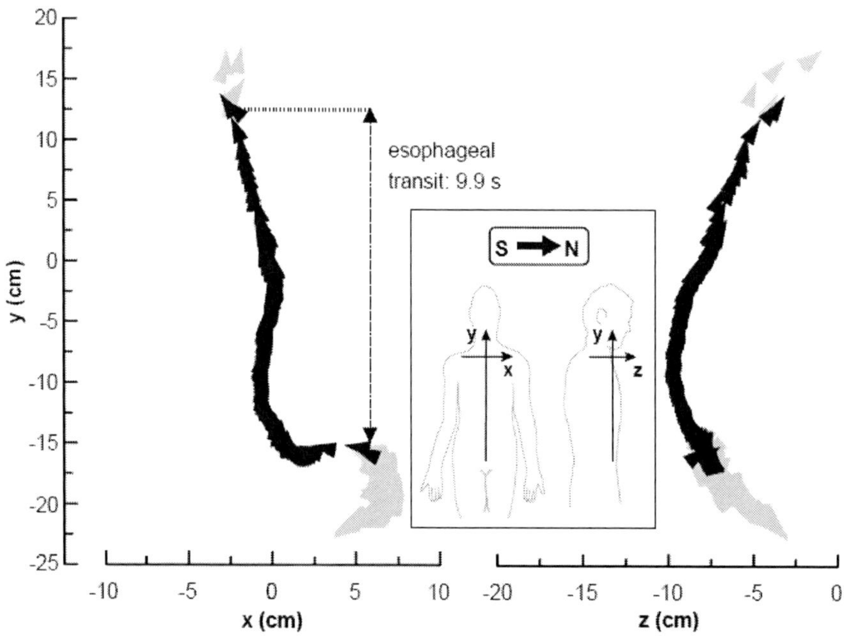

Figure 7. Magnetic monitoring of esophageal transit of a capsule. In the *inset* is represented the coordinate system and the orientation of the magnetization. (From Weitschies et al, 2005).

Another application of the magnetic measurement is the location of a solid dosage form in the human gastrointestinal tract. After the ingestion, components of the magnetic field can be continuously measured at different fixed positions above thorax or abdomen. Therefore, it is possible to monitor the esophageal transit, the gastric residence and the intestinal transit and to reconstruct location and orientation of the marker. In this case, considering that the dosage form does not disintegrate, the magnetic moment of the marker is constant and can be determined during its passage in the different gastrointestinal regions.

Due to its low permeability and transient nature, the esophagus is not a common site for drug delivery. Magnetic marker monitoring allows investigating the effects of exogenous and endogenous factors that influences the orogastric transit of solid dosage forms. Figure 7 shows the vertical component (z) and the horizontal components (x, y) in a typical example of the esophageal monitoring of a solid dosage form.

The intestinal transit time of magnetically marked dosage forms is characterized by an irregular sequence that alternates periods of quiescence, slow and rapid movements, as shown in Figure 8. The release rates from the dosage form and its location, as well as, the residence time in the different segments of the gastrointestinal tract are important variables.

Magnetic marker monitoring in combination with pharmacokinetic data provides a better understanding of the release properties of formulations and the plasma drug levels.

Despite of magnetic dipolar moments obtained for a magnetically marked dosage form be very weak, SQUID systems can measure easily since the sensors are in a magnetically shielded room in order to reduce environmental noise.

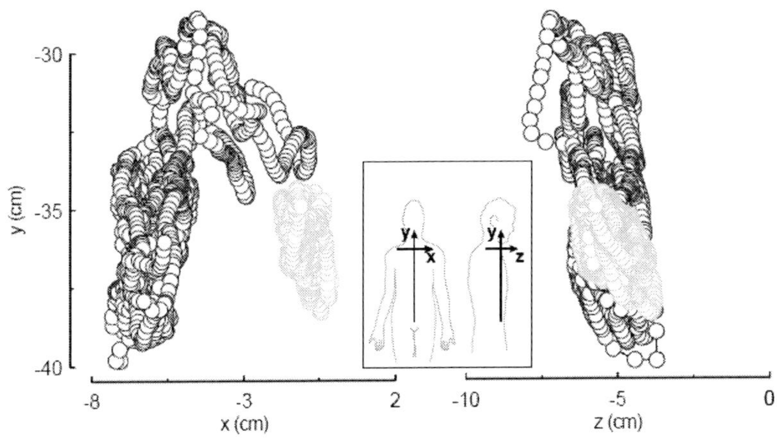

Figure 8. Magnetic monitoring of a non-disintegrating capsule in the small intestine. (From Weitschies et al., 2005).

Magnetoresistive Sensors

The magnetoresistive effect is the change of the electrical resistivity of a material due to a magnetic field. The sensors known as Anisotropic Magnetoresistive (AMR) require thin ferromagnetic films (e.g., permalloy) with a magnetic anisotropy. There is a hard axis with a high requirement of magnetization energy in one direction in the plane of the film, and, orthogonal to the hard axis in the plane of the film, which indicates the magnetic preference direction. AMR sensors have a high sensitivity at weak magnetic fields.

The method developed by Andrä et al (2000) is based on the measurement of the magnetic field of a permanent magnet which is repeatedly aligned by a vertically oriented pulsed magnetic field.

The permanent magnet is a homogeneously magnetized sphere, and then the magnetic field is a dipole determined by both two angles of orientation and three spatial coordinates of its magnetic moment. This property provides a real-time monitoring of the marker in the human gastrointestinal tract, since the three dipole field components are measured at multiple positions outside the body.

In the pharmaceutical assays, the position of a solid dosage form in a specific segment of the human gastrointestinal tract is essential for drugs with a narrow absorption window. Consequently, the development of a drug delivery system should take into consideration the time delayed in the region preceding and around the window.

Non-disintegrating dosage forms are monitored during the gastrointestinal transit time, since the magnetic dipole remains stable during the gastrointestinal passage. Hence, the magnetic moment has a constant value in the localization procedure. In Figure 9, the positions of the marker in the intestinal phantom simulated the propulsion and retropropulsion motion.

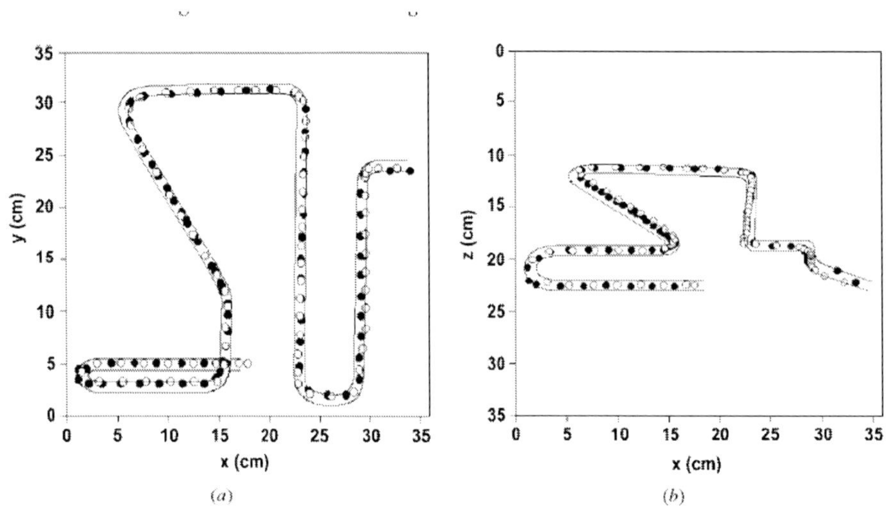

Figure 9. Magnetic monitoring of the marker positions in the intestinal phantom simulating the propulsion (open circles) and retropropulsion (full circles) motion . (*a*) top view and (*b*) side view. (From Andrä et al., 2000).

Alternatively, the disintegration process of magnetically marked tablets in relation to the temporal development of the magnetic moments also can be investigated (Weitschies et al, 2001). In this case, the magnetic moments of the magnetic particles of the tablets are aligned during magnetization into the direction of the magnetic field applied. Thus, a magnetically marked tablet is an ensemble of particles with a stable magnetic dipole moment. When the disintegration occurs, the particles are released from the tablet core and hence this dipole moment is reduced due to the disarrangement in the alignment of the particles, as shown in Figure 10.

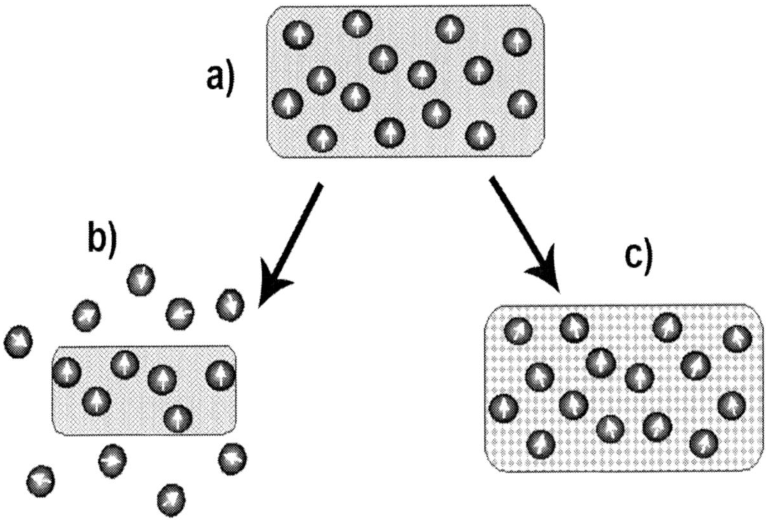

Figure 10. Representations of the magnetic dipole moments of magnetic particles. a) tablet after magnetization; b) disarrangement in the magnetic moment; c) decrease of the magnetic moment. (From Weitschies et al., 2001).

Once a magnetic dosage form can be located within the gastrointestinal tract, it would be useful to monitoring the drug release (Richert et al, 2005). With the magnetic marker monitoring, the drug release from a solid dosage form is achieved by magnetization losses or demagnetization by the use of decaying alternating magnetic field cycles.

Hall-Effect Sensors

Hall sensors are semiconductor active devices that produce a voltage signal proportional to the sensed magnetic field. Hall sensors feature low cost, small size, excellent linearity, and rotational measurement repeatability. Additional information on this sensor was reported by Popovic et al (2001) and Schlageter et al (2002).

For physiological or pharmaceutical purposes, Hall sensors are useful for tracking the position of a magnetic pill. The tracking system consists in an array of cylindrical sensors with integrated flux concentrators in order to convert locally the magnetic field and to increase the sensitivity (Stathopoulos et al, 2005).

The sensors measure the magnetic field in five coordinates, x, y, z (in mm) and two angles of rotation θ and φ (in degrees), as illustrated in Figure 11. The position of the magnetic marker is calculated with an iterative algorithm. The same approach is employed by SQUIDs and Magnetoresistive sensors.

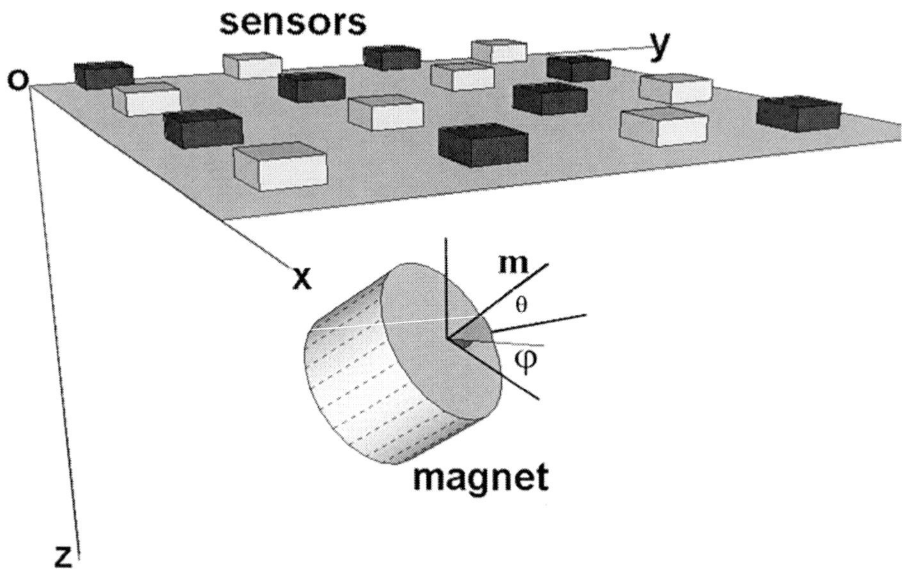

Figure 11. Magnetic tracking system. (Modified from Schlageter et al., 2002).

The magnetic tracking system seems to be an alternative for the gastrointestinal motility measurements. The trajectory of the magnet pill can be accomplished throughout entire digestive system from the oesophagus to the sigmoid colon. The system is sensitive to small variations in the position and orientation of the magnetic marker and therefore, is able to characterize the frequency of the rhythmic movements of the gastrointestinal tract.

Magnetic tracking offers an opportunity to study the effects of nutrients and drugs on specific segments of the gastrointestinal tract.

AC Biosusceptometry

Alternating Current Biosusceptometry (ACB) is an interesting and valuable tool for physiological and pharmaceutical research (Baffa et al, 1995; Corá et al, 2005). The AC Biosusceptometry bases its functioning on induction coils for recording the magnetic flux variation obtained from the response of a magnetic material. This material with a high magnetic susceptibility produces a strong response when an alternating magnetic field is applied on the biological system.

The principle behind Biosusceptometry is Faraday's Induction Law. Briefly, the induction occurs when two coils are close and a current is applied in one of the coils to generate a magnetic flux. Changing the current over time will generate a voltage in the other coil proportional to the rate of this change. The flux through the coil will change if the coil is in a magnetic field that varies with time, if the coil is rotated in a uniform field, or if the coil is moved through a nonuniform field. The flux changes generate an alternated electric current that produces its own magnetic field.

Essentially, an AC Biosusceptometer has two pairs of induction coils separated by a fixed distance (baseline), where each pair of coils is composed of an excitation coil (outer) and a detection coil (inner), in a first-order gradiometric configuration (Corá et al, 2003). The sensor is mounted as a couple of magnetic flux transformers with an air nucleus in which the pair (excitation/detection) that is located more distant from the magnetic material that will be detected acts as a reference transformer and the pair closest of the sample as a measurement transformer. Figure 12 illustrates the basic characteristics of the AC Biosusceptometer.

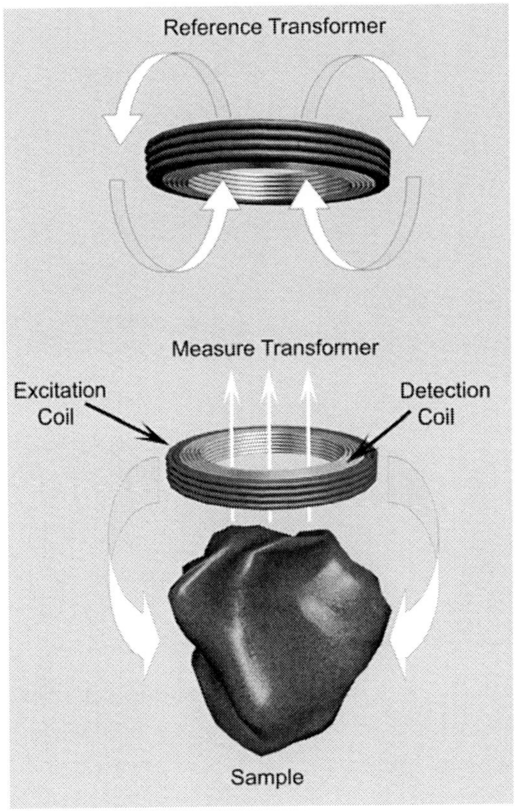

Figure 12. Functional diagram of the single sensor AC Biosusceptometer (Modified from Corá et al., 2006).

The excitation coil induces equal magnetic flux in the detection coil which is arranged in a first-order gradiometric configuration, to minimizing the output signal when there is no magnetic material near to the measure transformer. With the proximity of a magnetic sample an imbalance in the voltage occurs, due to the change in the differential flux between the detection coils. Hence, the gradiometric system detects the magnetic flux variation between the detection coils.

These concepts were then applied to a multisensor AC Biosusceptometry system that was developed to improve the spatial resolution and the sensitivity for pharmaceutical applications. The multisensor system has a pair of excitation coils and seven pairs of detection coils in a hexagonal configuration for acquisition of magnetic signals in distinct points, as shown in Figure 13.

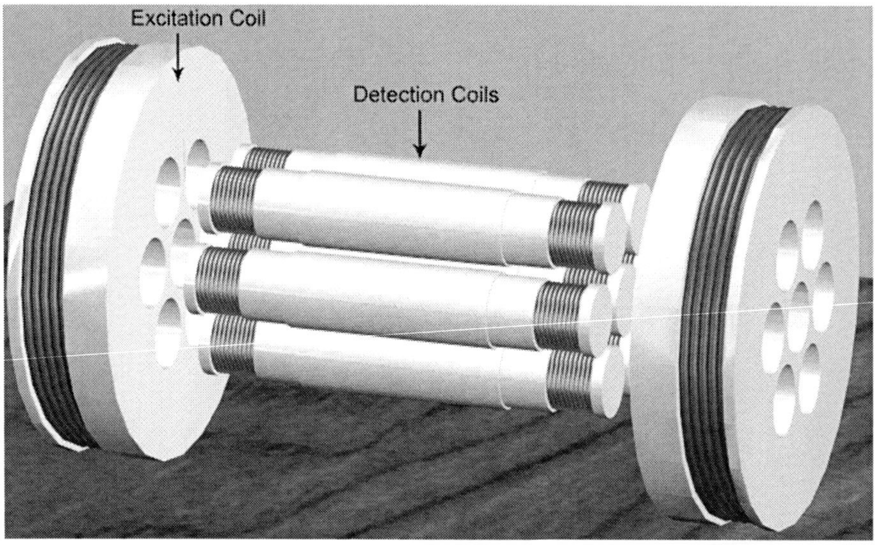

Figure 13. Multisensor AC Biosusceptometer system with the pairs of detection coils in hexagonal symmetry (Modified from Corá et al., 2006)

The signal detected by the Biosusceptometer depends on the area of the detection coil, the number of turns, the rate of change of the magnetic flux through this coil (i.e. applied field), the amount of ferromagnetic material, and the distance between the sensor and the magnetic material.

The AC Biosusceptometry system does not require magnetically shielded environment and due to its simplicity, has reasonably low implementation cost, when compared to the other biomagnetic techniques presented above. When applied to pharmaceutical dosage forms, the AC Biosusceptometry provides non-invasive real-time data on the drug delivery process. Moreover, for Biosusceptometry measurements, the magnetic markers are not previously magnetized.

In this section, we will discuss a wide range of applications of the AC Biosusceptometry in the pharmaceutical research.

Disintegration

The disintegration of the solid dosage forms promotes the drug release to the absorption in the gastrointestinal tract. Several approaches are currently developed by the pharmaceutical industry to deliver drugs at specific sites along the gastrointestinal tract aiming a more effective therapy. This includes the development of polymers or coating systems ensuring excellent performance for a product.

All these innovations require methods able to characterize the behavior of a pharmaceutical product in humans, since the gastrointestinal physiology exerts a critical influence on its performance. The AC Biosusceptometry is innovative in this research field and due to its versatility, has become an alternative to the conventional methods.

The Biosusceptometry was firstly proposed to evaluate the disintegration process of magnetic tablets in human stomach (Corá et al, 2003). Figure 14 shows typical examples of the magnetic signals recorded during the disintegration process of a tablet *in vitro* and in the human stomach.

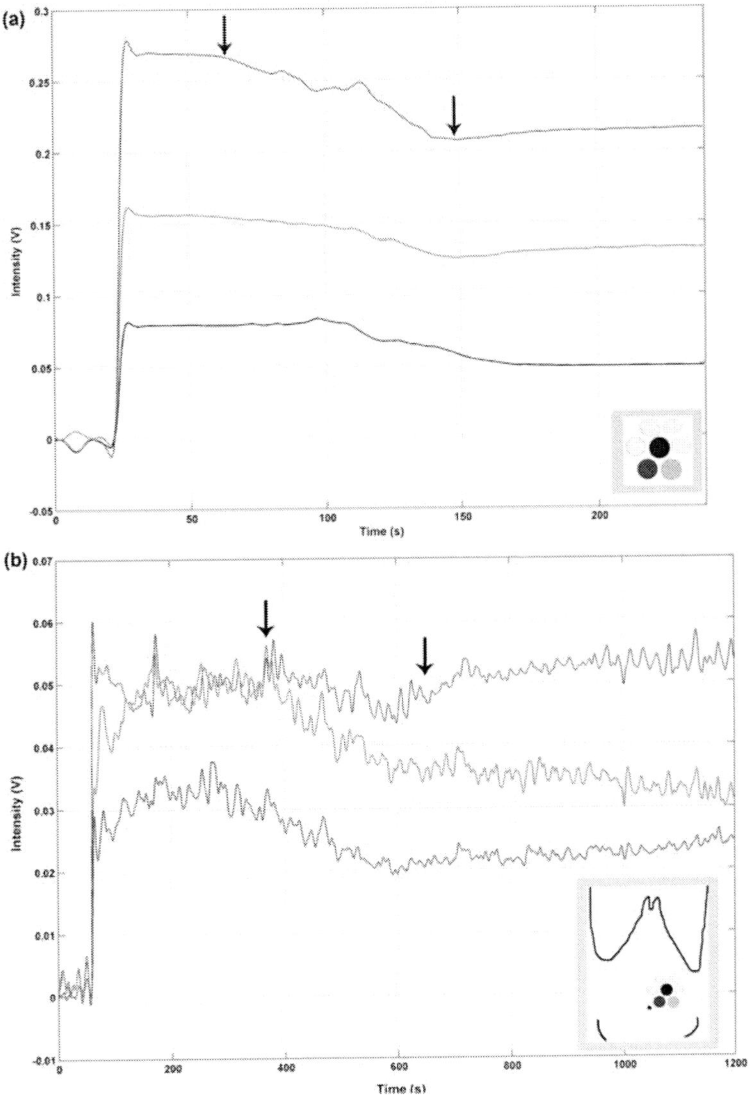

Figure 14. Magnetic signals of the disintegration process of a tablet recorded by the multisensor AC biosusceptometer. (a) *in vitro* measurement; (b) *in vivo* measurement. The *insets* represent the positioning of the multisensor system related with the magnetic signal recorded. The arrows indicate the onset and complete disintegration process, respectively.

The disintegration process for magnetic dosage forms is characterized by the transition between a magnetic marker (non-disintegrated dosage form) to a magnetic tracer (disintegrated dosage form). Generally, the ferrites ($MnFe_2O_4$) are the inert ferromagnetic material that is incorporated into the dosage forms since they present absence of toxicity and lack effects on the gastrointestinal tract (Frei et al, 1968).

Hence, when a volunteer ingests a magnetic dosage form, the biomagnetic signals generated from the response of the dosage form to an applied magnetic field are detected by the multisensor system.

AC Biosusceptometer is very sensitive to the movements of the gastric wall, and then the amplitude of the biomagnetic signals decreases when a gastric contraction occurs; it changes the distance between the sensors and the dosage forms within the organ. Simultaneously, in these biomagnetic signals there are information about the gastric activity contraction and the disintegration of the dosage form. This technique allows to monitor the disintegration process in real-time identifying the region where it is occurred.

Gastrointestinal Transit

The development of colonic delivery systems represents one of the most prominent approaches for the pharmacological treatment of inflammatory bowel diseases (IBD). However, because of the distal location of colon, a delivery system must overcome several physiological barriers along the gastrointestinal tract and prevent the drug release in the stomach and small intestine.

The knowledge of the gastrointestinal transit and how the physiological variables may interfere with the drug release and absorption is the major challenge for successful design of colon-specific delivery systems.

More reliable data are obtained when human studies are carried out, since the bioavailability of drugs from colonic dosage forms is dependent on gastric emptying, small intestinal transit time and drug release profile. AC Biosusceptometry has also gained importance in this kind of analysis (Corá et al, 2006a,b).

The motility pattern during the interdigestive period determines the residence time of a solid dosage form in a specific segment of the human gastrointestinal tract. Figure 15 illustrates the biomagnetic signals in the interdigestive activity following the administration of an enteric-coated dosage form.

It is interesting to notice that the colonic arrival time for a dosage form is influenced mainly by the gastric retention time that plays a dominating role in the overall transit of the dosage form. Conversely, the small intestine transit is not influenced by any physiological parameter or related to the pharmaceutical form. Figure 16 represents a gastrointestinal transit profile showing the gastric emptying time, the small intestinal transit time and the colonic arrival for a magnetic enteric-coated dosage form.

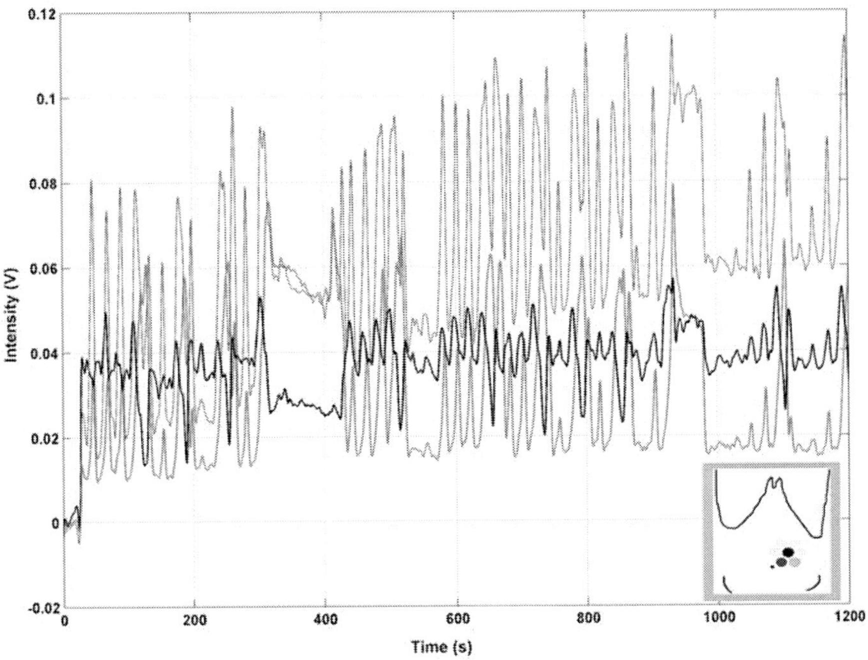

Figure 15. Magnetic signals recorded in the fasting state following the ingestion of an enteric-coated dosage form. The *inset* indicates the position of the multisensor AC Biosusceptometers in the human abdominal wall. (Modified from Corá et al., 2006.)

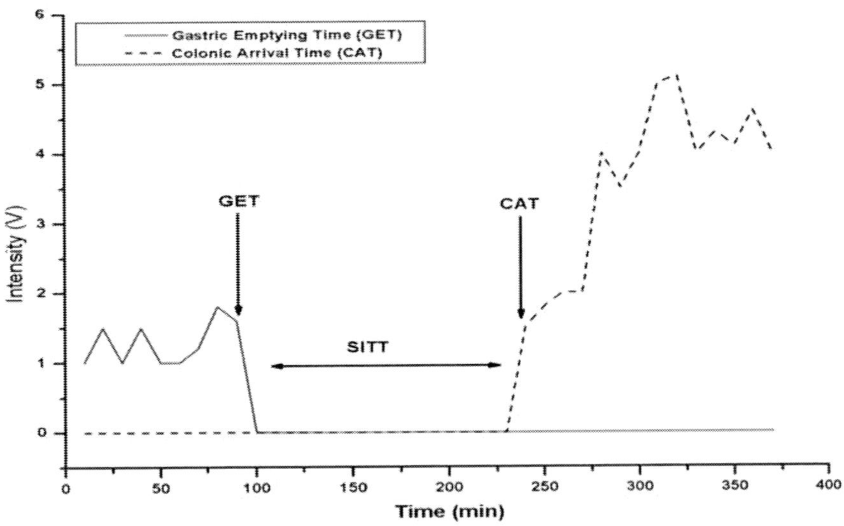

Figure 16. Gastrointestinal transit profile for a magnetic enteric-coated tablet. (Modified from Corá et al., 2005).

Magnetic Images

When applied to pharmaceutical dosage forms, medical imaging techniques provide non-invasive real-time data on the drug delivery process. Recently, the AC Biosusceptometry technique introduced a novel concept in imaging of the pharmaceutical processes.

Biomagnetic signals recorded by the multisensor AC Biosusceptometry system are represented by a time series matrix. From these signals it is possible to generate magnetic images of the solid dosage forms. The article by Corá and cols. (2005) provides a more detailed description of the principles of biomagnetic images for pharmaceutical applications.

Figure 17 shows a sequence of biomagnetic images of a tablet in the human stomach from the ingestion to it complete disintegration. In comparing the second image to the first, this corresponds to an increase of 50% in the number of pixels in the segmented image area. The disintegration process of solid dosage forms in the biomagnetic images is quantified when an increase of 50% in the number of pixels in the image area occurs.

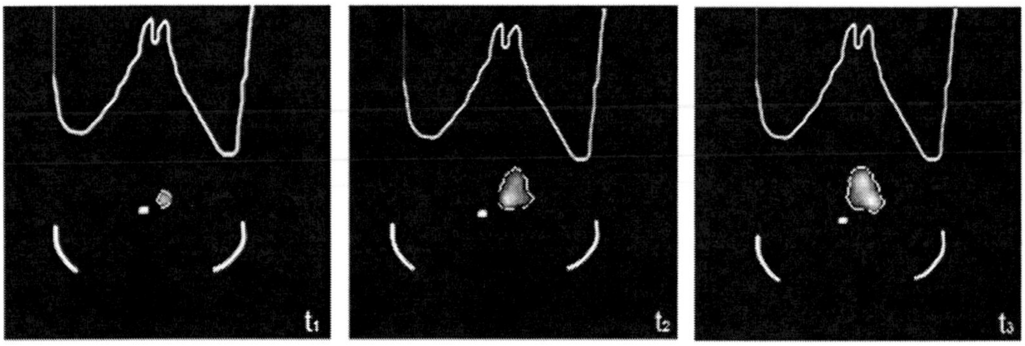

Figure 17. Magnetic images of the disintegration process of a tablet in the human stomach. 50% disintegration (t_{50}) is located between t_1 and t_2.

These studies may have many roles, according to their intended, and may be applied to a wide range of pharmaceutical technologies, including enteric-coated, gastroretentive and modified-release dosage forms. In Figure 18 an example of biomagnetic images of an enteric-coated hypromellose capsule and the release of the magnetic material in the human colon can be seen.

This monitoring for biomagnetic images is useful to the quality control to demonstrating the effectiveness of these formulations in the release of drugs in specific areas of the human gastrointestinal tract.

Controlled drug delivery systems

Several formulation strategies have been proposed for controlled drug delivery at specific sites of the human gastrointestinal tract. Controlled delivery systems are intended for release of drugs at an appropriate rate to avoid fluctuations in plasma drug concentrations. For controlled drug delivery technology, multiparticulate systems, such as microspheres or pellets, have several advantages in comparison to the conventional single unit.

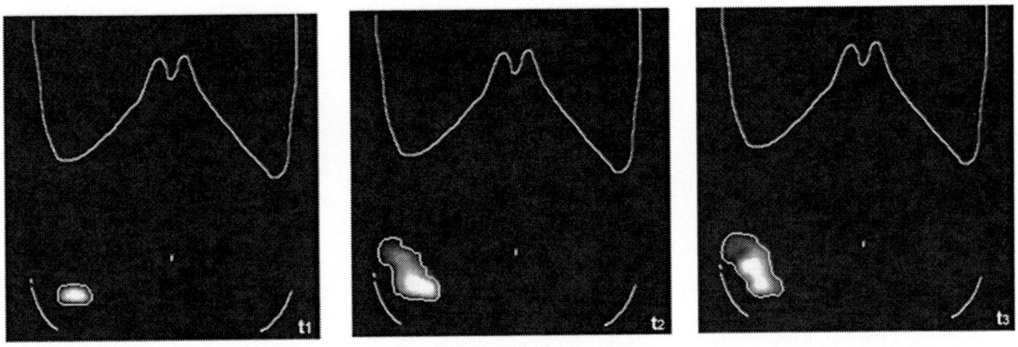

Figure 18. Magnetic images of the disintegration process of an enteric coated hypromellose capsule. In the instant t_1 is represented the arrival of the capsule at the colon; from t_2 occurs a gradual increase in the image area characterizing the spreading of the magnetic material by the disintegration process.

Drug targeting to the stomach is attractive for several reasons, particularly when there is an absorption window in the upper gastrointestinal tract. Gastroretentive dosage forms based on floating delivery systems are expected to prolong the gastric residence time increasing the bioavailability of these drugs.

AC Biosusceptometry is an interesting tool to investigate the in vivo performance of gastroretentive drug formulations. Figure 19 shows a typical example of the magnetic images of a floating delivery system.

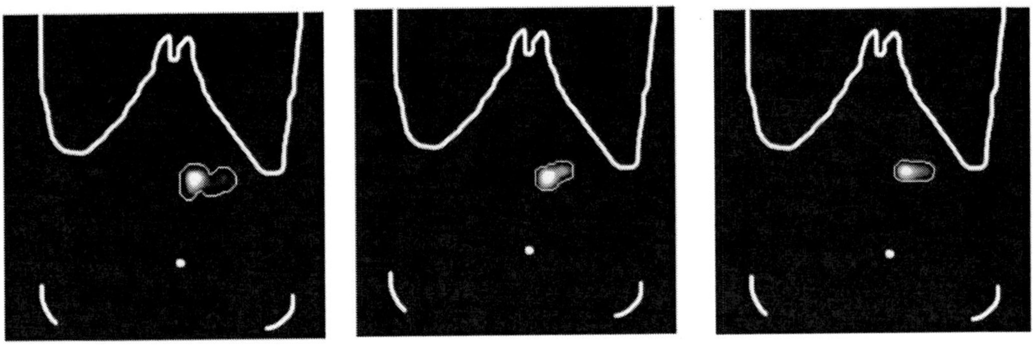

Figure 19. Magnetic gastroretentive delivery system based on floating property.

Likewise, the challenge of targeting drugs to the colonic region is to overcome the physiological variables and to provide a more reliable drug delivery. Due to their small particle size and the more uniform dispersion in the gastrointestinal tract, the multiparticulate dosage forms can reach the colon quickly and to remain retained longer in the proximal colon.

Figure 20 shows the biomagnetic images (a) and the gastrointestinal transit profile (b) of a multiparticulate formulation and its dispersion over time on the colonic region.

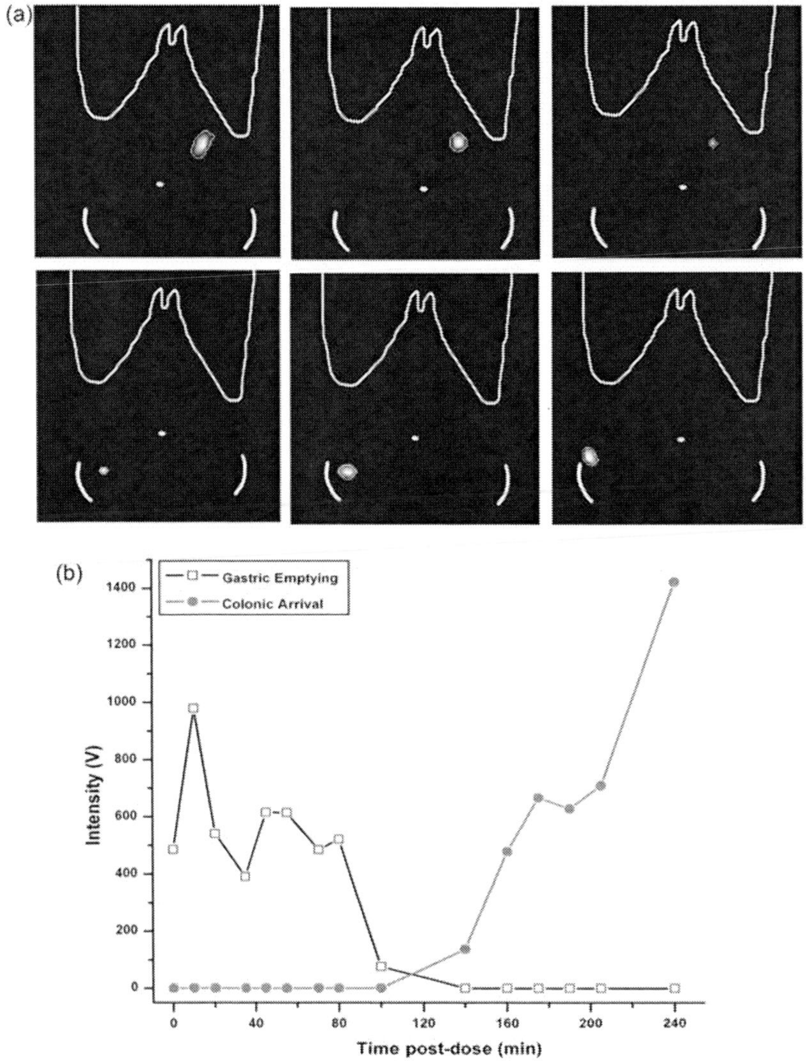

Figure 20. a) Magnetic images of a multiparticulate delivery system in the human stomach and ileocolonic region, respectively. b) Gastric emptying and colonic arrival profiles for the multi-units.

CONCLUSIONS

The idea of this chapter was to integrate the basic knowledge on the main biomagnetic techniques and the pharmaceutical research. The development of new technologies for delivery drugs requires techniques able to provide more detailed information about the behavior of solid dosage forms in the human gastrointestinal tract

In this context, biomagnetism plays an eminent role in a number of clinical researches, and more recently in the pharmaceutical field. Biomagnetism involves the detection of magnetic fields produced by the human body or due to magnetic markers previously ingested. As these magnetic fields are extremely weak, it is essential the use of highly sensitive sensors enable to record these fields.

Biomagnetic instrumentation based on SQUIDs systems allows to monitoring magnetically marked dosage forms with a high temporal and spatial resolution. Moreover, the three dimensional localization and orientation as well as the strength of the magnetic source can be reconstructed as a function of time.

On the other hand, the development of real time tracking systems based on magnetoresistive or hall-effect sensors allows the monitoring of strong magnetic markers. These systems are cheaper than SQUID and can be operated without magnetic shielding environment.

In contrast to the above mentioned techniques, AC Biosusceptometry is promising to evaluate accurately solid dosage forms in the human gastrointestinal tract. AC Biosusceptometry system represents a novel imaging tool able to characterize a number of parameters related to drug delivery, deserving the same importance as conventional techniques in pharmaceutical research.

Additionally, the AC Biosusceptometer system provides a more effective monitoring of the dosage form that can be accomplished in real-time and simultaneously in distinct points than those obtained employing SQUIDs, magnetoresistive or hall-sensors.

Considering this, the Biosusceptometry is versatile not only for human studies as well as to be used as a tool in quality control for pharmaceutical products. Moreover, this biomagnetic method is especially powerful when combined with classical pharmacokinetic data allowing monitoring the dosage form to correlate directly the drug release at specific sites along the gastrointestinal tract with the drug absorption in a new approach that could be coined: “magnetopharmacokinetic”.

REFERENCES

Amidon, GL; Lennernäs, H; Shah, VP; Crison, JR. A theoretical basis for a biopharmaceutic drug classification: the correlation of in vitro drug product dissolution and in vivo bioavailability. *Pharmaceutical Research*, 1995, v. 12, 413-420.

Andrä, W; Danan, H; Kirmße, W; Kramer, H-H; Saupe, P; Schmieg, R; Bellemann, ME. A novel method for real-time magnetic marker monitoring in the gastrointestinal tract. *Physics in Medicine and Biology,* 2000, v. 45, 3081-3093.

Andrä, W; Nowak, H. Magnetism in Medicine. 1st Ed. Berlin: Willey-VCH, 1998.

Arora, S; Ali, J; Ahuja, A; Khar, RK; Baboota, S. Floating drug delivery systems: a review. *AAPS Pharmaceutical Sciences and Technology*, 2005, v. 6, 372-390.

Baffa, O; Oliveira, RB; Miranda, JRA; Troncon, LEA. Analysis and development of AC biosusceptometer for orocaecal transit time measurements. *Medical and Biological Engineering and Computing*, 1995, v. 33, 353-357.

Bardonnet, PL; Faivre, V; Pugh, WJ; Piffaretti, JC; Falson, F. Gastroretentive dosage forms: overview and special case of *Helicobacter pylori*. *Journal of Controlled Release*, 2006, v. 111, 1 – 18.

Bradshaw, LA; Myers, A; Richards, WO; Drake, W; Wikswo, JP. Vector projection of biomagnetic fields. *Medical & Biological & Engineering & Computing*, 2005, v. 43, 85-93.

Camilleri, M. Integrated upper gastrointestinal response to food intake. *Gastroenterology*, 2006, v. 131, 640-658.

Caramella, C; Colombo, P; Conte, U; Ferrari, F; Gazzaniga, A; LaManna, A; Peppas, NA. A physical analysis of the phenomenon of tablet disintegration. *International Journal of Pharmaceutics*, 1988, v. 44, 177-186.

Chawla, G; Gupta, P; Koradia, V; Bansal, AK. A means to address regional variability in intestinal drug absorption. *Pharmaceutical Technology*, 2003, v. 27, 50-68.

Chourasia, MK; Jain, SK. Pharmaceutical approaches to colon target drug delivery systems. *Journal of Pharmacy and Pharmaceutical Sciences*, 2003, v. 6, 33-66.

Corá, LA; Américo, MF; Oliveira, RB; Baffa, O; Moraes, R; Romeiro, FG; Miranda, JRA. Disintegration of magnetic tablets in human stomach evaluated by alternate current Biosusceptometry. *European Journal of Pharmaceutics and Biopharmaceutics*, 2003, v.56, 413–420.

Corá, LA; Andreis, U; Romeiro, FG; Américo, MF; Oliveira, RB; Baffa, O; Miranda, JRA. Magnetic images of the disintegration process of tablets in the human stomach by AC Biosusceptometry. *Physics in Medicine and Biology*, 2005, v.50, 5523–5534.

Corá, LA; Romeiro, FG; Stelzer, M; Américo, MF; Oliveira, RB; Baffa, O; Miranda, JRA. AC biosusceptometry in the study of drug delivery. *Advanced Drug Delivery Reviews*, 2005, v.57, 1223– 1241.

Corá, LA; Romeiro, FG; Stelzer, M; Américo, MF; Oliveira, RB; Baffa, O; Stelzer, M; Miranda, JRA. Gastrointestinal transit and disintegration of enteric coated magnetic tablets assessed by AC Biosusceptometry. *European Journal of Pharmaceutical Sciences*, 2006, v.27, 1-8.

Corá, LA; Romeiro, FG; Paixão, FC; Américo, MF; Oliveira, RB; Baffa, O; Miranda, JRA. Enteric coated magnetic HPMC capsules evaluated in human gastrointestinal tract by AC Biosusceptometry. *Pharmaceutical Research*, 2006, v. 23, 1809-1816.

Coupe, AJ; Davis, SS; Wilding, IR. Variation in gastrointestinal transit of pharmaceutical dosage forms in healthy subjects. *Pharmaceutical Research*, 1991, v. 8, 360 – 364.

Davis, SS; Hardy, JG; Fara, JW. Transit of pharmaceutical dosage forms through the small intestine. Gut, 1986, v. 27, 886-892.

Davis, SS. Formulation strategies for absorption windows. *Drug Discovery Today*, 2005, v.10, 249-257.

Demírtürk, E; Öner, L. In vitro - In vivo correlations. *FABAD Journal of Pharmaceutical Sciences*, 2003, v. 28, 215 - 224.

Dressman, JB; Berardi, RR; Dermentzoglou, LC; Russel, TL; Schmaltz, SP; Barnett, JL; Jarvenpaa, KM. Upper gastrointestinal (GI) pH in young, healthy men and women. *Pharmaceutical Research*, 1990, v. 7, 756 – 761.

Emami, J. In vitro - In vivo correlation: from theory to applications. *Journal of Pharmacy and Pharmaceutical Sciences*, 2006, v. 9, 69-189.

Evans, DF; Pye, G; Bramley, R; Clark, AG; Dyson, TJ; Hardcastle, JD. Measurement of gastrointestinal pH profiles in normal ambulant human subjects. *Gut*, 1988, v. 29, 1035-1041.

Frei, EH; Gunders, E; Pajewsky, M; Alkan, WJ; Eshcher, J. Ferrites as contrast material for medical X-ray diagnosis. *Journal of Applied Physics*, 1968, v. 39, 99-101.

Frexinos, F; Delvaux, M. Colonic motility. In: Kumar, D; Wingate, D. (Eds.). *An Illustrated Guide to Gastrointestinal Motility*. London: Churchill Livingstone, 1993, 427– 448.

Guignet, R; Bergonzelli, G; Schlageter, V; Turini, M; Kucera, P. Magnetic tracking: a new tool for in vivo studies of the rat gastrointestinal motility. *Neurogastroenterology and Motility*, 2006, v. 18, 472-478.

Hobbie, RK. *Intermediate physics for medicine and biology*. 3. ed. New York: AIP Press, 2001.

Hasler, WL. The physiology of gastric motility and gastric emptying. In: Yamada, T. (Ed.). *Textbook of Gastroenterology*. Philadelphia: J.B. Lippincott, 1995, 181–206.

Hörter, D; Dressman, JB. Influence of physicochemical properties on dissolution of drugs in the gastrointestinal tract. *Advanced Drug Delivery Reviews*, 2001, v. 46, 75 – 87.

Irimia, A; Bradshaw, LA. Theoretical and computational methods for the noninvasive detection of gastric electrical source coupling. *Physical Review E*, 2004, v. 69, 051920-1 - 051920-7.

Jivraj, M; Martini, LG; Thomson, CM. An overview of the different excipients useful for the direct compression of tablets. *Pharmaceutical Science and Technology Today*, 2000, v. 3, 58-63.

Kleiner, R; Koelle, D; Ludwig, F; Clarke, J. Superconducting Quantum Interference Devices: state of the art and applications. *Proceedings of the IEEE*, 2004, v. 92, 1534-1548.

Kwiatkowski, W; Tumanski, S. The permalloy magnetoresistive sensors - properties and applications. *Journal of Physics E: Scientific Instruments*, 1986, v. 19, 502-515.

Levy, G; Impact of pharmacodynamics variability on drug delivery. *Advanced Drug Delivery Reviews*, 1998, v. 33, 201-206.

Lowenthal, W. Disintegration of tablets. *Journal of Pharmaceutical Sciences*, 1972, v. 61, pp. 1695-1711.

Martinez, MN; Amidon, GL. A mechanistic approach to understanding the factors affecting drug absorption: a review of fundamentals. *Journal of Clinical Pharmacology*, 2002, v. 42, 620-643.

Melia, CD; Davis, SS. Review article: mechanisms of drug release from tablets and capsules. I: disintegration. *Alimentary Pharmacology and Therapeutics*, 1989, v. 3, 223-232.

Quigley, EMM. Gastric and small intestinal motility in health and disease. *Gastroenterology Clinics of North America,* 1996, v. 25, 113– 145.

Pizzella, V; Della Penna, S; Del Gratta, C; Romani, GL. SQUID systems for biomagnetic imaging. *Superconductor Science and Technology*, 2001, v.14, R79–R114.

Popovic, RS; Randjelovic, Z; Manic, D. Integrated Hall-effect magnetic sensors. *Sensors and Actuators A*, 2001, v. 91, 46-50.

Rao, SSC, Schulze-Delrieu, K. The stomach, pylorus and duodenum. In: Kumar, D, Wingate, D (Eds.). *An Illustrated Guide to Gastrointestinal Motility*. London: Churchill Livingstone, 1993, 373–392.

Richert, H; Surzhenko, O; Wangemann, S; Heinrich, J; Görnert, P. Development of a magnetic capsule as a drug release system for future applications in the human GI tract. *Journal of Magnetism and Magnetic Materials*, 2005, v. 293, 497–500.

Romani, GL; Williamson, SJ; Kaufman, L. Biomagnetic instrumentation. *Review of Scientific Instruments*, 1982, v. 53, 1815-1845.

Rouge, N; Buri, P; Doelker, E. Drug absorption sites in the gastrointestinal tract and dosage forms for site-specific delivery. *International Journal of Pharmaceutics*, 1996, v. 136, 117-139.

Schareef, MA; Khar, RK; Ahuja, A; Ahmad, FJ; Raghava, S. Colonic Drug Delivery: an updated review. *AAPS Pharmaceutical Sciences*, 2003, v. 5, 1-25.

Schlageter, V; Drljaca, P; Popovic, RS; Kucera, P. A magnetic tracking system based on highly sensitive integrated hall sensors. *JSME International Journal Series C*, 2002, v. 45, 967-973.

Siegel, JA; Urbain, J-L; Adler, LP; Charkes, ND; Maurer, AH; Krevsky, B; Knight, LC; Fisher, RS; Malmud, LS. Biphasic nature of gastric emptying. *Gut*, 1988, v. 29, 85-89.

Stathopoulos, E; Schlageter, V; Meyrat, B; De Ribaupierre, Y; Kucera, P. Magnetic pill tracking: a novel non-invasive tool for investigation of human digestive motility. *Neurogastroenterology and Motility*, 2005, v. 17, 148–154.

Sternickel, K; Braginski, AI. Biomagnetism using SQUIDs: status and perspectives. *Superconductor Science and Technology*, 2006, v. 19, S160–S171.

Swithenby, SJ. SQUIDs and their applications in the measurement of weak magnetic fields. *Journal of Physics E: Scientific Instruments*, 1980, v. 13, 801-813.

Talukder, R; Fassihi, R. Gastroretentive Delivery Systems: a mini review. *Drug Development and Industrial Pharmacy*, 2004, v. 30, 1019–1028.

Yang, L; Watanabe, S; Li, J; Chu, JS; Katsuma, M; Yokohama, S; Fix, JA. Effect of colonic lactulose availability on the timing of drug release onset in vivo from a unique colon-specific drug delivery system (CODES™). *Pharmaceutical Research,* 2003, v. 20, 429-434.

Urquhart, J. Controlled drug delivery: therapeutic and pharmacological aspects. *Journal of Internal Medicine*, 2000, v. 248, 357-376.

Weitschies, W; Karaus, M; Cordini, D; Trahms, L; Breitkreutz, J; Semmler, W. Magnetic marker monitoring of disintegrating capsules. *European Journal of Pharmaceutical Sciences*, 2001, v. 13, 411–416.

Weitschies, W; Hartmann, V; Grützmann, R; Breitkreutz, J. Determination of the disintegration behavior of magnetically marked tablets. *European Journal of Pharmaceutics and Biopharmaceutics*, 2001, v. 52, 221-226.

Weitschies, W; Wedemeyer, J; Stehr, R; Trahms, L. Magnetic markers as a noninvasive tool to monitor gastrointestinal transit. *IEEE Transactions on Biomedical Engineering*, 1994, v. 41, 192-195.

Weitschies, W; Kosch, O; Mönnikes, H; Trahms, L. Magnetic Marker Monitoring: An application of biomagnetic measurement instrumentation and principles for the determination of the gastrointestinal behavior of magnetically marked solid dosage forms. *Advanced Drug Delivery Reviews*, 2005, v. 57, 1210– 1222.

Weitschies, W; Wedemeyer, RS; Kosch, O; Fach, K; Nagel, S; Söderlind, E; Trahms, L; Abrahamsson, B; Mönnikes, H. Impact of the intragastric location of extended release tablets on food interactions. *Journal of Controlled Release*, 2005, v. 108, 375–385.

Weitschies, W; Wedemeyer, J; Stehr, R; Trahms, L. Magnetically marked pharmaceutical dosage forms to monitor gastrointestinal transit by biomagnetic measurements. *Pharmaceutical and Pharmacological Letters*, 1991, v. 1, 45-48.

Weitschies, W; Kötitz R; Cordini, D; Trahms, L. High-resolution monitoring of the gastrointestinal transit of a magnetically marked capsule. *Journal of Pharmaceutical Sciences*, 1997, v. 86, 1218-1222.

Wilding, IR; Davis, SS; O'Hagan, DT. Optimizing gastrointestinal delivery of drugs. *Baillière's Clinical Gastroenterology*, 1994, v. 8, 255 – 270.

Williamson, SJ; Kaufman, L. Biomagnetism. *Journal of Magnetism and Magnetic Materials*, 1981, v. 22, 129-201.

In: Drugs: Approval and Evaluation, Delivery and Control ISBN: 978-1-60456-533-1
Editors: A.O. Hartmann, L.K. Neumann

Chapter 2

CORE-SHELL POLYMER NANOPARTICLE FORMULATIONS FOR THE ORAL ADMINISTRATION OF PEPTIDES AND PROTEINS

Irene Bravo-Osuna, Christine Vauthier* and Gilles Ponchel
Physicochimie, Pharmacotechnie et Biopharmacie
UMR CNRS 8612, Université de Paris XI
Faculté de Pharmacie, 5, Rue J.B. Clément, 92296 Chatenay-Malabry Cedex, France

SUMMARY

Innovation in pharmacology can be achieved designing polymer nanoparticles to rationalize drug delivery by enhancing the oral bioavailability of peptides and proteins. New types of formulations were designed during the last couple of years promoting interactions with the mucus for bioadhesion, with the gastro-intestinal fluids for decreasing antiprotease activity and possibly with cells constituting the epithelium to enhance permeability. As they will be presented in the present chapter, they result from the formation of core-shell poly(alkylcyanoacrylate) nanoparticles coated with chitosan and thiolated chitosan. The design and characterization of such core-shell polymer nanoparticles will be described in this chapter. Their evaluation as a tool to improve the bioavailability of peptides and proteins by the oral route will be discussed thanks to data obtained from different *in vitro* models and set ups. The more advanced research will then be presented on the last part of this chapter opening the conclusion and the discussion for future developments.

Keywords: chitosan, thiolated chitosan, poly(alkyl cyanoacrylate) (PACA), core-shell nanoparticles, bioadhesion, intestinal permeation, antiprotease activity, cation binding capacity.

* Corresponding author. E-mail: christine.vauthier@cep.u-psud.fr; Phone 33 1 46 83 56 03; Fax 33 1 46 83 53 12.

INTRODUCTION

Significant advances in biotechnology and biochemistry have led to the discovery of a large number of bioactive molecules and vaccines based on peptides and proteins (Jung et al., 2000, Morishita and Peppas, 2006). They have become the drugs of choice for the treatment of numerous diseases as a result of their selectivity and ability to provide effective and potent actions.

In comparison to other possible routes of administration, oral delivery of peptidic drugs has many advantages. It is non invasive and safe, it avoids complications arising from the need of sterile techniques including parenteral formulations. Moreover, it is convenient and easy dosage forms can be obtained at low preparation costs. Above all, it should encourage patient compliance (Pinto Reis et al., 2006). However, the suitable clinical exploitation of these pharmacologically active bio-engineered products including peptides by the oral route is seriously hampered by two main obstacles: their poor stability in the gastrointestinal tract (GIT), mainly due to enzymatic degradation (enzymatic barrier), and their limited transport across the intestinal epithelia (permeation barrier) (Zhou, 1994; Larionova et al., 1999; Madsen and Peppas, 1999; Ameye et al., 2000; Jung et al., 2000; Michael et al., 2000; Dorkoosh et al., 2002; Morishita and Peppas, 2006).

Most therapeutic peptides are still being administered by the parenteral route because of insufficient absorption from the gastrointestinal tract. It is clear that the development of suitable carrier systems enhancing drug delivery remains challenging for the pharmaceutical scientist but it is believed that it will make possible the oral delivery of peptides (Jung et al., 2000; Cox et al., 2001; Prego et al., 2005; Morishita and Peppas, 2006). The need to improve the administration of peptides by the oral route is not only focused on the increase of bioavailability of the pharmacologically active form of the therapeutic peptide such as insulin or calcitonin, but also includes the concept of mucosal vaccination which has become more prominent in the recent years. Oral dosage forms of vaccines would improve patient compliance and facilitate frequent boosting necessary to achieve an adequate protective immune response. Indeed, epithelia from mucosae are the entrance doors for many pathogens including viruses and bacteria hence mucosal immunity can be considered as an important protective barrier against infections (Jung et al., 2000; Le Buanec et al., 2001; Iqbal et al., 2003; Mansouri et al., 2004).

The aim of the present chapter is to highlight and discuss the advantages of recent innovations in pharmacology proposed to rationalize the oral delivery of therapeutic peptides and proteins. The first part will briefly summarize the different obstacles hampering so far peptide and protein therapies given by the oral route. The advantages of formulation strategies using nanoparticles will be discussed in the second part of the chapter. Recent results considering new types of formulations including core-shell poly(alkylcyanoacrylate) will be presented in the following 3 parts. First the synthesis of the nanoparticles will be described together with the physico-chemical characterization. The interactions of the chitosan-coated poly(alkylcyanoacrylate) nanoparticles with the mucosae will then be considered. Finally, results showing how these nanoparticles can modulate the intestinal permeation will be presented. The more advanced researches on core-shell poly(alkylcyanoacrylate) nanoparticles presented on the last part of this chapter will open the conclusion and the discussion for future developments.

Obstacles to the Oral Administration of Peptides and Proteins

Obstacles to the oral administration of peptides and proteins include many parameters. Parameters inherent of the therapeutic molecules include the high molecular weight shown by peptides and proteins and their hydrophilic natures. These two properties greatly compromise their absorption through the gut epithelium. Additional problems come from the very unfavourable conditions encountered in the gut generally resulting in the degradation of the therapeutic peptides and proteins. Moreover, once in the body, peptides are genrally characterised by high elimination rate constants, hence requiring constant feeding with large amounts of the peptides to ensure sustained therapeutic concentration levels and even sometime accordingly to very specific time-delivery pattern. To better understand the efforts made developing suitable delivery formulations for therapeutic peptides and proteins, this part of the chapter summarizes the different physiological and biochemical obstacles those compounds are facing when they are administered orally.

Physiological Obstacles

In human, the small intestine is 6 to 7 m long and is roughly divided into three sections: duodenum, jejunum and ileum, which comprise 5%, 50% and 45% of the total length respectively. The intestinal epithelium normally functions as a selective barrier with a surface area of about 500 m^2 in human (Balimane and Chung, 2005). It allows the absorption of nutrients, electrolytes and water but restricts the passage of larger potentially toxic compounds from the lumen into the systemic circulation. This restriction prevents the translocation of entire proteins like toxins and of bacteria eventually responsible for systemic infections (Usami et al., 2003). Approximately 90% of the all absorption occurs in the small intestinal region of the gastrointestinal tract (Balimane and Chong, 2005; Lee et al., 2005). The epithelium is covered by protective mucus composed of glycoproteins (mucins) and covering the mucosa as a continuous adherent blanket. The thickness of the mucus layer varies regionally throughout the gastrointestinal tract, decreasing distally from 50 to 500 μm in the stomach to 15 to 150 μm in the colon. Over the Peyer's patches, the mucus layer is much thinner than everywhere else in the intestine (Norris and Sinko, 1997; Ponchel and Irache, 1998).

To reach the epithelium where absorption takes place, molecules have to cross first the mucus layer. Mucoadhesive formulations are designed to adhere to the mucus layer hence delaying the transit of the associated molecule and prolonging its residence time in contact with the sites of absorption. When the formulation is engulfed in the gel formed by the mucins the established gradient of concentration in the drug between the delivery system and the epithelium is in favour to the absorption of the drug (Huang et al., 2000; Martinac et al., 2005; Morishita and Peppas, 2006).

In addition to the mucus layer, it is generally accepted that the main barrier for drug absorption is formed by the intestinal epithelium. Several routes can be followed to cross this epithelium (Mardones et al., 2004). Bio-engineered compounds including proteins and peptides are mostly large molecules which are highly hydrophilic in nature and do not partition to a large extent into cell membranes. They are consequently excluded from the transcellular transport pathway. The absorption of these compounds is for the most part limited to the alternative paracellular pathway (Tenhoor and Dressman, 1992), which occupies only a very small surface area of the intestine (around 1% of the total surface) compared to the transcellular route (Kotzé et al., 1998).

Epithelial cells of the intestinal mucosa are joined together at intercellular attachment zones by junctional complexes which represent 0.5 to 2 μm in length (Kriwet and Kissel 1996). The different elements of these complexes are known as *zonula occludens* or tight junctions, *zonula adherens* or intermediate junctions and *macula adherens* or spot desmosomes (Baker et al., 1991). The *zonula occudens* or tight junctions are located at the apical end of the lateral membrane of adjacent cells. They are continuous strand-like transmembrane proteins which interact with similar structures of adjacent cells. This interaction defines the paracellular permeability (Fasano and Nataro, 2004). They lead a pore with a range of 8 to 16 Å in diameter (Zhou, 1994) being the major restriction for the paracellular absorption of active molecules (Samanen et al., 1996).

Tight junctions are dynamic structures subjected to structural changes that dictate their functional status under a variety of developmental, physiological and pathological circumstances (Schulzke et al., 2005). To meet the many diverse physiological challenges to which the intestinal epithelial barrier is subjected, tight junctions must be capable of rapid and coordinated responses. This requires the presence of a complex regulatory system that orchestrates the state of assembly of the tight junction multi-protein network (Fasano and Nataro, 2004; Schulzke et al., 2005). Although these adaptive mechanisms and specific regulation of tight junctions are areas of active investigations, they still remain incompletely understood (Fasano and Nataro, 2004). It is well-known that the structure of the tight junctions is influenced by a variety of factors, e.g. protein kinase C, cytochalasin and hormones (Borchard et al., 1996; Cox et al., 2001; Usami et al., 2003). There are also evidences that tight junctions are linked to the cytoskeleton, so that intracellular processes might lead to change in their dynamic structure (Fasano and Nataro, 2004; Avadi et al., 2005). In addition, their intactness is linked to the presence of divalent cations, typically Ca^{2+} or Mg^{2+} (Borchard et al., 1996).

One approach to overcome the restriction of the paracellular transport pathway for active peptides and proteins delivery is the co-administration of *absorption-enhancing agents* regulating the integrity of the tight junctions by physicochemical interactions, either with the proteins of the tight junction or with environmental components such as extracellular calcium (Ameye et al., 2001; Roumi et al., 2001; Dorkoosh et al., 2002). The ideal enhancer will be non-toxic and act in a reversible way on the junctional complex maintaining it open just during the drug absorption. Currently, the search for safe and effective absorption enhancing agents is one of the major research fields in both academia and industry (Kotzé et al., 1998). Different absorption enhancers have been tested: calcium chelating agents (Boulenc et al., 1995a; Thanou et al., 2001; Schulzke et al., 2005), surfactants (Boulenc et al., 1995b), fatty acids (Michael et al., 2000; Usami et al., 2003), etc. Several cationic and anionic polymers have been also studied as absorption enhancers. Although the action mechanism of those polymers has not been totally elucidated, the mechanism proposed for cationic polymers (e.g. chitosan, poly-lysine, etc) was related to their ability to interact with tight junction proteins promoting their re-organization and subsequent opening (Ewan et al., 1993; Ranaedi et al., 2002). For anionic polymers, such as polyacrylic acid, a calcium binding mechanisms was suggested (Borchard et al., 1996; Kriwet and Kissel 1996; Jung et al., 2000). Both types of polymers can be used in the strategy to elaborate a carrier system aiming the improvement of the paracellular absorption of active molecules.

Enzymatic Barrier

The physiologic role of gastrointestinal proteases is to degrade dietary proteins into di- and tripeptides and aminoacids being absorbed by the small intestine. Obviously, these proteases represent a risk for the oral administration of therapeutic peptides resulting in the total loss of their biological activity. Generally, the intestinal route presents the largest enzymatic barrier to the absorption of peptides because intestinal tissues contain relatively high amount of soluble proteins (Zhou, 1994). According to their location, intestinal proteases can be divided into three main groups: luminal, brush border membrane-bounded and intracellular (cytosolic and lysosomal) enzymes (Lueβen et al., 1996; Langguth et al., 1997).

Luminal Enzymes

Once in the gastrointestinal tract, the first enzymes involved in protein degradation are the pepsins, secreted in the stomach lumen by the gastric pits. These proteases are mostly active at pH 2 to 3 and become inactive at a pH above 5 (Tenhoor and Dressman, 1992). Pepsins do not represent a real threat to orally administered pharmacologically active peptides because gastro-resistant coating materials can guarantee stability in the prevailing acidic conditions of the stomach. In contrast, the other important group of luminal enzymes including the pancreatic enzymes: trypsin, chymotrypsin, elastase and carboxypeptidases A and B represents a much serious risk for active peptides (Lueβen et al., 1996). They are highly active in the small intestine and are able to survive transit through the entire human digestive tract because their role is to transform proteins in assimilable molecules (e.i. di- or tri-peptides and even aminoacids).

Brush Border Membrane and Intracellular Proteases

Brush border membranes and intracellular proteases are present on all mucosal tissues. As pharmacologically active peptides will most likely choose the paracellular route rather than the permeation through the lipophilic cell membranes, the intracellular proteases have almost no influence in the active peptide stability. Conversely, membrane bound peptidases play the most prominent role in enzymatic degradation of active peptides (Quan et al., 1999; Ameye et al., 2000). Brush border membrane proteases are large glycoproteins facing toward from the membrane to hydrolyse peptides that come in contact with the cell surface. Examples of brush border proteases include aminopeptidases A and N, amino-oligopeptidase, dipeptidyl aminopeptidase IV, and angiotensin converting enzyme (Tenhoor and Dressman, 1992). Most of these enzymes, such as aminopeptidases, are metallopeptidases which need metal ions (Zn^{2+}, Co^{2+}, etc) as co-factors to be active (Sanderink et al., 1988; Taylor, 1993; Hooper, 1994).

Finally, it is also interesting to point out the metabolic activity of the microflora in the small and large intestine, especially in the colon. In the colon, it is composed of more than 500 species consisting of 10^{11} to 10^{12} bacteria per gram of gut content, and is capable of several metabolic reactions that can also influence peptide stability once they reach this part of the intestine (Pinto Reis et al., 2006).

Peptidic drugs can be absorbed through the gastrointestinal mucosa and enter the blood circulation in an intact form only if they are fully protected from enzymatic degradation down to their absorption site (Zhou, 1994; Larionova et al., 1999; Madsen and Peppas, 1999; Ameye et al., 2000). Because of the high variety of enzymes encountered, the many locations in the gut and the multiplicity of degradation sites in the peptide and protein structure it can be expected that there will be an upper limit to the percentage of an applied dose that will actually reach the absorption target site (Pinto Reis et al., 2006).

Some of the most important strategies tried to overcome the enzymatic barrier were: the design of drug delivery systems targeting a particular part of the gut where the luminal proteolytic activity is relatively low, typically the colon (Mackay et al., 1997), the structural modification peptides preventing proteolytic attack (Dass and Mahalakhmi, 1996; Jayawardene and Dass, 1999; Mizuma et al., 2000) or the use of protease inhibitors (Birk, 1985; Narayami, 2001). Although the use of protease inhibitors appeared to be an attractive strategy from a technological point of view, it raises serious problems of toxicity after simple co-administration of typical inhibitors, such as soybean trypsin inhibitor, aprotinin or Bowman-Birk inhibitor. Indeed, the toxic side effects of the inhibitors especially appeared during chronic therapy involving peptides because they can affect the digestion of dietary proteins (Lueβen et al., 1996; Morishita and Peppas, 2006). To prevent occurance of toxic effects due to the inhibitors, it was suggested to immobilize them in the pharmaceutical dosage form (Larionova et al., 1999; Madsen and Peppas, 1999). However, the inhibition of the proteases requires a direct interaction between the inhibitor and the enzyme. This is difficult to achieve when the inhibitor is immobilized on conventional dosage forms and the proteases are located in the mucus layer or at the apical membrane of the epithelial cells (Lueβen et al., 1996).

In the specific case of proteases requiring cations as co-factors (metallopeptidases) or to maintain their tridimensional structure (such as trypsin), one of the most effective inactivation approaches is to deplete the enzyme environment in this cation (Lueβen et al., 1996). This inhibition is interesting because it does not require a direct contact between the enzyme and the inhibitor (Lueβen et al., 1995). Indeed, it was demonstrated that chelating agents such as EDTA, EGTA, were efficient to inhibit different metallopeptidases. However, they must be immobilized in the pharmaceutical form to avoid toxic side effects (Bernkop-Schnürch and Krajicek, 1998; Bernkop-Schnürch and Kast, 2001). Some polymers showing intrinsic complexing properties, such as carbomers and polycarbophil, were able to inhibit trypsin activity thanks to a calcium depletion capability (Lueβen et al., 1995; 1996; Madsen and Peppas, 1999; Ameye et al., 2000; 2001).

Alternatively, another interesting approach is the use of *bioadhesive systems*. They are believed to be effective in enhancing the intestinal absorption of biologically active compounds vulnerable to proteolytic enzymes. Indeed, bioadhesive systems can minimize presystemic metabolism of peptide and protein drugs by the action of luminal peptidases during their transit throughout the intestine and during their transit between the delivery system and the membrane of the enterocytes (Mao et al., 2001; Iqbal et al., 2003; Mansouri et al., 2004; Vila et al., 2004; Salman et al., 2005; Morishita and Peppas, 2006).

Administration of Peptides and Proteins by the Oral Route Using Nanoparticles

From the previous section, it is obvious that peptides and proteins cannot overcome the gastrointestinal barriers by themselves. For instance, peptides of therapeutical interest such as TRH (Tyroïde Releasing Hormone) analogues, calcitonin or insulin are only poorly absorbed after oral administration. Their bioavailability remains very low being generally below 5%, 2% and 0.5% respectively (Smith et al., 1992; Tenhoor and Dressman, 1992).

Major efforts have been made to design effective and safe formulations for peptides and proteins using drug carriers. Several of the proposed strategies included the use of liposomes (Fukunaga et al., 1991; Takeuchi et al., 2005), emulsions (Matsuzawa et al., 1995; Silva Cunha et al., 1997), microcapsules (Morishita et al., 1992; Couvreur and Puisieux, 1993; Allémann et al., 1998) and nanoparticles (Couvreur et al., 1995; Couvreur et al., 2002; Panyam and Labhasetwar, 2003; Couvreur and Vauthier, 2006; Prego et al., 2006).

Nanoparticles may be defined as submicronic (< 1µm) colloidal systems. According to the process used for the preparation of nanoparticles, nanospheres or nanocapsules can be obtained. While nanospheres are matrix systems in which the drug is dispersed throughout the particles, nanocapsules are vesicular systems ("reservoir" systems) in which the drug is confined in an aqueous or oily cavity surrounded by a polymeric membrane (Alonso 2004; Couvreur et al., 2002). In many occasions, the literature has emphasized the importance of the size of the drug carrier and revealed the advantages of nanoparticles over microparticles (McClean et al., 1998; Zhi et al., 2005). It also emphasized the advantages of nanoparticles over liposomes because of their greater stability in biologic fluids as well as during storage (Soppimath et al., 2001).

Among the different kinds of nanoparticles that have been applied for drug delivery, polymeric nanoparticles were the most studied (Gupta et al., 2005). They present several characteristics that make them promising candidates to develop suitable carriers enhancing oral administration of bio-engineered drug products (Couvreur and Vauthier, 2006). The entrapment of active molecules within the polymeric nanoparticle would offer protection of the molecules against *in vivo* degradation after oral administration and control of the drug release. Moreover, due to their small size, they present an important specific surface area available for very define interactions with the absorptive epithelium and with tissues and cells (Zhou, 1994; Hillgren et al., 1995; Jung et al., 2000; Michael al., 2000; Dorkoosh et al., 2002; Mansouri et al., 2004; Morishita and Peppas, 2006; Pinto Reis et al., 2006; Prego et al., 2006).

The real utility of nanoparticles as carriers enhancing the oral delivery of drugs was demonstrated in many occasions in the scientific litterature. Briefly, nanoparticles have been used as oral drug carriers for several reasons: (I) improvement of the bioavailability for drugs with poor absorption characteristics, (II) prolongation of the residence time of drugs in the intestine, (III) high dispersion at the molecular level and consequently drastic decrease in the dissolution time for poorly soluble drugs, (IV) delivery of vaccine antigens to gut-associated lymphoid tissue, (V) control of the release rate of drugs, (VI) reduction of the gastrointestinal tract irritation caused by drugs and (VII) improvement of the stability of drugs in harsh conditions of the gastrointestinal tract (Pinto Reis et al., 2006).

Fate of the Nanoparticles in the Intestinal Tract

One approach enhancing oral delivery of therapeutic peptides and proteins using colloidal systems is to exploit the uptake of particles by the gastrointestinal tract (Hillery et al., 1996a; Florence, 2005). Indeed, nanoparticles administered orally can be absorbed, albeit in small quantities. Absorption not only occurs through the M- cells of the Peyer's patches in the gut-associated lymphoid tissues (GALT) (Hussain et al., 2001; Florence, 2005; Morishita and Peppas, 2006) but also through the enterocytes which represent the majority of the cells of the gut epithelium (Davda and Labhasetwar, 2002, Pinto-Alphandary et al., 2003, Florence, 2005).

According to Florence (2005), some of the most important factors affecting uptake and translocation of nanoparticles by the gut epithelium after oral administration are: (I) the diameter: Decrease in diameter below 1 μm increases the uptake of particles. With a diameter above 3 μm, particles are preferentially taken up by the Peyer's patches and remain there. (II) The surface charge: charged particles can be taken up but in a lower extend than non-ionic hydrophobic nanoparticles. (III) The presence of surface ligands: ligands selective to epithelial cell receptors enhance the affinity of the carriers for the cells hence promoting uptake but not necessarily translocation. (IV) The elasticity of the nanoparticles: the elasticity appears potentially important to allow nanosystems to cross capillaries with diameter smaller than the nanoparticle diameter once they have crossed the epithelium, and (V) the colloidal stability: the absence of flocculation and aggregation is a key issue for the absorption of nanoparticles. It is related to the particle size effect mentioned above.

Although the very small size of nanoparticles is in favour increasing the interactions of these types of formulations with the mucus due to the large specific surface area, the effect of mucus in nanoparticle uptake phenomena is controversial. On the one hand, it can inhibit the uptake of particles because of their engufment in the viscous glycoprotein gel hampering their access to the absorption sites. In this sense, Behrens et al. (2002) demonstrated that the presence of mucus was a major barrier to the absorption of hydrophobic polystyrene nanoparticles and showed an even stronger effect with hydrogel nanoparticles. On the other hand, it can be argued that entrapment of nanoparticles in mucus delay the transit of the nanoparticles along the gut bringing then closer to absorption sites for a longer period of time (Florence, 2005). Nevertheless, whatever the previous considerations were, nanoparticle uptake at the level of the gastrointestinal tract has been suggested to be responsible for the increased oral bioavailability observed for several peptides such as LHRH (Hillery et al., 1996b) and cyclosporin (Ford et al., 1999).

Plain Nanoparticles

Maybe some of the most popular polymeric nanocarrier for the oral administration of peptides are poly(alkyl cyanoacrylates) (PACA) nanocapsules and nanospheres. They have demonstrated to efficiently improve the oral bioavailability of peptides such as insulin (Damgé et al., 1988; Damgé et al., 1990; Lowe and Temple, 1994; Pinto-Alphandary et al., 2003), octeotride (Damgé et al., 1997), cyclosporine A (Allémann et al., 1998), calcitonin (Lowe and Temple, 1994) among other pharmacological peptides.

PACA nanoparticles can be prepared either by polymerisation of alkyl cyanoacrylate (ACA) monomers (Couvreur et al., 1979; Couvreur et al., 2002) or directly from PACA polymers and copolymers, by nanoprecipitation or emulsification solvent evaporation (Peracchia et al., 1997a; Couvreur et al., 2002). PACA are bioerodible polymers that are degraded in vivo mainly by esterases of the pancreatic juice in the intestinal tract or of serum in the blood. The degradation of PACA nanoparticles takes place in a couple of hours, depending on the alkyl side chain length, leading to degradation products (alkylalcohol and poly(cyanoacrylic acid)) that are soluble in water and easily eliminated (Vauthier et al., 2003b).

PACA nanoparticles can protect the active molecules and control their release by an erosion mechanism (Fawaz et al., 1997; Chattaraj et al., 1999; Dembri et al., 2001). There are evidences that PACA nanoparticles can be uptaken by M-cells (Michel et al., 1990), which might be favoured by the hydrophobic and anionic nature of PACA. The high esterase activity described along the M-cell apical side, might promote nanoparticle degradation and subsequent peptide release. PACA nanoparticles can also cross the epithelium by the paracellular pathway in some extent, releasing the peptide in the bloodstream after action of serum esterases. However, this mechanism is mainly limited to particles of small diameter (< 150μm) (Pinto-Alphandary et al., 2003). Finally, several authors have observed some tendency of PACA nanoparticles to develop intimate contact on large mucosal sites, evidencing the capture of PACA nanoparticles by the intestinal mucus (Ponchel et al., 1997; Dembri et al., 2001). Thus, the increase in bioavailability observed for active peptides administrated orally using PACA nanocarriers might be understood as a combination of several mechanisms: nanoparticle retention in the gastrointestinal mucus which creates a "reservoir" for peptide release and absorption, nanoparticle uptake by epithelium constituted by enterocytes and nanoparticle degradation at M-cell level (Damgé et al., 1990; Pinto-Alphandary et al., 2003)

Although it is not the aim of this chapter, it seems interesting to underline that PACA nanocarriers are also very promising tools in cancer therapy (for more detailed information audience is suggested to read Brigger et al., 2002; Vauthier et al., 2003a; Couvreur and Vauthier, 2006)

Other polymers of interest in the development of oral colloidal delivery systems are poly(lactic-co-glycolic acid) (PLGA) and poly(lactic acid) (PLA). They have gained some popularity mainly because of their noteworthy properties in terms of tissue compatibility and biodegradability (Anderson and Shive, 1997; Bilati et al., 2005). For example, Kim et al. (2002) demonstrated that a single administration of PLGA nanoparticles entrapping the peptide type II collagen was more efficient than repeated oral administrations of the peptide alone, in the induction of oral tolerance for the suppression of autoimmune rheumatoid arthritis. McClean et al. (1998) showed that about 10% of nanoparticles of PLA administered orally were adsorbed by the apical membrane of the gut in animals. No differences were found between the uptake patterns of tissues with and without Peyer's patches. The absorption mechanism was found to be size-dependent (nanoparticles better than microparticles) and predominately transcellular. However, the authors concluded that the surface of PLA nanoparticles could be modified to improve their use as vaccine delivery systems in the gut.

Other nanoparticles that have raised much attention during the last decade are those made of chitosan. Several methods of preparation of chitosan nanoparticles such as coacervation/precipitation methods, spray-drying, and gelation have been studied for conventional drug encapsulation. However, the cross-linking methods have been the most used for peptides and drug encapsulation (Agnihotri et al., 2004). Although this method guarantee the preparation of well defined and size controlled chitosan nanoparticles, the conventional cross-linking agents, including glutaraldehyde, must be avoided preventing both damage in the loaded peptide structure and cellular toxicity (Janes et al., 2001; Wang et al., 2006). As an interesting alternative way to produce chitosan nanoparticles, the use of anionic counterions like tripolyphosphate, dextran sulfate or alginate as cross-linking agents was proposed. With the so-called ionic gelation process, chitosan nano- and microparticles loaded with peptides can be produced in gentle conditions. This method has gained much attention because it is simple, non-toxic and involves the mixture of two aqueous solutions at room temperature avoiding the use of organic solvents (Calvo et al., 1997; Janes et al., 2001; Sarmento et al., 2006; 2007). Chitosan constituting the nanoparticles retains its cationic nature required for bioadhesion at the mucosae surface and permeation enhancing properties (Boonsongrit et al., 2006). Pan et al. (2002) have elaborated insulin loaded chitosan nanoparticles by ionotropic gelation with tripolyphosphate. The ability of these nanoparticles to enhance the intestinal absorption of insulin made possible the lowering of blood glucose levels for an extended period of time after oral administration. Ma et al (2005) observed similar results showing strong interactions between rat intestinal epithelium and chitosan nanoparticles several hours after oral administration which also promoted an increase in the peptide bioavailability.

The group of Ferreira also used insulin as model peptide to develop dextran sulfate/chitosan and alginate/chitosan nanoparticles, demonstrating in both cases a high insulin association efficacy and preserving the peptide activity. Current studies of this group are focused on the in vivo evaluation of such a systems (Sarmento et al., 2006; 2007).

Chitosan is a very promising candidate for designing carrier systems for oral vaccine delivery (Van der Lubben et al., 2001a). Using confocal laser scanning microscopy, Van der Lubben et al. (2001b) demonstrated the uptake of ovalbumin loaded chitosan microparticles by Peyer's patches after intragastric feeding of mice.

Core-shell Nanoparticles

According to Prego et al. (2006), the efficacy of polymeric nanocarriers to improve the absorption of labile macromolecules depends strongly on their composition. Polymers used should (I) provide the drug intact to the specific site of absorption, (II) preferentially prolong its residence time on the mucosa, and (III) reversibly and temporary increase the permeability of the mucosal epithelium to allow transport of macromolecular drugs to the blood circulation and/or to the lymphatic system. Additionally, a safety requirement should be that these excipients should not show adverse systemic effects, damage or exfoliate the epithelium (Thanou et al., 2001). It was suggested that a rational modification in the composition and structure of the nanoparticle surface, using safe materials, can increase the prospects of their usefulness for mucosal protein delivery and transport (Vila et al., 2002). Several modifications of nanoparticle surface were already proposed to improve the biopharmaceutical characteristics of the oral administration of peptides and proteins. One of the most promising consist in coating the nanoparticle surface with *poly(ethylene glycol)*

(PEG). Tobío et al. (2000) and Vila et al. (2002) observed an increment in the bioavailability of tetanus toxoid when poly(lactic acid) (PLA) loaded nanoparticles were coated with PEG. The PEG coating would compromise enzyme adsorption, thereby reducing the harsh conditions in which the particles are exposed until they reach the absorbing epithelium. Additionnaly, an increment of the bioadhesion of PLA nanoparticles was also suggested to occur in vivo after coating with PEG. Gref et al. (2001) analysed the benefit of PEG coating on PLA nanoparticles loaded with cyclosporin A. They noted that the presence of PEG not only improved the stability of nanoparticles in fluids medium and the peptide loading, but also performed a more adequate control of the release of the peptide *in vitro*.

The use of polysaccharides to coat nanoparticles was suggested to mimic the surface of cells, bacteria and viruses giving the nanoparticles new surface properties including the biological activity of the carbohydrate (Passirani et al. 1998a, Maruyama et al., 1999; Chauvierre et al., 2003c; Vauthier et al., 2007). In this view, the use of chitosan as coating material has been investigated. García-Fuentes et al. (2005a) prepared lipid nanoparticles coated with chitosan for the oral administration of calcitonin. The coating was performed by simple incubation of the lipid nanoparticle core in a chitosan solution thanks to the high affinity of chitosan for the lipid core. These nanoparticles showed a significant improvement of calcitonin oral bioavailability *in vivo*, which was attributed to the permeation enhancement properties already described for chitosan (García-Fuentes et al., 2005b). Prego et al. (2005) studied the permeation effect of chitosan coated nanosystems (lipid nanoparticles and oil nanodroplets) using a cell line developed as model of intestinal barrier representative of a monolayer of enterocytes (Caco-2 cell monolayer model). They observed that those chitosan-coated nanosystems caused a concentration-dependent opening of the tight junctions and particle internalisation in the cell monolayer. In subsequent *in vivo* studies performed in rats, it was suggested that this behaviour can explain the observed increased of intestinal absorption of calcitonin. In addition, the authors obtained more interesting results with the chitosan coated nanosystems than for nanoparticles elaborated exclusively with chitosan produced by ionotropic gelation (Prego et al., 2005).

With chitosan-coated submicron-sized liposomes, both the chitosan coating and the submicron size were key factors increasing enteral absorption of calcitonin as observed after oral administration to rats (Takeuchi et al., 2005). This mucoadhesive system is retained in the mucus partly owing the absorption by the intestinal epithelium.

Plain nanoparticles have almost no site-specificity in the gastrointestinal tract. To improve the specificity of nanosystems for the gastrointestinal mucosae, ligands binding to specific receptors shown by the gut were attached on the nanoparticle surface. This increased the binding specificity of the nanoparticles and decreased their elimination rate due to the mucus turnover. The most popular ligands used for this purpose included lectins, invasins and vitamine B12 (Nobs et al., 2004; Salman et al., 2005). *Lectins* raised special attention because they are involved in cell recognition mechanisms (Russell-Jones, 1999; Jung et al., 2000). Their specificity, multivalent featured, as well as their non-immunogenic properties render lectins appealing candidates for development of site-specific coated nanosystems as drug delivery carriers (Goldstein et al., 1980; Arangoa et al., 2000). For instance, Rodrigues et al. (2003) developed core (polyester)-shell (polysaccharide) nanoparticles with lectins at the surface as a tool for site-specific oral administration of peptides. Arangoa et al (2000) prepared surface modified nanoparticles by binding lectins improving the specificity of the drug delivery device for the colonic mucosa.

The literature is riched in examples demonstrating the benefit of nanoparticulate formulations in the oral delivery of therapeutic peptides and proteins. They were shown to protect peptides and proteins from degradation in a very efficient way. Bioadhesive formulations were demonstrated to promote the bioavailability due to an increase of residence time near absoption sites. Morover, nanoparticles were found to serve as shuttle transporting active peptides and proteins through the intestinal epithelium. None of the systems proposed so far combined the different functionalities in a single nanoparticle. Thus, the purpose of our work, presented in the next parts of this chapter, was to develop a new nanoparticulate formulation combining the different functionnalities based on the use of core-shell poly(alkylcyanoacrylate) nanoparticle technologies.

Elaboration of Core-shell Poly(Alkyl Cyanoacrylate) (PACA) Nanoparticles

Considering the potential of plain PACA nanoparticles for the efficent oral administration of labile molecules, and the interest of nanoparticle surface modifications, efforts have been made to further improve the characteristics of this system by modification of their surface properties. From a technological view point, most of the approaches used in the development of stable surface modified nanoparticles have been based on the synthesis of amphiphilic copolymers (Peracchia et al., 1997b; Uchegbu et al., 1998; Brigger et al., 2001; Rodrigues et al., 2003; Archambault and Brash, 2004, Lemarchand et al., 2004; Park et al., 2006). Generally, this requires the synthesis of a copolymer between the hydrophilic coating and the hydrophobic core materials. The copolymer is then formulated as nanoparticles using methods of nanoprecipitation or solvent evaporation for instance (Peracchia et al., 1997b; Gref et al., 2001; Lemarchand et al., 2004). To obtain surface-modified PACA nanoparticles, both copolymers and nanoparticles are synthesized in the same time by emulsion polymerization thanks to different mechanisms of initiation of the polymerization of alkylcyanoacrylate monomers. Those monomers are so reactive that any nucleophilic groups can initiate a spontaneous anionic polymerization. This results in covalent linkage of the growing polymer chains on the component having initiated the polymerization. In this way, PEG-coated nanoparticles were synthesized by initiating the polymerization of isobutylcyanoacrylate with the terminal hydroxyl groups of PEG. The PEG-coated nanoparticles were designed as stealth® nanoparticles to avoid non-specific uptake by macrophages and to show long circulating properties in the blood after intravenous administration. PACA nanoparticles coated with polysaccharides can also be obtained thanks such a mechanism of polymerization initiation induced by the nucleophilic groups beared on polysaccharide chains. Taking advantage of this polymerization, dextran and chitosan coated nanoparticles were prepared (Couvreur 1979, Douglas 1986, Zhang et al., 2003). The polysaccharide chains standed at the nanoparticles surface adopt a side-on conformation because several anchorage chains of poly(alkylcyanoacrylate) can be grafted on a single chain of polysaccharide due to the many nucleophilic polymerization initiator groups found on saccharide units.

Recently, Chauvierre et al. (2003a, 2003b, 2003c) developed a new method of polymerization for the elaboration of polysaccharide-coated poly(alkyl cyanoacrylate) nanoparticles. This method leading to poly(alkyl cyanoacrylate)-core polysaccharide shell nanoparticles can be coated with different polysaccharides, such as dextran, dextran sulphate, chitosan, heparin, and hyaluronic acid. The technique is based on a redox radical emulsion polymerisation of alkyl cyanoacrylate (ACA) monomers initiated on the carbohydrate structure by a radical polymerization. The copolymers which form during this polymerization showed a linear diblock structure which is quite different from the structure of the copolymer formed by the spontaneous anionic emulsion polymerization. Thus, a different conformation of polysaccharide chains on the nanoparticle surface can be obtained. While nanoparticles obtained by the anionic polymerization were characterized by a loop conformation of the polysaccharide chains arranged on the side-on position at the nanoparticle surface, radical polymerisation promoted brush like chain conformation thanks to the linear di-block structure of the copolymer formed (Bertholon et al., 2006a).

Polysaccharides grafted on the PACA nanoparticles did not only influence the physicochemical characteristics of the nanoparticles, such as surface charge or hydrodynamic diameter, but it also greatly affected their behaviour in physiological environments. For example, heparin gave antithrombic activity to particles (Chauvierre et al., 2006c) and dextran changed the response pattern of PACA particle interaction with blood opsonins typically responsible for the phagocytosis by macrophages after intravenous administration. Moreover, the interaction with proteins was demonstrated to be modulated by the polysaccharide molecular weight and the arrangement of the polysaccharide chains on the nanoparticle surface (Bertholon-Rajot et al., 2006a; 2006b).

Interest of Chitosan and Modified Chitosan in the Design of Surface Modified PACA Nanoparticles for the Oral Administration of Peptides and Proteins

Chitosan

Chitosan is a cationic high molecular weight heteropolysaccharide composed mainly of β-(1,4)-2-deoxy-2-amino-D-glucopyranose and secondary of β-(1,4)-2-deoxy-2-acetamido-D-glucopyranose. It is obtained from the natural polysaccharide chitin by partial deacetylation (Ding et al., 2003). Free amino groups of chitosan can undergo protonation hence making it soluble in aqueous acid solution (pH < 6.5) avoiding the use of hazardous organic solvents while handing (Agnihotri et al., 2004).

Because of a favourable biological profile including biodegradability, biocompatibility and absence of toxicity, chitosan has attracted attention in pharmaceutical and biomedical fields (Ravi Kumar, 2000; Agnihotri et al., 2004; Mao et al., 2004; Prego et al., 2005; 2006). Its cationic nature makes it an interesting candidate for DNA complexation involving electrostatic interactions and for proteins and vaccine encapsulation (Illum et al., 2001; Janes et al., 2001; Mao et al., 2001; Merdan et al., 2002; Li et al., 2003; Kim et al., 2004).

The inherent *bioadhesiveness* of chitosan has been denoted by many authors (Gaserod et al., 1998; Illum et al., 2001). Bioadhesive properties of chitosan involved electrostatic interactions with the negatively charged sialic acis groups on the mucus found at physiologic pH. It was demonstrated that chitosan can *enhance the intestinal absorption* of hydrophilic molecules. The mechanism behind this permeation enhancement effect seems to be based on the opening of the tight junction of the mucosal epithelium due to interactions of the positive charges of the polymer with tight junction-associated proteins therefore inducing a structural reorganization (Schipper et al., 1997; Jung et al., 2000; Leanes et al., 2004). Additionally, chitosan were found to bind divalent *cations* in neutral or weakly acid media, due to the free electronic doublet of nitrogen (Monteiro and Airoldi, 1999; Guibal et al., 2000; 2002; Lima and Airoldi, 2003). Thus chitosan may act as a cation scavenger interfering with the activity of cation-dependent proteases hence improving the chance for intact therapeutic peptides and proteins to be absorbed by the oral route. According to Lima and Airoldi (2003) the ion binding properties of chitosan is related to its high hydrophilicity owing to the large number of hydroxyl groups, the presence of a number of primary amino groups acting as potential base centers and the flexible polymeric chain structure which favours the adjustment of the cations dispersed in solution for complex formation.

All these characteristics make chitosan one of the most widely used biopolymers in development of nanoparticles for the oral administration of peptides (see the section: Plain Nanoparticles).

Modifiing Commercially Available Chitosan

Several types of modifications were considered to improve the properties of chitosan included in the formulation of drug delivery devices. Generally, the commercially available forms of chitosan are characterized by a high molecular weight (several hundred thousands g/mol) and by a certain degree of acetylation. In different works it was found that these characteristics are far from the optimal one. Thus several modifications of the commercial form of chitosan were undergone either to reduce the molecular weight of the initial compound or to introduce new chemical functions. As it will be explained bellow, there is a real benefice achieving such modifications. It generally allows to tune properties of the modified chitosan in such a way that the functionality of the polysaccharide is improved. For instance, the molecular weight of chitosan was influencing the stability of DNA/chitosan and peptides/chitosan complexes, the efficiency of cell uptake once in contact with the cellular membrane and the dissociation of active molecule from the complex after subsequent endocytosis. Reducing the size of chitosan to molecular weight ranging from 20,000 to 50,000 g/mol improved its transfection efficiency as demonstrated by Sato et al.(2001) and Lee et al. (2001). Vila et al. (2004) have demonstrated that tetanus toxin-loaded nanoparticles prepared with low molecular weight chitosan (28,000 g/mol and 38,000 g/mol) induced a stronger inmunoresponse towards the toxin at earlier times than the loaded nanoparticles elaborated with higher molecular weight chitosans.

Huang et al. (2004) developed an interesting method reducing the molecular weight of chitosan. This method is based on the oxidative degradation of the polysaccharide. It is performed by mixing an acidic solution of chitosan with different amounts of $NaNO_2$, because the molecular weight of the degraded chitosan will depend on the salt concentration. In our group, we have used this method to produce chitosans of different molecular weights from a commercial chitosan having a molecular weight of 400,000g/mol. The $NaNO_2$ concentrations were ranging from 7 to 1.5 mg/ml producing chitosan of molecular weight ranging from 10,000 to 100,000 g/mol respectively with a good production yield. All batches of low molecular weigh chitosan kept the same characteristics than the parent chitosan: general structure, degree of deacetylation, etc., (Bertholon-Rajot et al., 2006c; Bravo-Osuna et al., 2006; Bravo-Osuna et al., in press).

From an engineering point of view, the presence of hydroxyl and amino groups in the structure of chitosan make this polymer easy to modify introducing new chemical groups to modulate its characteristics and eventually to give it new properties (Kotzé et al., 1998; Zhang et al., 2003; Lemarchand et al., 2004; Sashiwa and Aiba, 2004). For example, several authors have modified chitosan by introducing diethyl or trymethyl groups in the structure. This increased the solubility of the polysaccharide at neutral pH (Thanou et al., 2001; Avadi et al., 2005) and gave the new polysaccharide potent intestinal permeation enhancement behaviour (van der Merwe et al., 2004a,b; Thanou et al., 2001; 2000). More recently, interesting peptide-chitosan polymers were created increasing the solubility of the chitosan derivatives over a wide range of pH (Batista et al., in press).

Another approach consists on copolymerising chitosan with other polymers. For instance, Prego et al. (2006) designed a new type of nanocapsules using chitosan chemically modified with PEG. The nanocapsules were obtained by the solvent displacement technique. Using the Caco-2 cell line model, it was observed that the pegylation of chitosan reduced the cytotoxicity of nanocapsules. In vivo studies showed that the capacity of the chitosan-PEG nanocapsules enhanced and prolonged the intestinal absorption of salmon calcitonin.

The group of Bernkop-Schnurch has introduced thiol groups in the structure of chitosan (Bernkop-Schnurch and Kast, 2001). The thiolated chitosans (chitosan-cysteine, chitosan-thioglycolic acid and chitosan-4-thiol-butyl-amidine) showed several interesting characteristics to be used for the development of pharmaceutical systems designed for the oral administration of drugs (Bernkop-Schnürch et al., 2004). Those products have improved mucoadhesive properties compared to chitosan because it can promote interactions with cysteine-rich domains of mucus glycoproteins resulting in the formation of disulphide bonds (Gum et al., 1992; Bernkop-Schnürch and Steininger, 2000; Bernkop-Schnürch and Kast, 2001; Kast and Bernkop-Schnürch, 2001; Marschutz and Bernkop-Schnürch, 2002; Roldo et al., 2004). Moreover, thiolated chitosans were found to develop additional mucosal permeation enhancing properties, which mechanism could be related with the gluthation (GSH) regeneration in the endothelial environment (Bernkop-Schnürch et al., 2003). Finally, as chitosan, thiolated chitosan can bind divalent cations including Zn^{2+} or Mg^{2+} suggesting that they will also have antiprotease activity (Bernkop-Schnürch and Kast, 2001; Bernkop-Schnürch et al., 2003; Bernkop-Schnürch et al., 2004; Roldo et al., 2004). The binding capacity was improved by the introduction of the thiol groups in the chitosan structure. Several possible binding mechanism were suggested: (I) the protonated form may bind divalent cations by ion pair formation thanks to an ion exchange mechanism; (II) the non protonated form of thiolated chitosan may bind cations via nitrogen and/or sulphur donor atoms by a coordination by ligand exchange mechanism; and (III) a more or like combination of the two previous mechanisms involving ion pair binding mechanism followed by slow ligand exchange. Among the different thiolated chitosan synthesized, those resulting from of the linkage of 2-iminothiolane (chitosan-4-thiol-butyl-amidine: chitosan-TBA) appeared the most promising in terms of stability. Moreover, the bioadhesive, permeation enhancement and antiprotease activity were also maximized with these compounds (Bernkop-Schnürch et al., 2003; Roldo et al., 2004).

In our group, we have prepared chitosan-TBA of different molecular weights. Both the total sulphur content and the free thiol groups were determined by elemental analysis and iodine titration respectively (Bravo-Osuna et al., submitted (1)). Interestingly, an inversed relationship between the molecular weight of chitosan and the percentage of amino groups involved in the reaction with 2-iminothiolane was observed suggesting a lower accessibility of those groups when the molecular weight of chitosan increased. In all cases, total sulphur content was higher than the amount of thiol groups suggesting the presence of intra- and/or inter disulfide bonds in the polymeric structure. This effect was increased with chitosan of high molecular weight reducing the solubility of the macromolecule (Bravo-Osuna et al., 2006; Bravo-Osuna et al., in press).

Thiolated chitosan have demonstrated their usefulness improving the oral bioavailability of several peptides. For instance, tablets and minitablets targeted towards the stomach prepared with thiolated chitosan were evaluated in vivo. Using such formulations, a moderate increment of bioavailability of encapsulated peptides (antide, calcitonin) was observed (Guggi et al., 2003; Bernkop-Schnürch et al., 2005). The use of these polymers in the elaboration of microparticles has also raised interest for the oral delivery of peptides and proteins. Krauland et al. (2006) developed thiolated chitosan microparticles loaded with insulin. They were administered by the nasal route showing moderate increment of peptide bioavailability. Very recently, formulations from the nanotechnologies were also investigated. Thiolated chitosan was conjugated with DNA forming particles in the nanometer-range. Transfection studies performed in Caco-2 cell culture evidenced a high transfection efficiency using these complexes making these systems promising new vectors for gene delivery (Schmitz et al., 2006).

According to these interesting results, the use of thiolated chitosan for the preparation of nanocarriers appears to be a very attractive tool and merit to be associated with nanotechnologies to formulate new carriers for the oral delivery of peptides and proteins.

Chitosan-coated PACA Nanoparticles

As other surface modified PACA naoparticles, chitosan-coated PACA nanoparticles were obtained by emulsion polymerization of the alkylcyanoacrylate monomers initiated by the anionic or the redox radical polymerization mechanisms (Zhang et al., 2003; Chauvierre et al., 2003c; Bertholon et al., 2006b, Bravo Osuna et al., in press), Chitosan-coated PACA particles obtained by redox radical emulsion polymerisation using commercial polysaccharide (400,000 g/mol), showed a diameter within the micrometer-range (hydrodynamic diameter of 59 μm). Chauvierre et al. (2003c). To reduce the size of the particle, Bertholon-Rajot et al. (2006c) and Bravo-Osuna et al. (2006; in press) suggested the use of depolymerised chitosan with molecular weight ranging between 10,000 and 200,000 g/mol. The nanoparticles obtained showed mean hydrodynamic diameters with values varying from 200 to 600 nm when increasing the molecular weight of chitosan. Slightly different diameters were shown by nanoparticles prepared by the anionic polymerization, suggesting a different copolymer arrangement of the copolymer within the nanoparticle structure. In all cases the presence of the cationic polysaccharide, chitosan, on the nanoparticles surface was demonstrated by ζ potential measurement, obtaining positive values. This has to be compared with the negative values characterizing PACA nanoparticles coated with dextran, a neutral polysaccharide. The stability of nanoparticles was evaluated in a wide range of pH (3-9) demonstrating that the covalent attachment of chitosan to the PIBCA core ensured no aggregation over the range of physiological pH encountered in the gastrointestinal tract. Thus the potential bioadhesive nature of the nanoparticles due to positively charged surfaces was also completed over the range of pH of the gastrointestinal tract.

In Figure 1, SEM and TEM micrographs showed the PIBCA nanoparticles coated with chitosan of molecular weights of 20,000 and 100,000 g/mol. Both microscopic methods showed spherical and individualised nanoparticles. A layer of polysaccharidic material standing at the nanoparticle surface was clearly highlighted by TEM for radical formulations, especially when the nanoparticles were prepared with high molecular weight chitosan (100,000 g/mol) (Bravo-Osuna et al., in press).

The versatility of the method of elaboration of core-shell nanoparticles based on anionic and redox radical polymerisation was demonstrated by modifying both core and surface compositions (Bravo-Osuna et al., 2006; Bravo-Osuna et al., in press).

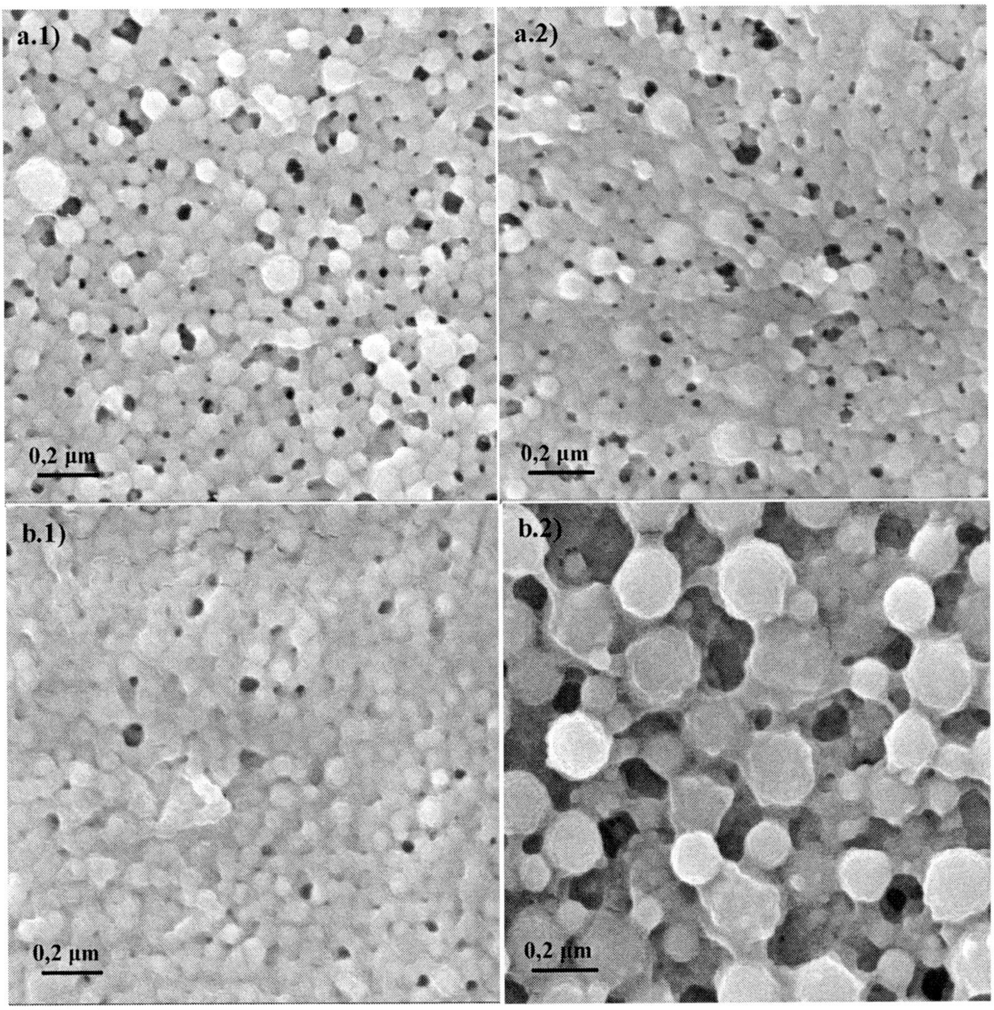

Figure 1. Scanning electron microphotographs of coated PIBCA nanoparticles elaborated with chitosan of 20,000 (a), and 100,000 (b) g/mol following anionic (1) or radical (2) polymerisation. Modified from Bravo-Osuna et al., in press.

The introduction of a second acrylic monomer in the formulation was investigated in order to modify the core properties, which can be useful for adjusting the core properties for drug encapsulation and control of the release kinetics of the drug. This can be also very usefull as a simple method for labelling the nanoparticles required for further biopharmaceutical evaluation. In this sense, the inclusion of moderate percentages of methylmethacrylate in the alkylcyanoacrylate monomer (5-10%) did not essentially modify the morphology of the nanoparticles obtained by both anionic and radical polymerization. In all cases, monodisperse suspensions of nanoparticles were obtained. The labelling of the nanoparticles by this method involved the copolymerization of isobutylcyanoacrylate with a fluorescent labelled acrylic monomer. This successful method allowed the covalent linkage of the rhodamine containing marker in the nanoparticle core during the polymerisation process (Bravo-Osuna et al., in press).

Nanoparticle surface modification was also evaluated by replacing chitosan by thiolated chitosan as shell component. As was previously pointed out, inclusion of thiolated polymers in the formulation should add several interesting characteristics to the nanocarrier systems that would improve their efficacy for the administration of biotechnology products by mucosal routes. To this aim, nanoparticles were elaborated using mixtures of chitosan and chitosan-TBA of different molecular weights in different proportions. Due to the lack of solubility of the high molecular weight chitosan-TBA (Bravo-Osuna et al., 2006), nanoparticles with a wide range of chitosan-TBA content was only obtained with the lower molecular weight analysed (Bravo-Osuna et al., in press). The presence of thiol groups on the nanoparticle surface was verified by the iodine titration method. This method allows the determination of thiol groups at acid pH promoting oxidation of thiol groups in presence of iodine (Bravo-Osuna et al., submitted (1)). The density of those "active" or "reactive" thiol groups at the nanoparticle surface increased with the percentage of chitosan-TBA used in the nanoparticle preparation. However, the incorporation of high percentages of chitosan-TBA in the formulation enhanced the formation of disulphide bonds, leading to a higher cross-linked structure of the shell of the nanoparticles and to an increase of the viscosity of the gel layer formed by these molecules at the nanoparticle surface (Bravo-Osuna et al., in press). For each series of nanoparticles, the hydrodynamic mean diameter of the nanoparticles increased with the percentage of chitosan-TBA, while the ζ potential values decreased.

Interaction of Chitosan-coated PACA Nanoparticles with the Intestinal Mucosa

Bioadhesion

When micro- or nanoparticles are administered orally in the form of a suspension, they diffuse into the liquid medium and they rapidly encounter the mucosal surface. The particles can be immobilized at the intestinal surface by an adhesion mechanism so-named "bioadhesion". More specifically, when adhesion is restricted to the mucus layer lining the mucosal surface, then the term "mucoadhesion" is employed. From a qualitative point of view, the following framework is generally accepted: After dilution in the gastrointestinal fluids, the mucoadhesiveness of a colloidal suspension depends basically (I) on the kinetics of the particles to diffuse into the suspension medium and (II) on the ability of the particles to interact with mucin glycoproteins or other mucus components being immobilized within the mucus layer (Durrer et al., 1994a; 1994b; Ponchel and Irache, 1998).

In recent works, we have evaluated the bioadhesiveness of several chitosan-coated PIBCA nanoparticles (Bertholon-Rajot et al., 2006c, Bravo-Osuna et al., submitted (2) submitted (3)) following a method developed by Durrer et al. (1994a; 1994b) and presented in Figure 2. Bertholon-Rajot et al. (2006c) evaluated different chitosan-coated PIBCA nanoparticles elaborated by anionic and radical polymerisation with chitosan of molecular weight ranging between 30,000 and 200,000 g/mol. They demonstrated that polysaccharides grafted at the nanoparticles surface in the brush conformation (radical polymerisation) appeared more favourable to promote interactions of nanoparticles with glycoproteins of mucus in comparison with more compact loop conformation of polysaccharide chains obtained by anionic polymerisation. Bravo-Osuna et al. (submitted (2) (3)) analyzed the bioadhesion behaviour of chitosan core-shell PIBCA nanoparticles elaborated by radical polymerisation using chitosan and thiolated chitosan of molecular weights between 20,000 and 100,000 g/mol. They observed that the presence of a cross-linked structure, due to the formation of intra- and interchains disulfide bonds, partially reduced the interaction with mucins. However, the presence of high amounts of free (reduced) thiol groups in the nanoparticle surface importantly increased the bioadhesion of the nanoparticles because covalent bonds with cysteine residues of glycoproteins of the mucus can be formed. In all cases, the presence of chitosan on the PIBCA nanoparticle surface importantly increased the bioadhesiveness of the system in comparison to PIBCA nanoparticles coated with dextran. This was in agreement with the bioadhesive nature of the chitosan used as coating material. The diffusibity of nanoparticles through the mucus hydrogel seemed to be mainly governed by their hydrodynamic diameter, so high bioadhesive capacity was observed for the nanoparticles of small hydrodynamic diameter (200-300 nm). These results were consistent with those of Durrer et al. (1994a; 1994b), who suggested that small particles can be considered as adsorbates penetrating into a porous adsorbent formed by the mucus layer.

Figure 3 presents the bioadhesion mechanism proposed for the chitosan-coated PIBCA nanoparticles (Bravo-Osuna et al., submitted (2)). In general, the deposition of model colloids on well-defined solid surface involves two steps: *transport* and *attachment*. In this work, the *transport* of the particles analysed was mainly governed by their particle size and the presence of hydrophilic chitosan on their surface. Different mechanisms can occur simultaneously in the *attachment* of the mucoadhesion process. Their intensity depends on the nanoparticle surface characteristics (Durrer et al., 1994a; Huang et al., 2000) (I) Non-covalent bonds can be created within the mucus-polymer interface (electronic and adsorption theory). For the systems analysed in this work, those non-covalent unions were improved by the presence of cationic chitosan. (II) The polymer and protein chains can interpenetrate (diffusion theory) and entangle together. This phenomenon depended on the chain conformation and on the degree of cross-linking in the gel layer formed by the polysaccharide on the nanoparticle surface. (III) Further non-covalent (physical) and covalent (chemical) bonds (electronic and adsorption theory) can be formed (Cilurzo et al., 2003; Dodou et al., 2005). In the case of thiolated nanoparticles, it can be expected that the presence of high amounts of reduced thiol groups on the nanoparticle surface should ensured the formation of covalent disulphide bonds with the mucus cysteine groups promoting the bioadhesion of the nanoparticles by covalent linkage.

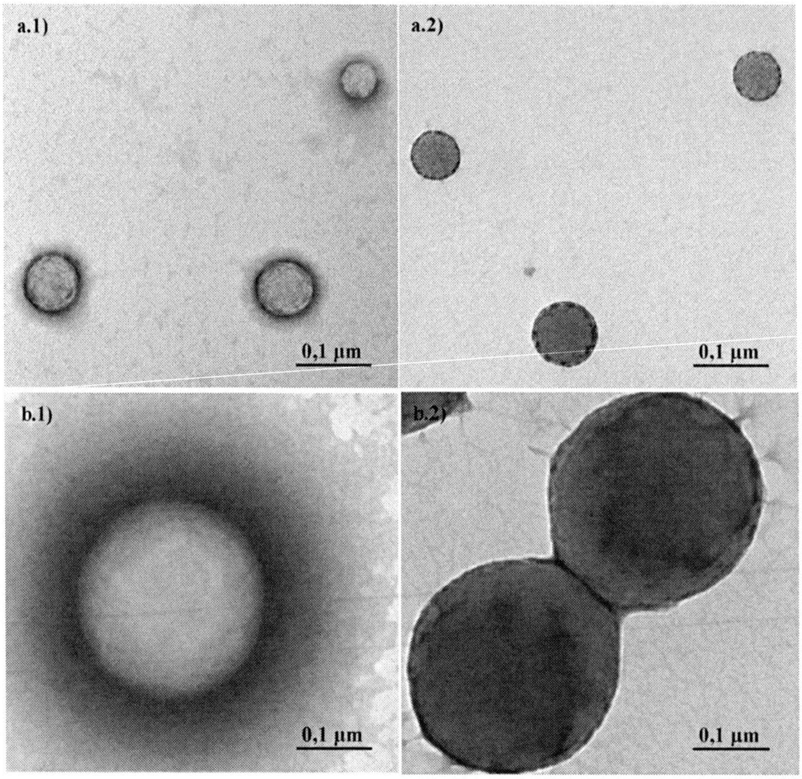

Figure 2. Transmission electron microphotographs of coated PIBCA nanoparticles elaborated with chitosan of 20,000 (a), and 100,000 (b) g/mol following anionic (1) or radical (2) polymerisation. Modified from Bravo-Osuna et al., in press.

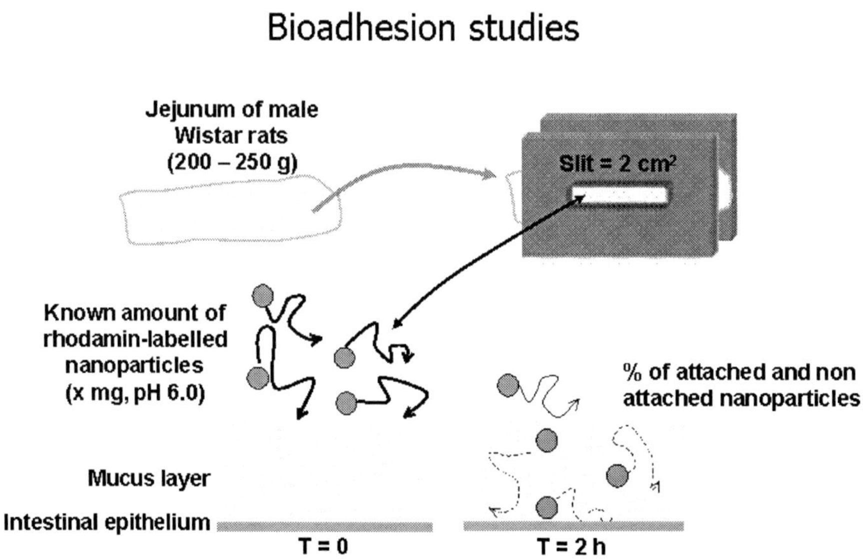

Figure 3. Scheme of *in vitro* bioadhesion studies according to the protocol developed by Durrer et al., (1994a; 1994b).

Ion binding Capacity

In the gastrointestinal tract, cations play an important role maintaining permeation properties of the epithelium and enzymatic activities. Thus potential cation binding capacity of colloidal systems might be an interesting tool for nanocarriers designed for the oral administration of pharmacologically active peptides because they may act as modulators of the enzymatic activity and permeation of the epithelium.

Thus, the cation binding capacity of chitosan and thiolated chitosan core-shell PIBCA nanoparticles was investigated (Bravo-Osuna et al. submitted (4), submitted (5)). Two cations of physiological interest calcium and zinc were selected as model ions. While calcium ions are necessary to maintain tight junction integrity and the tridimentional structure of several proteases such as trypsin, zinc ions are part of the active site of gastrointestinal metallopeptidases. With both cations, the binding capacity of chitosan appeared 2 to 3 folds higher when the polysaccharide was bound on the nanoparticle surface than when it was in solution. In agreement with data published by other authors, this demonstrated that physical changes in chitosan presentation (beads or films manufacturing) can improve the cation binding capacity of this polysaccharide (Chassary et al., 2004; Guibal 2004). According to Rhazi et al. (2002), this phenomenon can be explained by an increase of the accessibility of the free amine groups of chitosan when it is exposed at the nanoparticle surface. This accessibility to active sites was also limited by the formation of a cross-linked structure observed when thiolated chitosan was included in intermediate percentage. The negative effect of cross-linking structures on the binding capacity of polymer was clearly demonstrated by other authors (Madsen and Peppas, 1999; Becker et al., 2000; Dzul Erosa et al., 2001; Jeon and Holl, 2003; Guibal, 2004). However, the formulations with high percentage of free thiol groups on the nanoparticle surface allowed higher binding ability, overcoming the negative effect of the cross-linking structure assumed for the gel layer standing at the surface of these nanoparticles.

Antiprotease Activity

The inhibitory effect of chitosan and thiolated chitosan core-shell PIBCA nanoparticles was tested against two model metallopeptidases of the gastrointestinal tract: Carboxypeptidase A (CP A) and Leucine aminopeptidase M (LAP M) (Bravo-Osuna et al., submitted (5)).

Carboxypeptidase A is a prototypic zinc-containing proteolytic enzyme, representing a large family of physiologically important zinc proteases such as Angiotensin-Converting Enzyme (ACE) and matrix metallopeptidases. This enzyme catalyses the hydrolysis of the C-terminal amide bonds of peptide substrate (Chung and Kim, 2001; Park and Kim, 2004). As a representative zinc protease, the enzyme has received much attention as a model enzyme for devising design protocols of inhibitors that are effective against zinc proteases of medical interest (Lee and Kim, 2000; Li and Solomon, 2001; Cho et al., 2002). Removal of zinc leads to the formation of metal-free carboxypeptidase which is enzymatically inactive (Vallee et al., 1960; Li and Solomon, 2001; Phoon and Burton, 2005).

Leucine aminopeptidase M (EC.3.4.11.2.) is probably the aminopeptidase that has been studied the most extensively. It is located on the brush border of intestinal epithelial cells of the gastrointestinal tract, where it cleaves degraded small peptides in the final stages of protein digestion. Hence, the enzyme performs an important nutritional protein processing role (Sanderink et al., 1988). It is, for example, the main cause for degradation of insulin after administration by the oral route (Zhou, 1994). This membrane-bound enzyme is also a zinc-dependent metallopeptidase (Himmelhoch, 1969; Hooper, 1994) that can be inactivated by depletion in the cation (Bernkop-Schnurch and Krajicek, 1998).

The zinc binding capacity of chitosan and thiolated chitosan in solution was not high enough to develop effective ion depletion from the active site of CP A and LAP M. However, the same amount of the biopolymers presented as the coating material of nanoparticles showed inhibition capability against the two metallopeptidases. The inhibition factor values were higher than one, determined in the first five minutes of the study. The inhibition capacity decreased from nanoparticles elaborated with chitosan/chitosan-TBA proportions of 100/0 to 25/75, which is in total agreement with the zinc binding capacity previously observed. However, the high binding capacity observed for nanoparticles elaborated with 100% of chitosan-TBA did not correspond to the higher inhibitory effect expected. For this formulation, the affinity between polymer and ions was not high enough to induce sufficient ion depletion. Not only the zinc binding capacity of the biopolymer but also the biopolymer presentation on the nanoparticle surface clearly played a key role in the inhibitory effects observed on the peptidase activities.

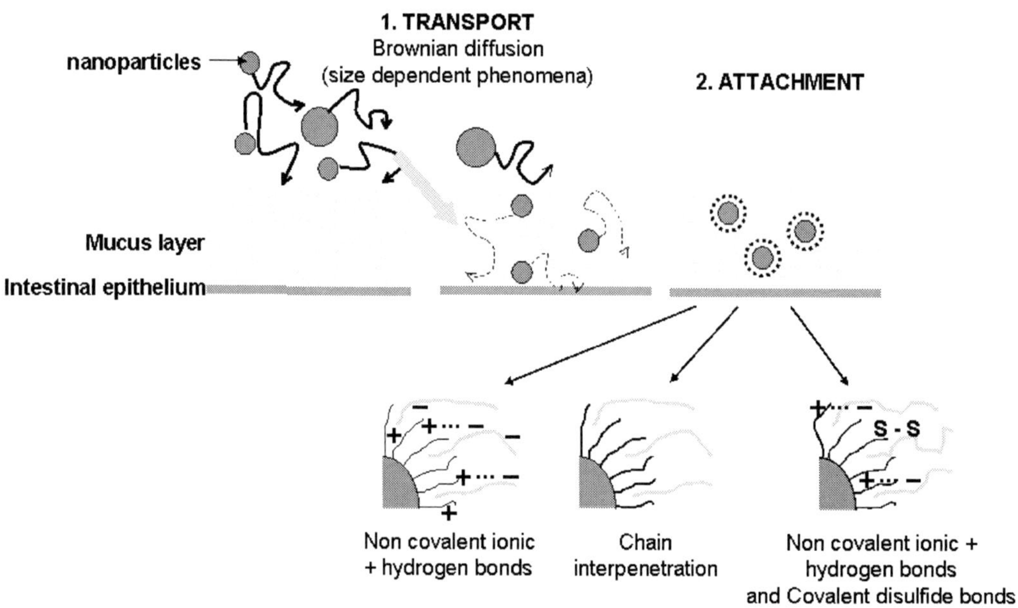

Figure 4. Suggested mechanisms describing the mucoadhesion of chitosan and thiolated chitosan-coated PIBCA nanoparticles. Mucin chains: yellow lines, chitosan and thiolated chitosan at the nanoparticle surface: black lines.

Modulation of the Intestinal Absorption of Active Molecules in Presence of Chitosan-coated PACA Nanoparticles

In vitro permeability studies are relevant approaches to evaluate the absorption enhancing effect of colloidal drug carrier systems (Hillgren et al., 1995; Lang et al., 1998; Watanabe et al., 2004). They offer many advantages over *in vivo* studies being performed more rapidly, involving fewer animals and simpler analytical procedures. They are also easier to standardised (Wadell et al., 1999). However, there is one restriction that must be considered concerning the viability and integrity of the tissue (Wadell et al., 1999). The feature of Ussing-like chambers is that they allow monitoring of the electrical parameters of the membrane during the course of the experiment assessing viability of tissues over the time course of the experiment (Hillgren et al., 1995; Samanen et al., 1996). In addition, the electrical parameters can be also used to determine the opening of tight junctions (Wadell et al., 1999) as complement of the monitoring of permeability of paracellular transport markers such as mannitol (Lang et al., 1998; Wadell et al., 1999; Boulenc et al., 1995a; Tanrattana et al., 2004).

The permeation enhancement properties of chitosan and thiolated chitosan coated PIBCA nanoparticles was evaluated using Ussing-type chambers and monitoring of the opening of tight junctions by both electrical and mannitol permeability measurements (Bravo-Osuna et al. submitted (3)). In a first set of experiments, the different formulations of core-shell nanoparticles were introduced in the donor compartment of the Ussing chamber allowing the direct contact of nanoparticles with the mucosal side. Surprisingly, the non-thiolated chitosan-coated nanoparticulate formulations did not show any enhancement of the paracellular pathway permeability during the study, considering the well-established enhancing permeation properties reported for chitosan in previous reports (Illum et al., 1994; Lueβen et al., 1997; Kotzé et al., 1998; Dodane et al., 1999). However, in agreement with other works, when the experiments were carried out with chitosan solutions at the same concentration than those used in the nanoparticles, an increment in the paracellular permeability was observed. Other authors have also reported a different behaviour between chitosan solutions and chitosan nanoparticles using the Caco-2 cell monolayer model (Prego et al., 2005). Similarly, they observed that chitosan solutions promoted a significant opening of the tight junctions, while the same amount of polymer formulated in nanoparticles did not lead to any significant permeation. Thus, our results confirmed that a different presentation of chitosan, in the form of a soluble solution or as solid nanoparticles, led to different permeation effects which can be explained considering the high interactions between particles and mucus observed in bioadhesion studies. Indeed, high interactions can decrease the possibility of direct contact between nanoparticles and epithelial cells requested to promote structural changes in the tight junction proteins responsible for the increase of the intestinal permeation.

Interestingly, thiolated formulations which were found to be far less bioadhesives demonstrated a higher tendency to induce paracellular permeation enhancement. This effect can be related to the bioadhesion mechanism of nanoparticles. Indeed, once in contact with the mucus layer, nanoparticles begin to diffuse in the three-dimensional gel. The higher they attached the mucus chains, the lower they can interact with the tight junction system to open it. The high mucus-nanoparticle interactions might also be the cause of the lack of correlation observed between the calcium binding capacity demonstrated for these nanoparticles in vitro and their permeation behaviour observed in the presence of the biological tissues.

A second set of experiments was performed in which the adhesion of nanoparticles on the mucosa was avoided by interposing a semi-permeable membrane between the tested formulations and the intestinal tissue. In this case, no permeation enhancement was obtained with any of the formulation tested. This undoubtedly confirmed that the absorption enhancing effect of the nanoparticles was intimately related to their bioadhesion on the mucosa.

From all the results presented in this study, the following sequence of events can be proposed to explain the permeation enhancing effect of chitosan or of thiolated-chitosan coated-nanoparticles: (I) The presence of chitosan (modified or non-modified) on the surface of nanoparticles promoted their bioadhesion with the mucus layer by electrostatic interactions. (II) The cross-linked structure due to the presence of disulphide bonds in the thiolated chitosan coating, might limit the development of strong interactions of the nanoparticles with the mucus components hence enhancing the interactions of the nanoparticles with endothelial cells. (III) At the level of the endothelial cells, the combination of both the remaining cationic nature of the particle surface and the presence of thiol groups, could promote the opening of the tight junctions (Bravo-Osuna et al. submitted (3)).

Conclusions and New Trends

Nanotechnology and more specifically nanoparticles is a very interesting approach for the oral administration of peptides and proteins. They can protect peptides from the harsh gastrointestinal environment and present a high surface area able to develop intimate contact with biological tissues. In addition, polymers used in their elaboration can give them useful additional characteristics to improve the bioavailability of active peptides and proteins. One of the most promising materials used with this objective are chitosan and some of their derivatives. They can modulate the gastrointestinal protease activity and can improve the peptide permeability across the intestinal epithelium.

Recent works focused on the elaboration of PACA nanoparticles allowed the development of an interesting method of preparation of PACA nanocarriers with modified surface based on emulsion polymerisation. The high versatility observed for this technique in the tuning of core-shell PACA nanoparticles opens a huge door for the development of such kind of nanocarriers with specific characteristics. The combination of this nanotechnology with the use of chitosan and their derivatives led to the creation of new nanoparticles having different advantageous functions required to promote the oral bioavailability of therapeutic peptides and proteins. There is no doubt that research will continue with approaches aiming to develop multifunctionnal drug delivery systems at the nanoscale size. In this view, the nanoparticles reported here are interesting platforms for multifunctional systems developments because they can be further modified by the introduction of new functions at the nanoparticle surface thanks to the easy chemistry that can be perfomed on chitosan and thiolated chitosan used as coating material.

REFERENCES

Agnihotri S.A., Mallikarjuna N.N., Aminabhavi T.M., 2004. Recent advances on chitosan-based micro- and nanoparticles in drug delivery. *J. Control. Release* 100, 5-28.

Allémann E., Leroux J.C., Gurny R., 1998. Polymeric nano- and microparticles for the oral delivery of peptides and peptidomimetics. *Adv. Drug Del. Rev.* 34, 171-189.

Alonso M.J., 2004. Nanomedicines for overcoming biological barriers. *Biomed & Pharmacotherapy* 58(3), 168-172.

Ameye D., Voorspoels J., Remon J.P., Demeester J., De Smedt S.C., 2000. Optimisation of an in vitro procedure for the determination of the enzymatic inhibition potency of multifunctional polymers. *J. Control. Release* 68, 413-417.

Ameye D., Voorspoels J., Foreman P., Tsai J., Richardson P., Geresh S., Remon J.P., 2001. Trypsin inhibition, calcium and zinc ion binding of starch-g-poly(acrylic acid) copolymers and starch/poly(acrylic acid) mixtures for peroral peptide drug delivery. *J. Control. Release* 75, 357-364.

Anderson J.M., Shive M.S., 1997. Biodegradation and biocompatibility of PLA and PLGA microspheres. *Adv. Drug Del. Rev.* 28, 5-24.

Arangoa M.A., Ponchel G., Orecchioni A.M., Renedo M.J., Duchene D., Irache J.M. 2000. Bioadhesive potential of gliadin nanoparticulate systems. *Eur. J. Pharm. Sci.* 11, 333-341.

Archambault J.C., Brash J.L., 2004. Protein resistant polyurethane surfaces by chemical grafting of PEO: amino-terminated PEO as grafting reagent. *Colloidal Surf. B: Biointerfaces* 25, 9-1.

Avadi M.R., Jalali A., Mir Mohammad Sadeghi A., Shamimi K., Bayati K.H., Nahid E, Dehpour A.R., Rafiee-Tehrani M., 2005. Diethyl methyl chitosan as an intestinal paracellular enhancer: ex vivo and in vivo studies. *Int. J. Pharm.* 293, 83-89.

Baker J., Hidalgo J., Borchardt R.T., 1991. Intestinal epithelial and vascular endothelial barriers to peptide and protein delivery. In *peptide and protein drug delivery.* Vincent H.L. Lee-Decker. New York, 359-390.

Balimane P.V., Chong S., 2005. Cell culture-based models for intestinal permeability: a critique. *Drug Discov. Today.* 10(5), 335-343.

Batista M.K.S., Pinto L.F., Gomes C.A.R., Gomes P. Novel highly-soluble peptide-chitosan polymers: Chemical synthesis and spectral characterization. Carbohydr. *Polymers.* In press

Becker T., Schlaak M., Strasdeit H., 2000. Adsorption of nickel(II), zinc(II) and cadmium(II) by new chitosan derivatives. React. & Funct. *Polymers* 44, 289-298.

Behrens I., Vila A.I., Alonso M.J., Kissel T., 2002. Comparative uptake studies of bioadhesive and non-bioadhesive nanoparticles in human intestinal cell lines and rats. The effect of mucus on particle adsorption and transport. *Pharm. Res.* 19, 1185-1193.

Bernkop-Schnürch A., Krajicek M.E., 1998. Mucoadhesive polymers as platforms for peroral peptide delivery and absorption: synthesis and evaluation of different chitosan-EDTA conjugates. *J. Control. Release* 50, 215-223.

Bernkop-Schnürch A., Kast C.E., 2001. Chemically modified chitosans as enzyme inhibitors. *Adv. Drug Del. Rev.* 52, 127-137.

Bernkop-Schnürch A., Steininger S., 2000. Synthesis and characterization of mucoadhesive thiolated polymers. *Int. J. Pharm.* 194, 239-247.

Bernkop-Schnürch A., Kast C.E., Guggi D., 2003. Permeation enhancing polymers in oral delivery of hydrophilic macromolecules: thiomer/GSH systems. *J. Control. Release* 93, 95-103.

Bernkop-Schnürch A., Hornof M., Guggi D., 2004. Thiolated chitosan. *Eur. J. Pharm. Biopharm.* 53, 9-17.

Bernkop-Schnürch A., Pinter Y., Guggi D., Kahlbacher H., Schöffmann G., Schuh M., Schmerold I., Del Curto N.D., D'Antonio M., Esposito P., Huck C., 2005. The use of thiolated polymers as carrier matrix in oral peptide delivery- Proof of concept. *J. Control. Release* 106(1-2), 26-33.

Bertholon I., Lesieur S., Labarre D., Bernard M., Vauthier C., 2006a. Characterization of dextran-poly(isobutylcyanoacrylate) copolymers obtained by redox radical and anionic emulsion polymerisation. *Macromolecules* 39, 3559-3567.

Bertholon I., Vauthier C., Labarre D., 2006b. Complement activation by core-shell poly(isobutyl cyanoacrylate) polysaccharide nanoparticles. *Pharm. Res.* 23(6), 1313-1323.

Bertholon I., Ponchel G., Labarre D., Couvreur P., Vauthier C., 2006c. Bioadhesive properties of poly(alkylcyanoacrylate) nanoparticles coated with polysaccharide. *J Nanosc. Nanotech.* 6, 3102-3109.

Bertholon-Rajot I., Labarre D., Vauthier C., 2005. Influence of the initiator system, cerium–polysaccharide, on the surface properties of poly(isobutylcyanoacrylate) nanoparticles. *Polymer* 46, 1407–1415.

Bilati U., Allémann E., Doelker E., 2005. Strategic approaches for overcoming peptide and protein instability within biodegradable nano- and microparticles. *Eur. J. Pharm. Biopharm.* 59, 375-388.

Birk Y., 1985. The Bowman-Birk inhibitor. Trypsin- and chymotrypsin-inhibitor from soybeans. *Int. J. Peptide Protein Res.* 25(2), 113-31.

Boonsongrit Y., Mitrevej A., Mueller B.W., 2006. Chitosan drug binding by ionic interaction. *Eur. J. Pharm. Biopharm.* 62(3), 267-74.

Borchard G., Lueβen H.L., de Boer A.G., Verhoef J.C., Lehr C.M., Junginger H.E., 1996. The potential of mucoadhesive polymers in enhancing intestinal peptide drug absorption III. Effect of chitosan-glutamate and carbomer on epithelial tight junction in vitro. *J. Control. Release* 39, 131-138.

Boulenc X., Roques C., Joyeux H., Berger Y., Fabre G., 1995a. Biphosphonates increase tight junction permeability in the human intestinal epithelial (Caco-2) model. *Int. J. Pharm.* 123, 13-24.

Boulenc X., Breul T., Gautier J.C., Saudemon P., Joyeux H., Roques C., Berger Y., Fabre G., 1995b. Sodium lauryl sulphate increases tiludronate paracellular transport using human epithelial Caco-2. *Int. J. Pharm.* 123(1), 71-83.

Bravo-Osuna I., Schmitz T., Bernkop-Schnürch A., Vauthier C., Ponchel G., 2006. Elaboration and characterization of thiolated chitosan-coated acrylic nanoparticles. *Int. J. Pharm.* 316, 170-175.

Bravo-Osuna I., Ponchel G., Vauthier C., Tuning of shell and core characteristics of chitosan-decorated acrylic nanoparticles. *Eur. J. Pharm. Sci.* In press.

Bravo-Osuna I., Teutonico D., Arpicco S., Vauthier C., Ponchel G., Characterization of chitosan thiolation and application to thiol quantification onto nanoparticles surface. Submitted for Publication in *Int. J. Pharm.* (1)

Bravo-Osuna I., Vauthier C., Farabollini A., Palmieri G.F., Ponchel G. Mucoadhesion mechanism of chitosan and thiolated chitosan-poly(isobutyl cyanoacrylate) core-shell nanoparticles" Submitted for Publication in *Biomaterials* (2)

Bravo-Osuna I., Vauthier C., Ponchel G. In-vitro biopharmaceutical evaluation of chitosan and thiolated chitosan-cyanoacrylic nanoparticles. Submitted for Publication in *Pharm. Res.* (3).

Bravo-Osuna I., Millotti G., Vauthier C., Ponchel G. In vitro evaluation of calcium binding capacity of chitosan and thiolated chitosan poly(isobutylcyanoacrylate) core-shell nanoparticles. Submitted for Publication in *Int. J. Pharm.* (4).

Bravo-Osuna I., Vauthier C., Farabollini A., Millotti G., Ponchel G. In vitro antiprotease activity of chitosan and thiolated chitosan-poly(isobutylcyanoacrylate) core-shell nanoparticles. Submitted for Publication in *Eur. J. Pharm. Sci.* (5).

Brigger I., Chaminade P., Marsaud V., Appel M., Besnard M., Gurny R., Renoir M., Couvreur P., 2001. Tamoxifen encapsulation within polyethylene glycol-coated nanospheres. A new antiestrogen formulation. *Int. J. Pharm.* 214, 37-42.

Brigger I., Dubernet C., Couvreur P., 2002. Nanoparticles in cancer therapy and diagnosis. *Adv. Drug Del. Rev.* 54, 631-651.

Calvo P., Remuñan-Lopez C., Vila-Jato J.L., Alonso M.J., 1997. Chitosan and chitosan/ethylene osyde-propylene oxide block copolymer nanoparticles as novel carriers for protein and vaccines. *Pharm. Res.* 14, 1431-1436.

Chassary P., Vincent T., Guibal E., 2004. Metal anion sorption of chitosan and derivative materials: a strategy for polymer modification and optimum use. *React & Funct. Poymers* 60, 137-149.

Chattaraj S.C., Rathinavelu A., Das S.K., 1999. Biodegradable microparticles of influenza viral vaccine: comparison of the effects of routes of administration on the in vivo immune response in mice *J. Control. Release* 58(2), 223-232.

Chauvierre C., Labarre D., Couvreur P., Vauthier C., 2003a. Radical polymerisation of alkylcyanoacrylates initiated by the redox system dextran-cerium (IV) under acidic aqueous conditions. *Macromolecules* 36, 6018-6027.

Chauvierre C., Labarre D., Couvreur P., Vauthier C., 2003b. Plug-in spectrometry with optical fibres as a novel analytical tool for nanoparticles technology: Application to the investigation of the emulsion polymerisation of the alkylcyanoacrylate. *J. Nano. Res.* 5, 365-371.

Chauvierre C., Labarre D., Couvreur P., Vauthier C., 2003c. Novel polysaccharide-Decorated poly(isobutyl cianoacrylate) nanoparticles. *Pharm. Res.* 20(11), 1786-1793.

Cho J.H., Kim D.H., Chung S.J., Ha N.C., Oh B.H., Choi K.Y., 2002. Insight into the stereochemistry in the inhibition of carboxypeptidase A with N-(hydroxyaminocarbonyl)phenylalanine: binding modes of an enantiomeric pair of the inhibitor to Carboxypeptidase A. *Bioorg. Med. Chem.* 10, 2015-2022.

Chung S.J., Kim D.H., 2001. N-(hydroxyaminocarbonyl)phenylalanine: A novel class of inhibitor for Carboxypeptidase A. *Bioorg. Med. Chem.* 9, 185-189.

Cilurzo F., Minghetti P., Casiraghi F.A., Montanari L., 2003. Polymethacrylate salts as new low-swellable mucoadhesive materials. *J Control. Release* 88(1), 43-53.

Couvreur P., Barratt G., Fattal E., Legrand P., Vauthier C., 2002. Nanocapsule Technology: A review. *Crit. Rev. Ther. Drug Carrier Syst.* 19(2), 99-134.

Couvreur P., Kante M., Roland P., Guiot P., Bauduin P., Speiser P., 1979. Polycyanoacrylate nanocapsules as intestinal lysosomatropic carriers: preparation, morphological and absorptive properties. *J. Pharm. Pharmacol.* 31, 331-332.

Couvreur P., Dubernet C., Puisieux F., 1995. Controlled drug delivery with nanoparticles: current possibilities and future trends. *Eur. J. Pharm. Biopharm.* 41, 2-13.

Couvreur P., Puisieux L.F., 1993. Nano- and microparticles for the delivery of polypeptides and proteins. *Adv. Drug Del. Rev.* 10, 141-162.

Couvreur P., Vauthier C., 2006. Nanotechnology: intelligent design to treat complex diseases. *Pharm. Res.* 23(7), 1417-1450.

Cox D.S., Gao H., Raje S., Scott K.R., Eddington N.D., 2001. Enhancing the permeation of marker compounds and enaminone anticonvulsants across Caco-2 monolayers by modulating tight junctions using zonula occludens toxins. *Eur. J. Pharm. Biopharm.* 51, 145-150.

Damgé C., Michel C., Aprahamian M., Couvreur P., 1988. New approach for oral administration of insulin with poly-alkylcyanoacrylate Nanocapsules as drug carrier. *Diabetes* 37, 246-251.

Damgé C., Michael C., Aprahamian M., Couvreur P., Devissaguet J.P., 1990. Nanocapsules as carriers for oral peptide delivery. *J. Control. Release* 13, 233-239.

Damgé C., Vonderscher J., Marbach P., Pinget M., 1997. Poly(alkylcyanoacrylate) Nanocapsules as a delivery system in the rat for octeotride, a long-acting somatostoatin analogue. *J. Pharm. Pharmacol.* 49, 949-954.

Dass C., Mahalakhmi P., 1996. Phosphorylation of enkephalins enhances their proteolytic stability. *Life Sci.* 58(13), 1039-1045.

Davda J., Labhasetwar V., 2002. Characterization of nanoparticle uptake by endothelial cells. *Int. J. Pharm.* 233, 51-59.

Dembri A., Montisci M.J., Gantier J.C., Chacun H., Ponchel G., 2001. Targeting of 3'-azido-3'-doxythymidine (AZT)-loaded poly(isohexylcyanoacrylate) nanospheres to the gastrointestinal mucosa and associated lymphoid tissues. *Pharm. Res.* 18(4), 1-7.

Ding W., Lian Q., Samuels R.J., Polk M.B., 2003. Synthesis and characterization of a novel derivative of chitosan. *Polymer* 44, 547-556.

Dodane V., Khan M.A., Merwin J.R., 1999. Effect of chitosan on epithelial permeability and structure. *Int. J. Pharm.* 182, 21-32.

Dodou D., Breedveld P., Wieringa P.A., 2005. Mucoadhesives in the gastrointestinal tract: revisiting the literature for novel applications. *Eur. J. Pharm. Biopharm.* 60(1), 1-16.

Dorkoosh F.A., Borchard G., Rafiee-Tehrani M., Verhoef J.C., Junginger H.E., 2002. Evaluation of superporous hydrogel (SPH) and SPH composite in porcine intestine *ex vivo*: assessment of drug transport, morphology effect, and mechanical fixation to intestinal wall. *Eur. J. Pharm. Biopharm.* 53, 161-166.

Durrer C., Irache J.M., Puisieux F., Duchêne D., Ponchel G., 1994a. Mucoadhesion of latexes. I. Analytical methods and kinetic studies. *Pharm. Res.* 11(5), 674-679.

Durrer C., Irache J.M., Puisieux F., Duchêne D., Ponchel G., 1994b. Mucoadhesion of latexes. II. Adsorption isotherms and desorption studies. *Pharm. Res.* 11(5), 680-683.

Dzul Erosa M.S., Saucedo Medina T.I., Navarro Mendoza R., Avila Rodríguez M., Guibal E., 2001. Cadmium sorption on chitosan sorbents: kinetic and equilibrium studies. *Hydrometal.* 61, 157-167.

Ewan G.M., Jepson M., Hirst B., Simmons N., 1993. Polycation-induced enhancement of epithelial paracellular permeability is independent of tight junctional characteristics. *Biochim. Biophys. Acta.* 1148, 51-60.

Fasano A., Nataro J.P., 2004. Intestinal epithelial tight junctions as targets for enteric bacteria-derived toxins. *Adv. Drug Del. Rev.* 56, 795-807.

Fawaz F., Guyot M., Lagueny A.M., Devissaguet J.P., 1997. Ciprofloxacin-loaded polyisobutylcyanoacrylate nanoparticles: Preparation and characterization . *Int. J. Pharm.* 154(2), 191-203.

Florence A.T., 2005. Nanoparticle uptake by the oral route: fulfilling its potential? *Drug disc. Today Techn.* 2, 75-81.

Ford J., Woolfe J., Florence A.T., 1999. Nanospheres of cyclosporin A. Poor oral abosrption in dogs. *Int. J. Pharm.* 183, 3-6.

Fukunaga M., Miller M.M., Deftos L.J., 1991. Liposome-entrapped calcitonin and parathyroid hormone are orally effective in rats. *Horm. Metab. Res.* 23, 166-167.

García-Fuentes M., Torres D., Alonso M.J., 2005a. New surface-modified lipid nanoparticles as delivery vehicles for salmon calcitonin. *Int. J. Pharm.* 296(1-2), 122-132.

García-Fuentes M., C. Prego, Torres D., Alonso M.J., 2005b. A comparative study of the potential of solid triglyceride nanostructures coated with chitosan or poly(ethylene glycol) as carriers for oral calcitonin delivery. *Eur. J. Pharm. Sci.* 25(1), 133-143.

Gaserod O., Jolliffe I.G., Hampson F.C., Dettmar P.W., Skjak-Braek G., 1998. The enhancement of the bioadhesive properties of calcium alginate gel beads by coating with chitosan. *Int. J. Pharm.* 175, 237-246.

Goldstein I.J., Hughes R.C., Mousigny M., Osawa T., Sharon N., 1980. What should be called a lectin? *Nature* 285, 66.

Gref R., Quellec P., Sanchez A., Calvo P., Dellacherie E., Alonso M.J., 2001. Development and characterization of CyA-loaded poly(lactic acid)-poly/ethylene glycol) PEG micro- and nanoparticles. Comparison with conventional PLA particulate carriers. *Eur. J. Pharm. Biopharm.* 5, 111-118.

Guggi D., Krauland A.H., Bernkop-Schnürch A., 2003. Systemic peptide delivery via the stomach: in vivo evaluation of an oral dosage form for salmon calcitonin. *J. Control. Release* 92(1-2), 125-135.

Guibal E., Vincent T., Navarro-Mendoza R., 2000. Synthesis and characterization of a thiourea derivative of chitosan for platinum recovery. *J. Appl. Polym. Sci.* 75, 199-134.

Guibal E., Von Offenberg Sweeney N., Vincent T., Tobin J.M., 2002. Sulfur derivatives of chitosan for palladium sorption. *React. Funct. Polym.* 50, 149-163.

Guibal E., 2004. Interactions of metal ions with chitosan-based sorbents: a review. *Sep. Purif. Techn.* 38, 43-74.

Gum J.R., Hicks J.W., Toribara N.W., Rothe E.M., Lagace R.E., Kim Y.S., 1992. The human MUC2 intestinal mucin has cysteine-rich subdomains located both upstream and downstream of its central repetitive region. *J. Biol. Chem.* 267, 21375-21383.

Gupta K., Ganguli M., Pasha S., Maiti S., 2005. Nanoparticle formation from poly(acrylic acid) and oppositely charged peptides. *Biophys. Chem.* 119, 302-305.

Hillery A.M., Toth I., Florence A.T., 1996a. Co-polymerised peptide particles II: Oral uptake of a novel co-polymeric nanoparticulate delivery system for peptides. *J. Control. Release* 42, 65-73.

Hillery A.M., Toth I., Florence A.T., 1996b. Biological activity of luteinizing hormone releasing hormone after oral dosing with a novel nanoparticle system: co-polymerised peptide particles. *Pharm. Sci.* 2, 281-283.

Hillgren K.M., Kato A., Borchardt R.T., 1995. In vitro systems for studying intestinal drug absorption. *Med. Res. Rev.* 15, 83-109.

Himmelhoch S.R., 1969. Leucine aminopeptidase: a zinc metalloenzyme. *Arch. Biochem. Biophys.* 134(2), 597-602.

Hooper N.M., 1994. Families of zinc metallopeptidases. *FEBS Lett.* 354, 1-6.

Huang M., Khor E., Lim L.Y., 2004. Uptake and cytotoxicity of chitosan molecules and nanoparticles: effects of molecular weight and degree of deacetylation. *Pharm. Res.* 21(2), 344-353.

Huang Y., Leobandung W., Foss A., Peppas N.A., 2000. Molecular aspects of muco- and bioadhesion: Tethered structures and site-specific surface. *J. Control. Release* 65, 63-71.

Hussain N., Jaitley V., Florence A.T., 2001. Recent advances in the understanding of uptake of microparticulates across the gastrointestinal lymphatics. *Adv. Drug Del. Rev.* 50, 107-142.

Illum, L., Jabbal-Gill, I., Hinchcliffe, M., Fisher, A.N., Davis S.S., 2001. Chitosan as a novel nasal delivery system for vaccines. *Adv. Drug Del. Rev.* 51, 81-96.

Illum L., Farraj N.F., Davis S.S., 1994. Chitosan nasal delivery system or peptide drugs. *Pharm. Res.* 11:1186-1189.

Iqbal M., Lin W., Jabbal-Gill I., Davis S.S., Steward M.W., Illum L., 2003. Nasal delivery of chitosan–DNA plasmid expressing epitopes of respiratory syncytial virus (RSV) induces protective CTL responses in BALB/c mice. *Vaccine* 21, 1478-1485.

Janes K.A., Calvo P., Alonso M.J., 2001. Polysaccharide colloidal particles as delivery systems for macromolecules. *Adv. Drug Del. Rev.* 47, 83-97.

Jayawardene D.S., Dass C., 1999. The effect of N-terminal acetylation and the inhibition activity of acetylated enkephalins on the aminopeptidase M-catalysed hydrolysis of enkephalins. *Peptides* 20, 963-970.

Jeon C., Holl W.H., 2003. Chemical modification of chitosan and equilibrium study for mercury ion removal. *Water Res.* 37, 4770-4780.

Jung T., Kamm W., Breitenbach A., Kaiserling E., Xiao J.X., Kissel T., 2000. Biodegradable nanoparticles for oral delivery of peptides: is there a role for polymers to affect mucosal uptake?. *Eur. J. Pharm. Biopharm.* 50, 147-160.

Kast C.E., Bernkop-Schnürch A., 2001 Thiolated polymers thiomers: development and in vitro evaluation of chitosan-thioglycolic acid conjugates, *Biomaterials* 22, 2345-2352.

Kim W.U., Lee W.K., Ryoo J.W., Kim S.H., Kim J., Youn J., Min S.Y., Bae E.Y., Hwuang S.Y., Park S.H., Cho C.S., Park J.S., Kim H.Y., 2002. Suppression of collagen-induced arthritis by single administration of poly(lactic-co-glicolic acid) nanoparticles entrapping type II collagen: a novel treatment strategy for induction of oral tolerance. *Arthritis Rheum.* 46(4) 1109-1120.

Kim T.H., Park I.K., Nah J.W., Choi Y.J., Cho C.S., 2004. Galactosylated chitosan/DNA nanoparticles prepared using water-soluble chitosan as a gene carrier. *Biomaterials* 25(17), 3783-3792.

Kotzé A.F., Lueβen H.L., Leeuw B.J., de Boer B.G., Verhoef J.C., Junginger H.E., 1998. Comparison of the effect of different chitosan salts N-trimethyl chitosan chloride on the permeability of intestinal epithelial cells (Caco-2). *J. Control. Release* 51, 35-46.

Krauland A.H., Guggi D., Bernkop-Schnürch A., 2006. Thiolated chitosan microparticles: A vehicle for nasal peptide drug delivery. *Int. J. Pharm.* 307(2), 270-277.

Kriwet B., Kissel T., 1996. Poly (acrylic acid) microparticles widen the intercellular spaces of Caco-2 cell monolayers: An examination by confocal laser scanning microscopy. *Eur. J. Pharm. Biopharm.* 42, 233-240

Lang S., Roten-Rutishauser B., Perriard J.C., Schmidt M.C., Merkle H.P., 1998. Permeation and pathways of human calcitonin (hCT) across excised bovine nasal mucosa. *Peptide* 19,599-607.

Langguth P., Bohner V., Heizmann J., Merkle H.P., Wolffram S., Amidon G.L., Yamashita S., 1997. The challenge of proteolytic enzymes in intestinal peptide delivery. *J. Control. Release* 46, 39-57

Larionova N.V., Ponchel G., Duchene D., Larionova N.I., 1999. Biodegradable cross-linked starch/protein microcapsules containing proteinase inhibitor for oral protein administration. *Int. J. Pharm.* 189, 171-178.

Leanes M.M., Nankervis R., Smith A., Illum L., 2004. Use of the ninhydrin assay to measure the release of chitosan from oral solid dosage forms. *Int. J. Pharm.* 271, 241-249.

Le Buanec H., Vetu C., Lachgar A., Benoit M.A., Gillard J., Paturance S., Aucouturier J., Gane V., Zagury D., Bizzini B., 2001. Induction in mice of anti-Tat mucosal immunity by the intranasal and oral routes. *Biomed. Pharmacother.* 55, 316-320.

Lee K.J., Johnson N., Castelo J., Sinko P.J., Grass G., Holme K., Lee Y.H., 2005. effect of experimental pH on the in vitro permeability in intact rabbit intestine and caco-2 monolayer. *Eur. J. Pharm. Sci.* 25, 193-200.

Lee M., Kim D.H., 2000. Hippuryl-α-methylphenylalanine and hyppuryl-α-methylphenyllactic acid as substrates for carboxypeptidase A. Synthesis, kinetic evaluation and mechanistic implication. *Bioorg, Med. Chem.* 8, 815-823.

Lee M., Nah J.W., Kwon Y., Koh J.J., Ko K.S., Kim S.W., 2001. Water-soluble and low molecular weight chitosan-based plasmid DNA delivery. *Pharm. Res.* 18(4), 427-431

Lemarchand C., Gref R., Couvreur P., 2004. Polysaccharide-decorated nanoparticles. *Eur. J. Pharm. Biopharm.* 58, 327-341.

Li X.W., Lee D.K.L., Chan A.S.C., Alpar H.O., 2003. Sustained expression in mammalian cells with DNA complexed with chitosan nanoparticles. *Biochimica et Biophysica Acta* 1630, 7-18.

Li X., Solomon B., 2001. Zinc-mediated thermal stabilization of carboxypeptidase A. *Biomol. Eng.* 18, 179-183.

Lima I.S., Airoldi C., 2003. Interaction of cooper with chitosan and succinic anhydride derivative- a factorial design evaluation of the chemisorption process. Colloidal Surf. A: Physicochem. *Eng. Aspects.* 229, 129-136.

Lowe P.J., Temple C.S., 1994. Calcitonin and insulin in isobutylcyanoacrylate nanocapsules: protection against proteases and effect on intestinal absorption in rats. *J. Pharm. Pharmacol.* 46, 547-552.

Lueβen H.L., Verhoef J.C., Borchard G., Lehr C.M., de Boer A.G., Junginger H.E., 1995. Mucoadhesive polymers in peroroal peptide drug delivery. II. Carbomer and polymcarbophil are potent inhibitors of the intestinal proteolytic enzyme trypsin. Pharm. *Res.* 12(9), 1293-1298.

Lueβen H.L., Leeuw B.J., Pérard D., Lehr C.M., de Boer A.G., Verhoef J.C., Junginger H.E., 1996. Mucoahdesive polymers in peroral peptide drug delivery. I. Influence of mucoadhesive excipients on the proteolytic activity of intestinal enzymes. *Eur. J. Pharm. Sci.* 4, 117-128.

Lueβen H.L., Rentel C.O., Kotzé A.F., Lehr C.M., de Boer A.G., Verhoef J.C., Junginger H.E., 1997. Mucoadhesive polymers in peroral peptide drug delivery. IV. Polycarbophil and chitosan are potent enhancers of peptide transport across intestinal mucosae in vitro. *J. Control. Release* 45, 15-23.

Ma Z., Lim T.M., Lim L.Y., 2005. Pharmacological activity of peroral chitosan-insulin nanoparticles in diadetic rats. *Int. J. Pharm.* 293, 271-280.

Mackay M., Phillips J., Hastewell J., 1997. Peptide drug delivery: Colonic and Rectal absorption. *Adv. Drug Del. Rev.* 28(2), 253-273.

Madsen F., Peppas N.A., 1999. Complexation graft copolymer networks: swelling properties, calcium binding and proteolytic enzyme inhibition. *Biomaterials* 20, 1701-1708.

Mansouri S., Lavigne P., Corsi K., Benderdour M., Beaumont E., Fernandes J.C., 2004. Chitosan-DNA nanoparticles as non-viral vectors in gene therapy: strategies to improve transfection efficacy. *Eur. J. Pharm. Biopharm.* 57, 1-8.

Mao H.Q., Roy K., Troung-Le V.L., Janes K.A., Lin K.Y., Wang Y., August J.T., Leong K.W., 2001. Chitosan-DNA nanoparticles as gene carriers: synthesis, characterization and transfection efficiency. *J. Control. Release* 70, 399-421.

Mao S., Shuai X., Unger F., Simon M., Bi D., Kissel T., 2004. The depolymerisation of chitosan: effects on physicochemical and biological properties. *Int. J. Pharm.* 281, 45-54.

Mardones P., Andrinolo D., Csendes A., Lagos N., 2004. Permeability of human jejunal segments to gonyautoxins measured by the Ussing chamber technique. *Toxicon* 44, 521-528.

Martinac A., Filipović-Grčić J., Voinovich D., Perissutti B., Franceschinis E., 2005. Development and bioadhesive properties of chitosan-ethylcellulose microspheres for nasal delivery. *Int. J. Pharm.* 291(1-2), 69-77.

Maruyama A., Ishihara T., Kim J.S., Kim S.W., Akaike T., 1999. Design of multi-layered nanoparticles as a DNA carrier. Colloids and Surfaces A: *Physiochemical and Engineering Aspects* 153, 439-443.

Marschutz M.K., Bernkop-Schnürch A., 2002. Thiolated polymers: self-crosslinking properties of thiolated 450 kDa poly(acrylic acid) and their influence on mucoadhesion. *Eur. J. Pharm. Sci.* 15, 387-394.

Matsuzawa A., Morishita M., Takayama K., Nagai T., 1995. Absorption of insulin using water-in-oil-in-water emulsion from enteral loop in rats. *Biol. Pharm. Bull.* 18, 1718-1723.

McClean S., Prosser E., Meehan E., O'Malley D., Clarke N., Ramtoola Z., Brayden D., 1998. Binding and uptake of biodegradable poly-DL-lactide micro- and nanoparticles in intestinal epithelia. *Eur. J. Pharm. Sci.* 6, 153-163.

Merdan T., Kopecek J., Kissel T., 2002. Prospects for cationic polymers in gene and oligonucleotide therapy against cancer. *Adv. Drug Del. Rev.* 54(5), 715-758.

Michael S., Thöle M., Dillmann R., Fahr A., Drewe J., Fricker G., 2000. Improvement of intestinal peptide absorption by a synthetic bile acid derivative, cholylsarcosine. *Eur. J. Pharm. Sci.* 10(2), 133-140.

Michel C., Aprahamian M., Defontaine L., Couvreur P., Damgè C., 1990. The effect of site of administration in the gastrointestinal tract on the absorption of insulin from nanocapsules in diabetic rats. *J. Pharm. Pharmacol.* 43, 1-5.

Mizuma T., Koyanagi A., Awazu S., 2000. Intestinal transport and metabolism of glucose-conjugated kyotorphin and cyclic kyotorphin: metabolic degradation is crucial to intestinal absorption of peptide drugs. *Biochim. Biophys. Acta* 1475, 90-98.

Morishita I., Morishita M., Takayama K., Machida Y., Nagai T., 1992. Hypocalcemic effect of novel oral microspheres of insulin with protease inhibitor in normal and diabetic rats. *Int. J. Pharm.* 78, 9-16.

Monteiro O.A.C., Airoldi C., 1999. Some thermodynamic data on copper-chitin and copper-chitosan biopolymer interactions. *J. Colloidal Interface Sci.* 212, 212-219.

Morishita M., Peppas N.A., 2006. In the oral route possible for peptide and protein drug delivery? *Drug. Disc. Today* 11(19/20), 905-910.

Narayani R., 2001. Oral delivery of insulin-making needles needless. *Trends Biomater. Artif. Organs.* 15(1) 12-16.

Nobs L., Buchegger F., Gurny R., Allémann E., 2004. Current methods for attaching targeting ligands to liposomes and nanoparticles. *J. Pharm. Sci.* 93, 1980-1992.

Norris D.A., Sinko P.J., 1997. Effect of size, surface charge, and hydrophobicity on the translocation of polystyrene microspheres through gastrointestinal mucin. *J. Appl. Polym. Sci.* 63(11), 1481-1492.

Pan Y., Li Y.J., Zhao H.Y., Zheng J.M., Xu H., Wei G., Hao J.S., Cui F.D., 2002. Bioadhesive polysaccharide in protein delivery systems: chitosan nanoparticles improve the intestinal absorption of insulin in vivo. *Int. J. Pharm.* 249(1-2), 139-147.

Panyam J., Labhasetwar V., 2003. Biodegradable nanoparticles for drug and gene delivery to cell and tissues. *Adv. Drug Del. Rev.* 55, 329-347.

Park J.D., Kim D.H., 2004. Sulphamide derivatives as transition state analogue inhibitors for carboxypeptidase A. *Bioorg. Med. Chem.* 12, 2349-2356.

Park J.H., Kwon S., Lee M., Chung H., Kim J.H., Kim Y.S., Park R.W., Kim I.S., Seo S.B., Kwon I.C., Jeong S.Y. 2006. Self-assembled nanoparticles based on glycol chitosan bearing hydrophobic moieties as carriers for doxorubicin: In vivo biodistribution and anti-tumor activity. *Biomaterials* 27, 119-126.

Passirani C., Barratt G., Devissaguet J.P., Labarre D., 1998a. Interactions of nanoparticles bearing heparin or dextran covalently bound to poly(methyl methacrylate) with the complement system. *Life Sci.* 62(8), 775-785.

Passirani C., Barratt G., Devissaguet J.P., Labarre D., 1998b. Long-circulating nanoparticles bearing heparin or dextran covalently bound to poly(methyl methacrylate). *Pharm. Res.* 15(7), 1046-1050.

Peppas N.A., Huang Y., 2004. Nanoscale technology of mucoadhesive interactions. *Adv. Drug Del. Rev.* 56, 1675-1687.

Peracchia M.T., Vauthier C., Passirani C., Couvreur P., Labarre D., 1997a. Complement consumption by poly(ethylene glycol) in different conformations chemically coupled to poly(isobutyl 2-cyanoacrylate) nanoparticles. *Life Sci.* 61(7), 749-61.

Peracchia M.T., Desmaële D., Couvreur P., d'Angelo J., 1997b. Synthesis of a novel poly(MePEG cyanoacrylate-*co*-alkyl cyanoacrylate) amphiphilic copolymer of nanoparticle technology. *Macromolecules* 30(4), 846-851.

Peracchia M.T., Harnisch S., Pinto-Alphandary H., Gulik A., Dedieu J.C., Desmaële D., d'Angelo J., Müller R.H., Couvreur P., 1999. Visualization of in vitro protein-rejecting properties of PEGylated stealth® polycyanoacrylate nanoparticles. *Biomaterials* 20, 1269-1275

Phoon L., Burton A., 2005. Assessment of a mechanism for reactive inhibitors of carboxypeptidase A with QM/MM methods. *J. Mol. Graphics Modell.* 24, 94-101.

Pinto-Alphandary H., Aboudakar M., Jaillard D., Couvreur P., Vauthier C., 2003. Visualization of insulin-loaded nanocapsules: in vitro and in vivo studies after oral administration to rats. *Pharm. Res.* 20(7), 1071-1084.

Pinto Reis C., Neufeld R.J., Ribeiro A.J., Veiga F., 2006. Nanoencapsulation II. Biomedical applications and current status of peptide and protein nanoparticulate delivery systems. Nanomed. Nanotechn. *Biol. Med.* 2, 53-65.

Ponchel G., Montisci M.J., Dembri A., Durrer C., Duchene D., 1997. Mucoadhesion of colloidal particulate systems in gastrointestinal tract. *Eur. J. Pharm. Biopharm.* 44, 25-31.

Ponchel G., Irache J.M., 1998. Specific and non-specific bioadhesive particulate systems for oral delivery to the gastrointestinal tract. *Adv. Drug Del. Rev.* 34, 191-219.

Prego C., García M., Torres D., Alonso M.J., 2005. Transmucosal macromolecular drug delivery. *J. Control. Release* 101, 151-162.

Prego C., Torres D., Fernández-Megía E., Novoa-Caballal R., Quínoa E., Alonso M.J., 2006. Chitosan-PEG Nanocapsules as new carriers or oral peptide delivery. Effect of chitosan pegylation degree. *J. Control. Release* 111, 299-308.

Quan Y.S., Fujita T., Tohara D., Tsuji M., Kohyama M., Yamamoto A., 1999. Transport kinetics of leucine enkephalin across caco-2 monolayers: quantitative analysis for contribution of enzymatic and transport barrier. *Life Sci.* 64(14), 1243-1252.

Ranaedi G., Marigliano I., Verpignani I., Peroxxi G., Sambuy Y., 2002. The effect of chitosan and other polycations on tight junction permeability in the human intestinal Caco-2 cell line. *J. of Nutritional Biochem.* 13, 157-167.

Ravi Kumar M.N.V., 2000. A review of chitin and chitosan applications. *Reactive & Functional Polymers* 46, 1-27.

Rhazi M., Desbrières J., Tolaimate A., Rinaudo M., Vottero P., Alagui A., El Meray M., 2002. Influence of the nature of metal ions on the complexation with chitosan. Application to the treatment of liquid waste. *Eur. Polym. J.* 38, 1523-1530.

Rodrigues J.S., Santos-Magalhaes N.S., Coelho L.C.B.B., Couvreur P., Ponchel G., Gref R., 2003. Novel core(polyester)-shell(polysaccharide) nanoparticles: protein loading and surface modification with lectins. *J. Control. Release* 92, 103-112.

Roldo M., Hornof M., Caliceti P., Bernkop-Schnürch A., 2004. Mucoadhesive thiolated chitosans as platforms for oral controlled drug delivery: synthesis and in vitro evaluation. *Eur. J. Pharm. Biopharm.* 57, 115-121.

Roumi M., Kwong E., Deghenghi R., Locatelli V., Marleau S., Souich P.D., Béliveau R., Ong H., 2001. Permeability of peptidic GH secretagogues hexarelin and EP51389 across rat jejunum. *Peptides* 22, 1229-1138.

Russell-Jones G., 1999. Use of bioconjugates for the oral delivery of peptides, proteins and immunogens. *S.T.P. Pharma Sci.* 9(1) 47-59.

Salman H., Gamazo C., Campanero M.A., Irache J.M., 2005. Salmonella-like bioadhesive nanoparticles. *J. Control. Release* 106 (1-2), 1-13.

Samanen J., Wilson G., Smith P.L., Lee C.P., Bondinell W., Ku T., Rhodes G., Nichols A., 1996. Chemical approaches to improve the oral bioavailability of peptidergic molecules. *J. Pharm. Pharmacol.* 48(2), 119-135.

Sanderink G.J., Arthur Y., Siest G., 1988. Human aminopeptidases: A review of the Literature. *J. Clin. Chem. Clin. Biochem.* 26, 795-807.

Sarmento B., Ferreira D.C., Jorgensen L., van de Weert M., 2007. Probing insulin's secondary structure after entrapment into alginate/chitosan nanoparticles. *Eur. J. Pharm. Biopharm.* 65, 10-17.

Sarmento B., Ribeiro A., Veiga F., Ferreira D., 2006. Development and characterization of new insulin containing polysaccharide nanoparticles. *Coll. Surf. B Biointerf.* 53, 193-202.

Sashiwa H., Aiba S.I., 2004. Chemically modified chitin and chitosan as biomaterials. *Prog. Polym. Sci.* 29, 887-908.

Sato T., Ishii T., Okahata Y., 2001. In vitro gene delivery mediated chitosan. Effect of pH, serum, and molecular mass of chitosan on the transfection efficiency. *Biomaterials* 22, 2075-2080.

Schmitz T., Bravo-Osuna I., Ponchel G., Vauthier C., Loretz B., Bernkop-Schnürch A., 2006. Thiomers: Development and in vitro Evaluation of a nanoparticulate gene delivery system. In press *Biomaterials*

Schipper N.G.M., Olsson S., Hoogstraate J.A., de Boer A.G., Varum K.M., Artursson P., 1997. Chitosans as absorption enhancers for poorly absorbable drugs. 2: mechanism of absorption enhancement. *Pharm. Res.* 14, 923-929.

Schulzke J.D., Gillet A.H., Mankertz J., Spiegel S., Seidler U., Amasheh S., Saitou M., Rsukita S., Fromm M., 2005. Epithelial transport and barrier function in occluding-deficient mice. *Biochim. Biophys. Acta* 1669, 34-42.

Silva Cunha A., Grossiord J.L., Puisieux F., Séller M., 1997. Insulin in w/o/w multiple emulsions: preparation, characterization and determination of stability towards proteases in vitro. *J. Microencapsulation* 14, 311-319.

Soppimath K.S., Aminabhavi T.M., Kulkarni A.R., Rudzinski W.E., 2001. Biodegradable polymeric nanoparticles as drug delivery devices. *J. Control. Release* 70, 1-20.

Smith P.L., Wall D.A., Gichoco C.H., Wilson G., 1992. Oral absorption of peptides and proteins. *Adv. Drug Del. Rev.* 8(2-3), 253-290.

Takeuchi H., Matsui Y., Sugihara H., Yamamoto H., Kawashima Y., 2005. Effectiveness of submicron-sized, chitosan-coated liposomes in oral administration of peptide drugs. *Int. J. Pharm.* 303(1-2), 160-170.

Tanrattana C., Charoenphandhu N., Limlomwongse L., Krishnamra N., 2004. Prolactin directly stimulated the solvent drug-induced calcium transport in the duodenum of female rats. *Biochim. Biophys. Acta 1*665, 81-91.

Taylor A., 1993. Aminopeptidases: towards a mechanism of action. T*rends. Biochem. Sci.,* 18(5) 167-171.

Tenhoor C., Dressman J., 1992. Oral absorption of peptides and proteins. *S.T.P. Pharma. Sci.* 2, 301-312.

Thanou M.M., Verhoef J.C., Junginger H.E., 2001. Chitosan and its derivatives as intestinal absorption enhancers. *Adv. Drug Del. Rev.* 50, S91-S101.

Thanou M.M. Kotzé A.F., Scharringhausen T., Lueβen H.L., de Boer A.G., Verhoef J.C., Junginger H.E., 2000. Effect of degree of quaternization of N-trimethyl chitosan chloride for enhanced transport of hydrophilic compounds across intestinal Caco-2 cell monolayer. *J. Control. Release* 64(1-3), 15-25.

Tobío M., Sánchez A., Vila A., Soriano I., Evora C., Vila-Jato J.L., Alonso M.J., 2000. The role of PEG on the stability in digestive fluids and in vivo fate of PEG-PLA nanoparticles following oral administration. Colloids and Surfaces B: *Biointerfaces* 18, 315-323.

Uchegbu I.F., Schatzlein A.G., Tetley L., Gray A.I., Sludden J., Siddique S., Mosha E., 1998. Polymeric chitosan-based vesicles for drug delivery, *J. Pharm. Pharmacol.* 50, 453-458.

Usami M., Komurasaki T., Hanada A., Kinoshita K., Ohata A., 2003. Effect of γ-linolenic acid or docosahexaenoic acid on tight junction permeability in intestinal monolayer cells and their mechanism by protein kinase C activation and/or eicosanoid formation. *Nutrition,* 19, 150-156.

Vallee B.L., Rupley J.A., Coombs T.L., Neurath H., 1960. The role of zinc in carboxypeptidase. *J. Biol. Chem.* 235(1), 64-69.

Van der Lubben I.M., Verhoef J.C., Borchard G., Junginger H.E., 2001a. Chitosan for mucosal vaccination. *Adv. Drug Del. Rev.* 52, 139-144.

Van der Lubben I.M., Konings F.A.J., Borchard G., Verhoef J.C., Junginger H.E., 2001b. In vivo uptake of chitosan micorparticles by murine Peyer's patches: visualization studies using confocal laser scanning microscopy and immuno-histochemistry. *J. Drug Target.* 9, 39-47.

Van der Merwe S.M., Verhoef J.C., Verheijden J.H.M., Kotzé A.F., Junginger H.E., 2004a. Trimethylated chitosan as polymeric absorption enhancer for improved peroral delivery of peptide drugs. *Eur. J. Pharm. Biopharm.* 58, 225-235.

Van der Merwe S.M., Verhoef J.C., Kotzé A.F., Junginger H.E., 2004b. N-Trymethyl chitosan chloride as absorption enhancer in oral peptide drug delivery. Development and characterization of minitablet and granule formulation. *Eur. J. Pharm. Biopharm.* 57(1), 85-91.

Vauthier C., Dubernet C., Chauvierre C., Brigger I., Couvreur P. 2003a. Drug delivery to resistant tumors: the potential of poly(alkyl cyanoacrylates) nanoparticles. *J. Control. Release* 93, 151-160.

Vauthier C., Dubernet C., Fattal E., Pinto-Alphandary H., Couvreur P., 2003b. Poly(alkylcyanoacrylates) as biodegradable materials for biomedical applications. *Adv. Drug Del. Rev.* 55(4), 519-548.

Vauthier C., Bertholon I., Labarre D., 2007. Integrated development of glycobiologics: from discovery to applications in the design of nanoparticular drug delivery systems. In *Handbook of Pharmaceutical Biotechnology.* Ed Shayne, Cox Gad, Willey and son, Inc.

Vila A., Sánchez A., Tobío M., Calvo P., Alonso M.J., 2002. Design of biodegradable particles for protein delivery. *J. Control. Release* 78, 15-24.

Vila A., Sánchez A., Janes K., Berhrens I., Kissel T., Vila Jato J.L., Alonso M.J., 2004. Low molecular weight chitosan nanoparticles as new carriers for nasal vaccine delivery in mice. *Eur. J. Pharm. Biopharm.* 57, 123-131.

Wadell C., Bjork E., Camber O., 1999. Nasal drug delivery-evaluation of an in vitro model using porcine nasal mucosa. *Eur. J. Pharm. Sci.* 7(3):197-206.

Wang L.Y., Gu Y.H., Su Z.G., Ma G.H., 2006. Preparation and improvement of released behaviour of chitosan microspheres containing insulin. *Int. J. Pharm.* 311(1-2),187-95.

Watanabe E., Takahashi M., Hayashi M., 2004. A possibility to predict the absorbability of poor water-soluble drugs in humans based on the rat intestinal permeability assessed by an in vitro chamber method. *Eur. J. Pharm. Biopharm.* 58, 659-665.

Zhang C., Ping Q., Zhang H., Shen J., 2003 Synthesis and characterization of water-soluble Q-succinyl- Chitosan. *Eur. Polymer J.* 39, 1629-1624.

Zhi J., Wang Y., Luo G., 2005. Adsorption of diuretic furosemide onto chitosan nanoparticles prepared with a water-in-oil nanoemulsion system. *Reactive & Functional Polymers* 65, 249-257.

Zhou X.H., 1994. Overcoming enzymatic and absorption barriers to non-parenterally administered protein and peptide drugs. *J. Control. Release* 29(3), 239-252.

In: Drugs: Approval and Evaluation, Delivery and Control ISBN: 978-1-60456-533-1
Editors: A.O. Hartmann, L.K. Neumann

Chapter 3

EXCIPIENTS AS MODULATORS OF DRUG-CARRIER MEDIATED ABSORPTION IN THE INTESTINE

Stefan Grube and Peter Langguth
Department of Biopharmaceutics and Pharmaceutical Technology, School of Pharmacy, Johannes Gutenberg-University, Staudingerweg 5, 55099 Mainz, Germany

ABSTRACT

Over the past years the awareness of the importance of intestinal drug transporters for the bioavailability of certain drugs has grown steadily. More and more drugs are being identified as substrates or inhibitors of one or another transporter. Aside from drugs, however, numerous excipients have been found to modulate the functioning of drug transporters, too. Thus, they might also interfere with the absorption of drugs on a physiological level either enhancing or decreasing their absorption.

For developing rational drug formulations it is important to take into account such effects when conceiving a new formulation or redesigning existing formulations. In the first case, choosing the right excipient might result in higher bioavailability or even allow for absorption in the first place. In the second case unwanted changes of the performance of the redesigned dosage form might be prevented. The knowledge of such excipients is also important from a drug regulatory point of view in order to evaluate post-approval changes in the formulation.

This article will review the current findings on excipients with modulatory potential on intestinal transporters. With respect to excipients the article will mainly discuss Cremophor EL, Tocopheryl Polyethylenglycol Succinate (TPGS), Polysorbate 80, Pluronic P85, Polyethyleneglycol (PEG), Solutol HS15 and Labrasol. In addition, a comprehensive table of excipients with modulatory effects on drug transporters will be included. With respect to intestinal drug transporters the article will concentrate on interactions between excipients and two important members of the ABC-transporter family (P-glycoprotein and MRP) as well as two members of the solute carrier family (PEPT1 and the monocarboxylate transporter).

The article shall serve both as an introduction and reference for those active in the field of drug formulation or drug regulatory affairs.

1. Introduction

Absorption of drugs via the intestinal epithelium can be brought about by either passive or carrier-mediated transport. The dominant force of passive transport is diffusion which enables transport by the paracellular or transcellular pathway along the concentration gradient of a compound. A special case of passive transport is the so called facilitated transport which is mediated by carrier systems in the cell membrane and allows accelerated transfer of a compound (e.g. fructose) across the membrane along its concentration gradient without consumption of energy. Active transport requires the presence of a transport protein and consumption of energy which can be provided either directly by ATP-hydrolysis or indirectly by an ion gradient (e.g. H^+, K^+, Na^+) which has been generated by the use of energy or eventually ATP-hydrolysis. Transport proteins relying directly on ATP-hydrolysis are referred to as pumps and their action is also called primary active transport. Transporters working by ion gradients are also referred to as carriers and can be further classified into cotransporters and countertransporters. They use energy provided by the downhill transport of one substrate to propel the uphill transport of another substrate. In the case of cotransport both substrates flow in the same direction, in the case of countertransport the flux of the two substrates is in opposite directions.

In the past diffusion, has been regarded as the prevalent mechanism of absorption. But in recent years more and more transport proteins have been discovered and recognized to affect absorption or secretion of physiological substrates, drugs and their metabolites in liver, kidney, blood-brain barrier, placental barrier, tumor tissue and the intestine. These include P-glycoprotein [1], multi-drug-resistant protein [2], peptide transporter [3, 4], organic cation transporter [5] and the monocarboxylate transporter [6, 7].

Meanwhile drug-carrier mediated absorption and secretion across intestinal cell monolayers like Caco-2 and isolated or perfused rat tissue has been shown to be a relevant factor for a variety of drugs. These include celiprolol [8], digoxin [9], ranitidine and cimetidine [10], saquinavir [11] and fluorquinolone antibiotics [12] as well as enalapril [13] and valacyclovir [14]. Furthermore, secretion of intravenously administered digoxin and its inhibition by quinidine, a P-gp inhibitor, has been observed in the human intestine [15] which points out the in vivo relevance of drug-carrier mediated transport.

Drug carriers and pumps are proteins in nature and their action is influenced by various factors. On the transcriptional level higher expression could change activity, posttranscriptionally stabilization or destabilization of mRNA could play a role, translation itself, posttranslational events and trafficking of the protein to membranes can influence the actual amount of protein present in the membrane at any one time. Once in the membrane the protein activity can be altered by competitive, noncompetitive, or uncompetitive inhibitors or allosteric effectors. The functioning of the ABC-transporters, like P-gp and the MRPs, depends on ATP and the activity of the secondary-active transporters, like PEPT or MCT of the solute carrier family, is influenced by the ion-gradient of the propelling moiety. For example, a variety of inhibitors are already known for P-gp, besides the above mentioned quinidine, verapamil, vinblastine and GF120918 may be mentioned. Pretreatment of Caco-2 cells with verapamil or vinblastine [16] or in situ of rats with vinblastine and rifampin [17] can also increase P-gp expression and protein levels. Furthermore, propranolol and verapamil were shown to cause a rapid induction of P-glycoprotein in colonic cells in vitro [18].

Polymorphisms are known for some of the drug carriers and pumps e.g. MDR-1 [19] and might account for inter-individual differences in drug absorption.

Interfering with the expression or activity of drug carriers and pumps might thus provide an opportunity to increase absorption of such drugs, that are substrates of these transport proteins. E.g. in the case where there is a secretory transporter inhibition or down-regulation could lead to increased absorption and in the case where there is an absorptive transporter, enhancing its activity and expression could lead to higher absorption.

This is not just hypothetical, since e.g. rifampin enhanced intestinal secretion of talinolol by induction of P-glycoprotein in humans [20]. Of course, one would need to find less toxic compounds or compounds devoid of systemic action in order to make use of these properties in the treatment of otherwise healthy patients.

Not only drugs can influence drug carriers and drug pumps. There are now quite a few publications available which describe excipients as modulators of drug-carrier activity in vitro and in vivo. For the most part, these excipients have been used for years in pharmaceutical formulations and thus when administered orally their toxicity is considered to be very low, their systemic availability poor and no relevant systemic effects are known. So they might be potentially valuable for modulation of intestinal drug carriers in those cases where bioavailability is limited by drug-carrier mediated efflux or absorption.

This review shall give an overview of excipients which have already been tested for their modulatory actions on intestinal drug carriers and pumps. It includes a list with several of those excipients but we do not claim completeness. Further discussion will concentrate on some selected excipients, since it is not possible to cover all of them in this review.

2. Drug Transporters in the Intestine

A variety of intestinal drug transporters has been described and we refer to reviews dealing exclusively with this topic [21]. Here, we will focus on some transporters that have been dealt with in the literature with regard to interaction with excipients. These transporters fall into two families: the solute carrier family (SLC), which uses ion gradients as driving force or functions by the principle of facilitative transport, and the ABC (ATP binding cassette) family, which uses energy from ATP-hydrolysis. Steffanssen et al. [22] give a fairly comprehensive overview of the absorptive solute drug carriers found in the intestine and Chan et al. [1] provide insight into ABC-tranporters and their regulation in intestine and liver.

For the SLC family we will consider the peptide transporter and the monocarboxylate transporter and for the ABC familiy P-glycoprotein (MDR-1) and multi drug resistance protein (MRP).

Table 1. Substrates, inhibitors and inducers of MDR-1, MRP1, MRP2, MRP3 and BCRP

Substrate	MDR-1	MRP1	MRP2	MRP3	BCRP
2,4-Dinitrophenyl-S-glutathione		S [35]	S [36]	S [37]	S [38]
Adefovir			S [39]		
Aldosterone	S [40]				
Amiodarone	I [41]				
Amitryptiline	S [42]				
Amprenavir	S [43] ; U [44]				
Atorvastatin	S/I [45, 46]				
Bisantrene					S [47]
Bromocriptine	I [48]				
Carvedilol	I [49]				
Celiprolol	S [8]				
Chloropromazine	I [50]				
Cidofovir			S [39]		
Cimetidine	S [51]				
Cisplatin	N [52]	N [53]	S [54]		
Clarithromycin	I [55]				
Colchicine	S [11]				
Cortisol	S [40]				
Cyclosporin	S [32, 56]				
Daunorubicin	S [27]	S [57]		N [58]	S [59]
Dehydroepiandrosterone sulphate		S [60]	N [60]	N[60]	
Dexamethasone	S [40] U [61-63]				
Diethylstilbestrol					I [64]
Digoxin	S [34, 65]		N [66]		
Diltiazem	I [67]				
Docetaxel	S [68]				
Domperidon	S [69]				
Doxorubicin	S [27] ; U [70]		S[54]	N [58]	S [59]
Epirubicin					S [71]
Erythromycin	S/I [72]				
Estradiol-17-β-glucuronide	S [73]	S [74, 75]	S [75]	S [37]	
Etoposide	S [76]		S [54]	S [58]	S [76]
Fexofenadine	S [77]				
Flavopiridol					S [78]
Fluoxetine	I [79]				
Furosemid			I [80]		
Glibenclamid		I [81]	I [81]		
Grepafloxacin	S [12, 28, 82]	S [28]	S [12]		
Indinavir	S [29] ; U [83]	N [84]	S [84]	N [84]	N [84]
Itraconazole	S/I [85]				
Ketoconazole	N/I [86]				
Lamivudin					S [87]
Lansoprazol	S/I [88]				

Substrate	MDR-1	MRP1	MRP2	MRP3	BCRP
Leukotriene C4		S [35]	S [36]	S [37]	
Levofloxacin	S [82]				
Loperamide	S [69]				
Losartan	S [89]				
Methadone	I [90]				
Methotrexat	S [91]	S [92]	S [93, 94]	S [92, 95]	S [96, 97]
Mitoxantrone	S [98]	S [99]			S [47]
Morphine	S [90] , U [100]				
Nelfinavir	S [29] ; U [83]				I [101]
Octreotide	S [102]		S [102]		
Omeprazole	S/I [88]				I [103]
Ondansetron	S [69]				
Paclitaxel	S [26]	N [53]		N [58]	
Pantoprazol	S/I [88]				S/I [103]
Pentazocine	I [90]				
Phenytoin	S [69]				
Prazosin					S [47]
Probenecid			I [80]		
Quinidine	S/I [104]				
Ranitidine	S [10]				
Reserpine	I [105, 106]; U [106]				
Retinoic acid	U [107]				
Rhodamine 123	S [108]	S [109]			S [59]
Rifampin	S [110]; U [106]		S [111]		
Ritonavir	S [29]; U [83]		S [84]		I [101]
Saquinavir	S [29, 31] ; U[83]		S [84]		I [101]
Sertraline	I [112]				
Simvastatin	I [113]				
Spironolactone	I [114]				
St John´s wort	U [115]				
Tacrolimus	S [32]; I [116]				
Talinolol	S [33]				
Taurodeoxycholate-3-sulphate			S [117]	S [118]	
Teniposide				S [95]	S [76]
Terfenadine	S [86]				
Tetracycline	S [119]				
Topotecan	S [120]				S [47]
Verapamil	S/I [11]				
Vinblastine	S [68]		S [121]		
Vincristine	S [122]	S [123]	S [54]; U [124]	S [58] ; U [124]	

S = substrate.

I = inhibitor.

U = induction (Up-regulation).

N = no substrate.

2a. P-glycoprotein (P-gp)

P-gp is a MDR-1 gene product and belongs to the ABC-transporter family. It is localized in the apical cellular membrane and exerts a secretory function. In the human intestine P-gp expression increases from proximal to distal (small intestine to colon) [23]. Several authors suggest a coordinate response of P-gp and Cyp P450 to exposure of cell to xenobiotics [24, 25]. Its substrate specificity is rather broad and includes drugs from a range of different therapeutic groups e.g. anticancer agents such as taxol [26] or doxorubicin [27], antibiotics e.g. grepafloxacin [28], HIV-protease inhibitors [29-31] and immunosuppressive agents as cyclosporin A [32] , drugs used in cardiovascular disease as talinolol [33] and digoxin [34]. Additionally, verapamil is not only a substrate but also acts as a potent inhibitor of P-gp [11]. Table 1 illustrates the large number of compounds interacting with P-gp in one or another way.

Talinolol and digoxin are often chosen as substrates for transport studies because of their metabolic stability, such that metabolic influences in absorption studies can be excluded. Furthermore, the fluorescent dye rhodamine 123 is a P-gp substrate and has often been used in transport studies for its relatively easy detection by fluorescence.

2b. Multi-drug-resistance Protein (MRP)

MRPs belong to the ABC-transporter family. Only MRP2, MRP3 and perhaps MRP1 are known to be relevant for intestinal transport. They are all secretory tranporters. While MRP2 is located in the apical membrane MRP1 and MRP3 are routed to the basolaterol membrane [1, 2]. The basolateral location of MRP1 and MRP3 prevents direct exposure to excipients on the luminal side, whereas MRP2 could possibly interact directly with high excipient concentrations. Substrates of MRP2 and MRP3 are shown in Table 1. Some of the substrates of MRPs show or affinity to P-gp (see Table 1); thus using them in transport studies might yield ambiguous results.

MRP1-3 might play a role in the secretion of anionic compounds generated during metabolism by conjugation with glutathione or sulphate as can be seen by their substrates (Table1) dehydroepiandrosterone sulphate (MRP1), taurodeoxycholate-3-sulphate (MRP2 and MRP3) and leukotriene C4 (MRP1-3).

2c. Peptide Transporter (PEPT)

A couple of peptide transporters have been described by now including PEPT1, PEPT2 and peptide/histidine transporter PHT (reviewed by Steffansen et al. [22]). Not much is known about PHT and PEPT2 is not expressed in the intestine. So it will only be dealt with PEPT1.

PEPT1 belongs to the SLC15A gene family and is systematically referred to as SLC15A1 gene product. It is a secondary active H^+-co-transporter and is expressed in human intestinal epithelial cells as well as in Caco-2 cells [3, 125]. The transporter is found in the apical membrane and acts as an absorptive transporter. Typical substrates of PEPT1 are di- and tripeptides. Additionally, further substrates have been identified e.g. the ACE-Inhibitor enalapril [13], some β-lactam antibiotics e.g. cyclacillin and ceftibuten from the group of the cephalosporines [126]. Furthermore peptidyl-prodrugs have been shown to increase bioavailability in comparison to the simple parent drug e.g. L-valine aciclovir [14] or biphosphonate-peptide drugs [127] and are thought to be substrates of the peptide transport system.

2d. Monocarboxylate Transporter (MCT)

Eight members (MCT1-MCT8) of the family of monocarboxylate transporters have been identified until today. Most is known about MCT-1, which is involved in the uptake of weak organic acids such as benzoic acid, lactate, pravastatin or salicylate. Additionally, atorvastatin has been recognized as a MCT substrate by Wu et al. [45].. MCT1 is encoded by the gene SLC16A1 and has been characterize in Caco-2 cells and rat small intestine. It has been detected predominantly in the basolateral membrane of rat enterocytes [128] but also in apical membrane vesicles from pigs and humans [129, 130].

3. Modulation of Drug-carrier Activity by Excipients

3a. Overview

Modulatory potential of excipients on drug carriers has first been discovered by reversal of drug resistance, which is at least in part due to drug efflux pumps, of multi-drug resistant cancer cells. One of the first reports by Woodcock et al. [131] about excipient inhibition of drug efflux was in cancer cells using Cremophor EL. They pointed out its potential usefulness as an additive in cancer therapy to overcome drug resistance of cancer cells.

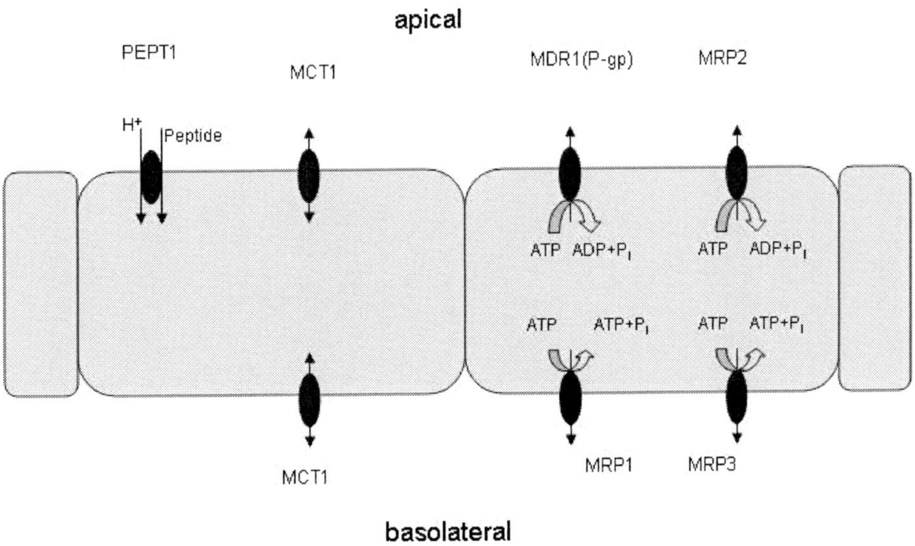

Figure 1. Transporters in intestinal epithelium; detailed explanation in the text.

Table 2. Excipients that showed modulatory effects on drug-carrier-mediated transport for the substrates, models and concentrations indicated

Excipient	Concentration	Test model	Substrate	Parameter	Reference
Acconon E	0,05-0,5% [w/v]	Everted rat gut sac	Digoxin	1	[135]
Cremophor EL	0,05-0,5% [w/v]	Everted rat gut sac	Digoxin	1	[135]
	ca. 0,05-2,5% [w/v] (0,02-1mM)	Caco-2	Rhodamine 123	2	[136]
	0,1% [w/v]	Caco-2	^{3}H-Taxol	2	[137]
	0,10%	Rat intestinal membrane	Rhodamine123	2	[138]
Imwitor 742	0,1-0,5% [w/v]	Everted rat gut sac	Digoxin	1	[135]
	0,5% [w/v]	Everted rat gut sac	Celiprolol	1	[135]
Labrasol	0,05-0,5% [w/v]	Everted rat gut sac	Digoxin	1	[135]
Miglyol	0,05-0,5% [w/v]	Everted rat gut sac	Digoxin	1	[135]
MO-310 (Tetraglycerol monooleate)	0,03% [w/v]	BBMVesicles	Ceftibuten	1	[139]
MS-310 (Tetraglycerol monostearate)	0,03% [w/v]				
MS-500 (Hexaglycerol monostearate)	0,03% [w/v]				
n-dodecyl-β-D-malto-pyranoside	0,10%	Rat intestinal membrane	Rhodamine123	2	[138]
PEG 300	20% [m/v]	Caco-2	^{3}H-Taxol	2	[137, 140]
	20% [m/v]	MDR1-MDCK	^{3}H-Taxol	2	
PEG 400	1-10% [w/v]	Rat jejunal tissue	Digoxin	3	[141]
Pluronic L61	0.04% [w/v]	LLC-MDR1	^{3}H-Vinblastine	2	[57]
Pluronic L43/L61/L62/ L64/ L81/ L92/ L101	below corresponding CMC	KBv cells	Rhodamine 123	1	[142]
Pluronic P85	0,1% [w/v]	Rat jejunal tissue	Digoxin	3	[141]
	0,01%-1%	Caco-2	Fluorescein	2	[143]
	0,1-1%	Caco-2	Doxorubicin	2	
	0,01% ; 1%	Caco-2	Etoposide	2	
	0,01-1%	Caco-2	^{3}H-Taxol	2	
	0,01-1%	Caco-2	Azidodeoxythymidine	2	
	0,01-1%	Caco-2	Loperamide	2	
	0,01%	BBMEC cells	Fluorescein	2	
	0,1%-1%	BBMEC cells	Doxorubicin	2	
	0,01%-1%	BBMEC cells	^{3}H-Taxol	2	
	0,1-1%	BBMEC cells	Azidodeoxythymidine	2	

Excipient	Concentration	Test model	Substrate	Parameter	Reference
Pluronic P103/P104/P123	below corresponding CMC	KBv cells	Rhodamine 123	1	[142]
Polysorbate 20	0,5% [w/v]	Everted rat gut sac	Digoxin	1	[135]
	0,03% [w/v]	BBMVesicles	Ceftibuten	1	[139]
Polysorbate 40	0,03% [w/v]	BBMVesicles	Ceftibuten	1	
Polysorbate 80	1,8mg/ml	Caco-2	Ranitidine	2b	[134]
	1,8mg/ml	Caco-2	Furosemide	2	
	1,8mg/ml	Caco-2	Cimetidine	2	
	1,8mg/ml	Caco-2	Hydrochlorothiazide	2	
	0,5%[w/v]	Everted rat gut sac	Digoxin	1	[135]
	ca. 0,015-0,6% [w/v] (0,025 - 1mM)	Caco-2	Rhodamine 123	2	[136]
	0,05% [w/v]	Caco-2	^{3}H-Taxol	2	[137, 140]
	0,10%	Rat intestinal membrane	Rhodamine123	2	[138]
Sodium lauryl sulfate	0,04mg/ml	Caco-2	Ranitidine	2	[134]
	0,04mg/ml	Caco-2	Furosemide	2a	
	0,04mg/ml	Caco-2	Cimetidine	2a	
	0,04mg/ml	Caco-2	Hydrochlorothiazide	2	
	0,04mg/ml	Caco-2	Acyclovir	2	
Softigen 767	0,5% [w/v]	Everted rat gut sac	Celiprolol	1	[135]
	0,5% [w/v]	Everted rat gut sac	Digoxin	1	[135]
Solutol HS 15	0,05-0,5% [w/v]	Everted rat gut sac	Digoxin	1	[135]
Sucrose stearate palmitate (7:3) monoester	0,03% [w/v]	BBMVesicles	Ceftibuten	1	[139]
SS-500 (Hexaglycerol sesquistearate)	0,03% [w/v]	BBMVesicles	Ceftibuten	1	[139]
TPGS 1000	0,05-0,5% [w/v]	Everted rat gut sac	Digoxin	1	[135]
	0,5% [w/v]	Everted rat gut sac	Celiprolol	1	[135]
	0,01 %-0,02%	Caco-2	Talinolol	2	[144]
	0,04%	Human	Talinolol	4	
TGPS 800	ca. 0,01-0,4% [w/v] (0,025-0,75mM)	Caco-2	Rhodamine 123	2	[136]
TS-500 (Hexaglycerol tristearate)	0,03% [w/v]	BBMVesicles	Ceftibuten	1	[139]
TS-750 (Decaglycerol tristearate)	0,03% [w/v]	BBMVesicles	Ceftibuten	1	

Note: Parameter 1 = increased uptake; 2 = increased transport; 3 = inhibition of efflux; 4 = increased AUC.

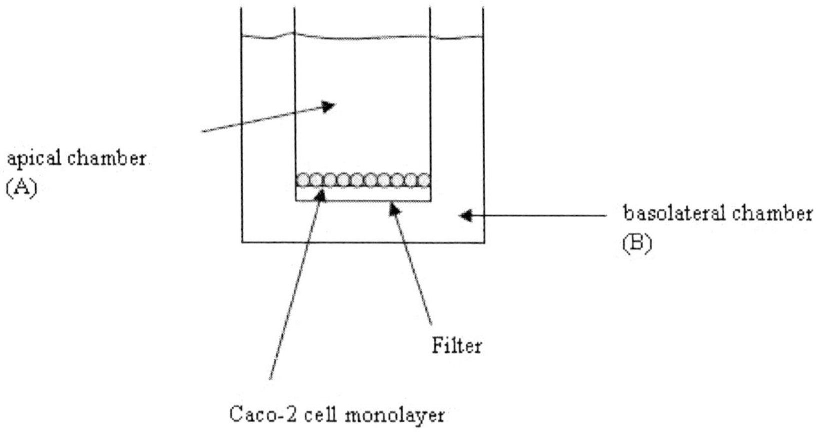

Substrate and excipient can be given either to the apical or basolateral chamber or to both and face the apical or basolateral membrane of the cells. Active transport will be different from A→B than from B→A if secretory or absorptive transport takes place. If only diffusion takes place, transport should be the same for A→B and B→A.

Figure 2. Transport studies - principle.

Nerurkar and Borchardt [132] expanded that idea by outlining the potential usefulness of excipients for increasing absorption of drugs which are substrates for drug efflux pumps in the intestine.

Until today several excipients have been screened for their potential to modulate drug carrier mediated transport in cancer cells, intestine or other epithelial tissue. Studies have been conducted using in vitro, in situ and in vivo models such as cell culture (Caco-2, NIH3, MDCK), BBMV (brush border membrane vesicles), isolated rat tissue mounted in diffusion chambers or perfusion models. Only few clinical trials have been undertaken.

As a tendency rather nonionic than ionic surfactants have been examined with respect to inhibition of P-gp as can be seen in Tables 2 and 3, probably because of lower toxicity. Furthermore, ionic surfactants such as sodium dodecyl sulfate often enhanced paracellular transport possibly by changing permeability of tight junctions, thus indicating another mechanism than modulation of drug carriers [133, 134].

Table 3. Excipients without positive effects on carrier-mediated transport for the substrates, models and concentrations indicated

Excipient	Concentration	Test model	Substrate	Reference
Acconon E	0,05-0,5% [w/v]	Everted gut sac	Celiprolol	[135]
Anhydrous cherry flavor	0,006% [v/v]	Caco-2	Acyclovir, furosemide, hydrochlorothiazide	[134]
Cremophor EL	0,05-0,5% [w/v]	Everted gut sac	Celiprolol	[135]
	0,1% [w/v]	MDR1-MDCK	[^{3}H]taxol	[137]
	0-1mM	Caco-2	Gly-Sar	[136]
	0,10%	Rat intestinal tissue	Gly-Sar	[138]
	0,10%	Rat intestinal tissue	3-O-methylD-glucose	

Excipient	Concentration	Test model	Substrate	Reference
Docusate sodium	0,02mg/ml	Caco-2	Ayclovir, atenolol, hydrochlorothiazide, ranitidine	[134]
EDTA	0,06mg/ml	Caco-2	Ayclovir, atenolol, cimetidine, ranitidine	
F-140 (sucrose stearate palmitate(7:3)polyester)	0,03%	BBMVesicles	Ceftibuten	[139]
F-160 (sucrose stearate palmitate(7:3)polyester)	0,03%	BBMVesicles	Ceftibuten	
Gelucire 44/14	0,05-0,5% [w/v]	Everted rat gut sac	Digoxin	[135]
Hexadecyltrimethyl ammonium bromide	0,10%	Rat intestinal tissue	Rhodamine123	[138]
HPMC	0,12 mg/ml	Caco-2	Acyclovir, atenolol, ranitidine	[134]
Imwitor 370	0,05-0,5% [w/v]	Everted rat gut sac	Digoxin	[135]
Labrafil M1944CS	0,05-0,5% [w/v]	Everted rat gut sac	Digoxin	
Lactose	2mg/ml	Caco-2	Acyclovir, atenolol, ranitidine	[134]
ML-310 (Tetraglycerol monolaureate)	0,03%	BBMVesicles	Ceftibuten	[139]
ML-500 (Hexaglycerol monolaureate)	0,03%	BBMVesicles	Ceftibuten	
ML-750 (Decaglycerol monolaureate)	0,03%	BBMVesicles	Ceftibuten	
MO-500 (Hexglycerol monooleate)	0,03%	BBMVesicles	Ceftibuten	
MO-750 (Decaglycerol monooleate)	0,03%	BBMVesicles	Ceftibuten	
N-octylglycoside	0,034mM	Caco-2	Benzoci acid, gly-sar, rhodamine 123	[136]
PEG 400	1,5% [v/v]	Caco-2	Acyclovir, atenolol, ranitidine	[134]
PEG 400	0,05-0,5% [w/v]	Everted rat gut sac	Digoxin	[135]
Plurol oleic	0,05-0,5% [w/v]	Everted rat gut sac	Digoxin	
Poloxamer 188	0,80%	Caco-2 cells/ human	Talinolol	[145]
Polysorbate (Tween 21)	0,03%	BBMVesicles	Ceftibuten	[139]
Polysorbate (Tween 60)	0,03%	BBMVesicles	Ceftibuten	
Polysorbate (Tween 80)	0,03%	BBMVesicles	Ceftibuten	
Polysorbate (Tween 81)	0,03%	BBMVesicles	Ceftibuten	
Propylenglycol	0,05-0,5% [w/v]	Everted rat gut sac	Digoxin	[135]
Propylenglycol	1.5 % [v/v]	Caco2	Cimetidine, furosemide	[134]
Span 20	0,03%	BBMVesicles	Ceftibuten	[139]
Span 30	0,03%	BBMVesicles	Ceftibuten	
Span 80	0,03%	BBMVesicles	Ceftibuten	
Span 85	0,03%	BBMVesicles	Ceftibuten	
Sucroester 15	0,05-0,5% [w/v]	Everted rat gut sac	Digoxin	[135]
Sucroester 7	0,05-0,5% [w/v]	Everted rat gut sac	Digoxin	
TPGS-1000	0,01% [w/v]	Rat intestinal tissue	Digoxin	[141]
TPGS-800	0-0,75mM	Caco-2 cells	Gly-Sar	[136]
TPGS-800	0-0,75mM	Caco-2 cells	benzoic acid	

Not all of the excipients given in the list will be covered in this review. Instead we have selected some interesting examples which will be discussed in more detail.

3b. Cremophor EL

Cremophor EL is used in several oral pharmaceutical formulations containing paclitaxel, cyclosporine A or ritonavir. It mediates solubilization of theses drugs and thus enhances their bioavailability. However, recently more and more evidence appeared that bioavailability enhancement might also be due to inhibition of P-glycoprotein-mediated secretion for such drugs that are P-gp substrates. Evidence came from in vitro and in vivo transport studies. Most of the studies found positive effects on absorption or transport, however some studies did not which triggered controversial discussion.

Shono et al [138] investigated the use of Cremophor EL as an inhibitor of drug-carrier mediated uptake of rhodamine 123 in a diffusion chamber with rat jejunal intestinal tissue. They used a concentration range from 0.005-1%[w/v] Cremophor EL and found increased transport in the absorptive and decreased transport in the secretory direction at concentrations as low as 0.05% [w/v]. At higher concentrations the effect diminished. Equilibrium studies with dialysis membranes with rhodamine 123 and Cremophor EL showed that the amount of micelle-bound dye increased remarkably above Cremophor EL concentrations of 0.05%[w/v]. This seems a reasonable explanation for the waning effects at higher excipient concentration, since the free drug concentration and thus the amount of rhodamine 123 available for transport is reduced and so would be absorption. The CMC of Cremophor EL was given as 0.0095% [m/V] but had not been adapted to the chamber condition and a higher CMC in the presence of cell tissue might well be possible because of partitioning of Cremophor EL monomers into membranes.

Rege et al [136] found increased permeability of rhodamine across Caco-2 monolayers in the apical-to-basolateral direction and a substantial decrease of permeability in basolaterol-to-apical direction in the presence of Cremophor EL (0.02-1 mM or ca. 0.005-0.25% estimated by a molecular weight of ~2500 Da), However, they did not find a decline of Cremophor EL effect at higher concentrations (> 0.25%) as was described by Shono. Bogman et al [145] determined the CMC of Cremophor EL in HBSS buffer in the presence of cells as 0.03% [w/v] . The differences might be due to the different models, buffers or rhodamine 123 concentrations used (rat jejunal tissue, Krebs Ringer Bicarbonate Solution pH 7.4 vs. Caco-2 monolayers and HBSS/HEPES buffer pH 6.8) .

The phenomenon of decreasing apparent permeability at very high excipient concentrations has already been described by Nerurkar et al. [146]. They carried out transport studies in Caco-2 cell monolayers with a peptide drug which showed P-gp like mediated transport when Cremophor EL was present in the apical chamber and demonstrated that permeability reaches a minimum for basolateral-to-apical transport in the proximity of the CMC of Cremophor EL and that for apical-to-basolateral transport a maximum is reached which starts to decrease again at higher surfactant concentrations. The concentration at which this occurs will be dependent on the substrate´s affinity to the surfactant micelles. The higher its affinity the faster should be the onset of permeability decrease above the CMC. Furthermore, whether or not the substrate´s permeability will be higher in the presence of surfactant also depends on its likeliness to associate with micelles. Therefore, depending on the substrate, micelle formation might not always exert a negative effect on transport.

The study of Nerurkar et al. further suggested that it is primarily the surfactant monomers which increase drug permeability, since increases above the CMC did not yield in higher permeability. The monomer concentration remains about the same above the CMC (and then is about equal to the CMC) and therefore no further enhancement would be expected if the monomers are the species contributing to the permeability enhancement.

Using rhodamine 123 as substrate primarily aims at analysing P-gp mediated transport since it is a known P-gp substrate. However, rhodamine 123 is also known as MRP [109] and BCRP [59] substrate. So, if those carriers were also present in the cell lines or rat tissue used, the overall effect on rhodamine transport might be the consequence of their common action.

MRP1 and MRP3 are secretory transporters and located at the basolateral membrane. Shono et al. added Cremophor EL to the basolateral side of cell tissue and no transport inhibition was observed suggesting that MRP1 and MRP3 either do not play a role in the transport of rhodamine in rat tissue or that Cremophor EL does not alter their transport activity. MRP2 is a secretory transporter present in the apical membrane, as well as BCRP. Currently, it is not clear to which extent these carriers are involved in drug secretion in the intestine.

Other substrates have been used in order to investigate the effects of Cremophor EL on peptide transporters and the monocarboxylate transporter in Caco-2 cell monolayers. Rege et al. [136] used gly-sar (substrate of PEPT1) and benzoic acid (substrate of MCT) but did not find altered transport of these substrates in the presence of 0.01-1 mM Cremophor EL.

This might indicate that the effect of Cremophor EL is transporter specific.

Cornaire et al. [135] used the P-gp substrates digoxin and celiprolol to investigate Cremophor EL effects on absorption in rats in-vivo (1 mg/kg) and by ussing chamber technique with rat intestine in-vitro (0.05-0.5% [w/v]). Cremophor EL enhanced uptake of digoxin (10μM) in vitro but not of celiprolol. Celiprolol (100μM) was used at concentrations ten times higher than digoxin (10μM) therefore it is possible that active secretion at this concentration is neglible compared to passive transport and not rate-limiting for absorption. The concentration dependence of carrier-mediated absorption reflects in the Michaelis-Menten-equation and has been reported for talinolol by Wagner et al [147] and for vinblastine [148].

However, celiprolol absorption could be effectively increased by verapamil, a competitive P-gp inhibitor. Furthermore, TPGS was shown to enhance both absorption of celiprolol and digoxin in the same study, though for absorption enhancement of celiprolol higher TPGS concentrations than for digoxin were needed. Therefore, different inhibitory mechanisms might also be involved and sensitivity of transport inhibition may also depend on the substrate itself. Another explanation could be the participation of other drug-carriers like MRP or BCRP together with specific inhibition of only P-gp or MRP/BCRP, respectively. Digoxin has been shown to be a substrate of P-gp and it has been shown that it is not a substrate for MRP2. Nevertheless, Lowes et al. remarked that besides P-gp another transporter might be involved in digoxin secretion [66]. For celiprolol it is not known whether it has or has no affinity to MRP2 or other transporters. Supposed it had, selective inhibition of P-gp might not suffice to stop secretion of digoxin efflux because of the efflux mediated by another transporter.

Neither of the authors (Cornaire, Nerurkar, Rege, Shono) observed relevant decreases of cell viability either measured by LDH release or trypan blue assay or increases in paracellular transport as measured by mannitol transport. So the effects of Cremophor EL are not due to cell death or changes in paracellular transport.

In in vivo trials [135] in rats with Cremophor EL and digoxin the AUC was reduced and t_{max} shifted to later times indicating diminished permeability of digoxin in the presence of the non-ionic surfactant. This is contrary to what would be expected from in vitro experiments. In this experiment 1 mg/kg Cremophor EL together with digoxin was administered by gavage in a mixture of water/propyleneglycol/ethanol. The use of cosolvents can change the CMC of surfactants, normally decreasing it and thus also lowering monomer concentration which might decrease the inhibitory effect. If the surfactant concentration was too high micellar incorporation of digoxin might have reduced the free drug concentration and thus drug absorption. However, the actual concentration at the epithelial boundary layer as well as the CMC of Cremophor EL under in-vivo conditions are currently unknown and therefore one can only speculate about possible mechanisms.

In a clinical trial Cremophor EL was administered up to 5000 mg [149]. Cremophor EL in single daily doses of 100, 1000 and 5000 mg together with 600 mg saquinavir (Invirase ®), which is also a P-gp substrate, was given to fasted volunteers. Doses of 100 mg and 1000 mg slightly increased $AUC_{0-\infty}$ by 1.4 fold compared to placebo. 5000 mg led to 5-fold increases. The effect of 5000 mg Cremophor EL on saquinavir pharmacokinetics was said to be similar to an opulent breakfast. In this regard, metabolic effects, solubilization by bile salts and altered intestinal and hepatic blood flow may be contributing. Furthermore, AUC_{0-4h} was 2-3 times enhanced by 100 mg or 1000 mg and 13 times enhanced by 5000 mg Cremophor EL. This shows an increased uptake in the early phase of absorption up to four hours after drug administration. The purpose of the study was to evaluate dose-dependant effects of Cremophor EL on saquinavir absorption and not to elucidate the possible mechanism. Besides P-gp inhibition CYP3A4 inhibition, i.e. decreased metabolism, favourable dissolution or solubility, might also play a role. Furthermore, the viscosity of gastric or intestinal fluid might be changed and thus the ability of the drug to diffuse freely.

Besides Cremophor EL Cremophor RH40, a structurally related compound, has also been assessed for its potential to enhance absorption of the P-gp substrate digoxin in humans. A 19-22% increase in AUC_{0-3h} was observed [150].

Cremophor EL is already used as an absorption enhancer in marketed products. To which extent enhancement is mediated by improvement of solubilization, P-gp inhibition or other physiological effects such as metabolism or changing gastric fluid viscosity remains to be determined.

As to whether high concentrations of surfactants (above CMC) rather hamper than enhance absorption depends on the substrate.

Bardelmeijer and Malingré [151, 152] as well as Chiu [153] reported that Cremophor EL might actually lower the intrinsic permeability of paclitaxel and cyclosporine A, respectively, in humans because of its association with Cremophor EL micelles whereas Nerurkar et al. [146] found a decrease in permeability for their peptide drug only at very high surfactant concentrations (100-1000 times higher than CMC) in studies conducted with Caco-2 cell monolayers.

In vitro experiments strongly suggest a role of P-gp inhibition (or other carriers) as shown e.g. with the metabolically stable substrate digoxin in Caco-2 cell monolayers. Most publications report an approximately twofold increase in permeability [135, 136, 138]. Flux is not only dependent on permeability but also on the concentration that remains on the luminal side. Thus effects might attenuate faster in-vivo because unlike in in-vitro experiments surfactant and drug pass along the intestine and surfactant concentration continuously decreases over time [154] . However, in-vitro only little amounts of drug are transported so that drug and surfactant concentration remain virtually constant in the donor chamber. On the other hand in vivo mRNA levels of P-gp have been shown to be higher in duodenal enterocytes than in Caco-2 cells [155]. However, in the jejunum expression levels of P-gp have been shown to be equal or somewhat lower than in Caco-2 cells [156] and the jejunum is regarded as the more important absorption site. It is not possible to directly correlate in vitro and in vivo experiments and therefore the relevance of modulatory effects on drug-carriers and pumps can only be shown by in vivo experiments.

As a conclusion, Cremophor EL employed at appropriate concentrations with a suitable drug might be a useful absorption enhancer of drug-carrier substrates but it should be kept in mind that enhancing solubility by micellization can counteract an effect mediated by P-gp inhibition depending on the drug´s affinity to the micelles. If it is low however, then the P-gp inhibition produced by surfactant (monomers) might further increase permeability and yield a synergistic effect together with micellar solubilization.

Whether P-gp inhibition by Cremophor EL might play a substantial role in absorption of P-gp substrates in humans remains to be shown. In-vitro evidence, however, suggests such a role.

3c. Tocopheryl-polyethyleneglycol-1000-succinate (TPGS)

TPGS is used as water-soluble form of vitamin E to treat vitamine E deficiency. Furthermore, it has been shown to enhance absorption of drugs e.g. amprenavir [157], cyclosporine A [158] and vitamine D in chronic cholestatic liver disease of infancy and childhood [159]. TPGS is listed as an excipient in the USP24 and is used as an embedding agent for the formulation of soft-gelatine capsules.

Dintaman and Silverman [160] observed that TPGS added to both sides of an using chamber simultaneously may inhibit basolateral-to-apical transport of rhodamine 123 (13 μM) and paclitaxel (0.1 μM) in Caco-2 and HCT-8 cells in concentrations from 0.001 to 0.005%, i.e. well below its CMC of 0.02% [w/w]. Furthermore, they showed that TPGS was able to reverse multi-drug resistance in NIH 3T3 G185 cells towards the P-gp substrate doxorubicin to the level of drug-sensitive NIH 3T3 cells whereas no such effect was observed using the non P-gp substrate 5-fluorouracil.

Cornaire et al. [135] observed a 2.5-fold increase mucosal to serosal digoxin transport using the everted rat gut model at a TPGS concentration of 0.05%[w/v]. Transport was still enhanced at concentrations of 0.1% (2.4-fold) and 0.5% (1.9-fold) but to a smaller extent than at 0.05%. The digoxin concentration used was 10 μM.

In a study by Johnson et al. [141] no reduction in serosal to mucosal digoxin flux across isolated rat jejunum was found at concentrations of 0.01% TPGS and 1 mM digoxin, which is twofold higher than that used in Caco-2 cell transport studies by Dintaman and Silverman, but would still be in accordance with the results of Cornaire et al..

However, the different experimental set-ups (e.g. different subtrates, substrate concentrations and transport models) do not allow a direct comparison

Chiu et al. [153] found a reduction of basolaterol-to-apical and apical-to-basolateral transport of cyclosporin A (0,4 µg/ml, corresponding to approximately 3.3 µM) across Caco-2 cell monolayers at TPGS concentrations of 0.02% and 0.2% [w/v]. In their method TPGS was used together with cyclosporin A either in the donor or acceptor chamber. Therefore these results indicated rather a sequestration of cyclosporin A into TPGS micelles to be the underlying mechanism for decreased transport as opposed to transporter inhibition as this might have lowered the free drug concentration. If TPGS is not present on the apical cell side no P-gp inhibition should take place since P-gp is expressed predominantly on the apical side and movement of TPGS to the apical membrane via the epithelium is restricted by tight junctions whereas transcellular transport should be negligible. Therefore, no reduction should have been expected. Nevertheless, one cannot absolutely deny concurrent inhibition of TPGS on P-gp in these experiments, since one has to consider the fact that in this study TPGS concentrations were equal or higher to the CMC of TPGS and thus association with micelles might have dominated over any other possibly observable inhibition of P-gp. Nevertheless, it indicates that TPGS similar to Cremophor EL might be more useful below or equal to its CMC for increasing bioavailability by inhibition of P-gp for certain substrates.

In vivo rat studies by Cornaire et al. [135] using TPGS at a concentration of 1 mg/kg did not enhance the $AUC_{0\text{-}480min}$ of digoxin, though the $AUC_{0\text{-}40min}$ was significantly higher. This shows that TPGS has a potential to modify the absorption of a drug and indicates that TPGS might be more effective in enhancing the rate of absorption rather than the extent.

None of the authors found significant cell toxicity or increases in paracellular transport with TPGS demonstrating its non-toxicity on rat tissue and cell cultures.

Varma and Panchagnula [161] showed that TPGS at concentrations of 0.1 mg/ml was superior to 1 mg/ml in enhancing the permeability of paclitaxel in in situ rat experiments, although at 1 mg/ml TPGS permeability was still significantly higher than in the control experiment. Moreover, they demonstrated that solubility of paclitaxel substantially increased above the CMC and that therefore improved solubility of paclitaxel could not be the reason for enhanced transport at the lower TPGS concentration.

An in vivo study in rats using the substrate colchicine in a 10% [v/v] TPGS solution showed a more than twofold increase in colchicine´s AUC. Colchicine has good inherent solubility leading the authors of the study to conclude that the solubilizing effect alone could not account for the increase in AUC [162].

TPGS effects on talinolol absorption have recently been studied with regard to P-gp-inhibition in humans [144]. The study was designed to exclude absorption phenomena mediated by improved solubility, dissolution, wetting or other generally surfactant-associated effects by using a non-P-gp inhibiting excipient, poloxamer 188, as a control and administration of solutions via nasogastral tubes. Possible metabolic effects on bioavailability were excluded by the use of talinolol as substrate as it can be considered as metabolically stable. The study provided good evidence that oral TPGS is able to enhance the bioavailability of talinolol and that this effect is due to inhibition of P-glycoprotein. The $AUC_{0\text{-}\infty}$ of talinolol was reported to augment by 39% compared to talinolol administered in the control vehicle.

Collnot et al. [163] studied the effect of polyethyleneglycol chain length of TPGS on absorptive transport of rhodamine 123 with the Caco2-cell model. The chain length of TPGS was varied from 200-6000 and it was shown that TPGS-1000 has the optimal chain length with respect to enhancement of rhodamine 123 transport.

Brouwers et al. [154] measured the TPGS concentration in duodenum and jejunum after administration of TPGS-containing amprenavir soft gelatine capsules. TPGS concentration reached levels as high as four mM in the jejunum and as high as eight mM in the duodenum. This is in the range of 0.01 to 0.1% , concentrations which have been shown to be effective in inhibiting P-gp in vitro as well.

In conclusion, there is broad evidence that TPGS can enhance bioavailability of P-gp substrates such as digoxin, talinolol and paclitaxel by both enhancing their solubility and inhibiting their efflux in the intestine. Evidence comes from in vitro, in situ and clinical trials. The efficacy of TPGS has been shown for different substrates. Thus TPGS might be a useful excipient in particular for increasing bioavailability of P-gp substrates.

3d. Polysorbate 80

Polysorbate 80 (Tween 80) is a non-ionic surfactant used as an emulsifier in O/W emulsions and as solubilizing agent. Furthermore it is used in mixture with other excipients in some formulations with self emulsifying properties containing e.g. cyclosporin A (Gengraf®) and sirolimus (Rapamune®) [164].

Nerurkar et al. [146] performed mechanistical studies on the effect of Polysorbate 80 on P-gp-mediated transport of a peptide drug in Caco-2 cell monolayers. The maximum decrease in basolateral-to-apical permeability was attained already below the CMC of Polysorbate 80 (given as 50 μM) indicating again the monomer and not micelle as the active moiety. Apical-to-basolateral permeability was enhanced by increasing Polysorbate concentrations up to 30 μM. The effect remained constant up to a concentration of about 25 times higher than the Polysorbate CMC. Then, like for Cremophor EL, permeability decreased suggesting associaton of relevant amounts of the peptide drug with surfactant micelles.

In a study by Rege et al. [134] it was demonstrated that Polysorbate 80 at concentrations of 1.8 mg/ml increased the overall permeability of furosemide, ranitidine and cimetidine in Caco-2 cell monolayer. Furthermore they showed that Tween 80 increased apical-to-basolateral permeability and decreased basolateral-to-apical permeability of rhodamine 123 in Caco-2 cell monolayers at concentrations ranging from 0.01 mM to 1 mM in a dose-dependent manner [136]. Membrane fluidization (DPH anisoptropy) was observed at a concentration as low as 0.025 mM. Polysorbate 80 also decreased apical-to-basolateral permeability of gly-sar, suggesting inhibition of the absorptive peptide transporter.

In Caco-2 cell monolayers ^{3}H-Taxol transport was increased at a concentration of 0.05% [w/v] without increasing mannitol transport measured as a marker of passive paracellular transport. The onset of transfer enhancement at 0.05% [w/v] correlated with the onset of membrane fluidization as observed by fluorescence anisotropy of DPH whereas no change occurred in Trimethylammonuiumphenyl-DPH (TMA-DPH) anisotropy [137].

Furthermore Polysorbate 80 increased the digoxin transfer across isolated rat jejunal tissue by 1.8-fold at a concentration of 0.5% [w/v] [135, 165] without enhancing LDH release measured as a marker of cell toxicity.

Zhang et al. [166] examined the effects of Polysorbate 80 on digoxin absorption in rats. Digoxin was given orally in solutions containing 1% and 10% Polysorbate 80. Moreover digoxin was given intravenously while Tween 80 was administered orally to estimate the effect of oral Tween 80 on extraintestinal P-gp in liver and kidney. For 1% Polysorbate 80 the AUC_{0-10h} increased by 30%, for 10% Polysorbate 80 by 61%. C_{max} climbed to about 160% for both. No influence of orally administered Polysorbate 80 on the AUC of intravenous digoxin was found. Therefore the increased AUC is most probably due to inhibition of intestinal P-gp by Polysorbate 80.

Seeballuck et al [167] addressed a different aspect of Polysorbate 80. They demonstrated that it can enhance chylomicron secretion in Caco-2 cell monolayers and thus might be able to enhance lymphatic transport of lipophilic drugs. This would result in a synergistic effect for lipophilic P-gp substrates.

Oral formulation of paclitaxel with Polysorbate 80 results in higher bioavailability than with Cremophor EL as shown by Malingré et al. [152]. Less paclitaxel was found in faeces when formulated with Polysorbate 80 than with Cremophor EL. Moreover, the amount of paclitaxel in the faeces was correlated to the Cremophor EL concentration in the Cremophor EL formulation.

Though modulation of drug carriers by Polysorbate 80 has not yet been directly shown in vivo the results of in vitro studies strongly suggest it. Together with its potential as a solubilizing agent and perhaps its capability of enhancing lymphatic transport it seems a valuable excipient for increasing bioavailability of low-solube, lipophilic drugs with affinity to P-gp and P-gp like transporters. However, Polysorbate 80 may inhibit PEPT1 and therefore possibly decrease the uptake of substrates of absorptive carriers.

3e. Pluronic P85 (and Other Pluronics)

Pluronics (also called poloxamers) are ABA block copolymers which are built from polyoxypropylene and polyoxyethylene. The hydrophobic polyoxypropylene chain (B) takes a central position and is flanked by two polyoxyethylene chains (A) on either side. Pluronics can be used for different purposes e.g. as O/W- type emulsifiers, to increase viscosity or for surfactant gels. A review about the use of pluronics as novel polymer therapeutics for drug and gene delivery is given by Kabanov et al. [168].

Batrakova et al. [169] studied the effects of Pluronic P85 on drug permeability in BBMEC (Bovine brain microvessel endothelial cells) and Caco-2 cells using rhodamine 123 as substrate. They found that at a concentration of 22 μM (CMC ~ 67μM) Pluronic P85 effectively eliminated polarized transport of rhodamine 123 across Caco-2 cell monolayers, i.e. flux in basolateral-to-apical direction and apical-to-basolateral direction practically equals each other, whereas without P85 apical-to-basolateral flux was 7.8-times higher than basolateral-to-apical flux. The effect was only seen when P85 was included on the apical cell side. This implies the involvement of an apical efflux transporter like P-gp, whose activity was inhibited by Pluronic P85.

Like the non-ionic surfactants discussed above, here again the monomers (or unimers) and not micelles are the active moiety, since inhibition was observed well below the CMC.

Working with a P85 concentration of 11 mM (i.e. above the CMC) on the apical side decreased apical-to-basolateral transport as compared to buffer plus rhodamine 123 only (control). Basolateral-to-apical flux was decreased likewise when P85 was added to the basolateral side. With no inhibition of drug transporters on the apical side, one would have expected increased transport because of accelerated efflux. At a P85 concentration of 11 mM about 50% of rhodamine 123 was associated with micelles indicating that decreased transport was due to decreased concentration of free rhodamine 123. Earlier, Batrakova et al. had shown that P85 at concentrations slightly above the CMC can still mediate P-gp inhibition by free unimers. However, when concentrations were further increased uptake of rhodamine 123 can be inhibited as compared to control (assay buffer + rhodamine 123 only). Similar phenomena were observed for Pluronic L81 and F68 [170].

The authors also described endocytosis of whole micelles into cells, but suggested that micelles were then routed back to the apical membrane and recycled out of the cell so that they do not positively contribute to uptake or transport of rhodamine 123 in Caco-2 cells [169]. Furthermore, it was shown in Caco-2 (and BBMEC) cell monolayers that not only rhodamine 123 transport can be enhanced by Pluronic P85 but also transport of fluorescein and drugs including doxorubicin, taxol, etoposide, azidodeoxythymidine, loperamide and valproic acid [143, 171]. Fluorescein is regarded as MRP substrate [172, 173] though its affinity to other drug carriers is not well defined. Nevertheless, it might be possible that Pluronic P85, as well as the other surfactants, can modulate activity of more than one drug carrier or pump.

The effects of Pluronic P85 on MRP1 and MRP2 overexpressing MDCK cells were studied and increased accumulation of vinblastine and doxorubicin was found suggesting that P85 is capable of inhibiting MRP1 and MRP2 [174]. On the other hand Evers et al. [57] studied effects of Pluronic L61, a compound structurally related to P85, on vinblastine transport in MDCK2-MRP transfected cells and concluded that neither vinblastine transport by MRP1 nor MRP2 were significantly inhibited by Pluronic L61. However, it is not known how important MRPs are for the intestinal absorption of drugs and not many conclusions can be derived from experiments in MRP overexpressing cells since they do not reflect MRP expression and activity in the human intestine.

Pluronic P85 (0.001%-1% [w/w]) has been shown to inhibit P-gp ATPase activity (also MRP1 and MRP2 ATPase activity but to a smaller extent) with concomitant increase of membrane fluidity in BBMEC cells. At high concentrations (> 0.01%) P85 also depletes intracellular ATP stores to a certain level [175-177]. Both actions, P-gp ATPase inhibition and ATP-depletion contribute to efflux inhibition of rhodamine 123.

Rhodamine 123 uptake was increased twofold by P85 concentrations from 0.001%-0.01% in BBMEC cells. At higher concentrations uptake was lowered again because of micelle formation. Thus the onset of enhanced uptake falls together with inhibition of P-gp, whereas at higher concentrations ATP-depletion adds up to the effect and at concentrations higher than the CMC (~ 0.03%) uptake enhancement levels off again because of the incorporation of drug into micelles resulting in lower free drug concentrations.

Transport studies have been performed with ^{3}H-P85 in LLC-MDR1 and MDCK-MRP2 and no directionality of transport was found indicating that ^{3}H-P85 is not a substrate of P-gp and MRP2 [177] and it was therefore concluded that inhibition rather operates by conformational changes of the transporter induced by membrane fluidization or by sterical hindrance of the drug binding site by P85.

Batrakova et al. [178] also reported inhibiton of MCT1, probably by inhibition of H^+-ATPase in BBMEC cells. However, BBMEC cells are model cells for blood brain endothelial cells and might show other physiology, expression levels and transporter activity than intestinal epithelial cells. The same study also investigated toxicity of Pluronic P85 administered intravenously but did not find histological or immunohistochemical difference as compared to control.

Batrakova et al. [142] studied several pluronics with varying content of polyoxyethylene and polyoxypropylene. It was concluded that with increasing polypropylenoxide content and higher hydrophobicity, compounds had higher potency in efflux inhibition. However, higher hydrophobicity also went along with lower CMCs, i.e. lower concentrations of Pluronic monomers. Since therefore the concentration of the free monomers decreases, so does efflux inhibition. Therefore at a certain point, further increasing compound hydrophobicity will counteract efflux inhibition. Pluronic P85 turned out to be a compound with near optimal properties with respect to polypropyleneoxide content, hydrophobicity and CMC. No efflux inhibition was found for Pluronics with high HLB (above 20), i.e. with high polyoxyethylene content.

In conclusion, several of the more hydrophobic Pluronics can inhibit P-gp and probably other ATP-dependant carriers as MRP1 and MRP2, whereas hydrophilic Pluronics (HLB higher than 20) do not seem to have such properties. Investigations have mainly focussed on Pluronic P85, because it turned out to be one of the most potent pluronics with respect to modulation of carrier-mediated transport.

Pluronic P85 might also inhibit MCT1, but no studies are available for intestinal cells. Enhanced transport of several substrates including doxorubicin, taxol and etoposide was demonstrated for Pluronic P85. Its toxicity seems to be low in mice even if administered intravenously. As for the surfactants the monomers are the active moiety. The mechanism of inhibition includes P-gp ATPase inhibition and at higher concentration ATP-depletion. Data is available mainly from in vitro studies. Until now, in vivo experiments in humans dealing with drug-carrier mediated transport have not been conducted to our knowledge.

3f. PEG 400 and PEG 300

Polyethyleneglycols are polymers made by polymerization of ethyleneoxide. They are good solvents for several drugs though some incompatibilities e.g. with phenols are known.

Wagner et al. [147] reported on the effects of PEG 400 and other surfactants on radioligand binding of ^{3}H-talinolol in a Caco-2 cell suspension. The IC50 of PEG400 was determined as 56.25 mM while IC50 values of the surfactants Cremophor EL and Tween 80 were as low as 0.41 mM and 0.23 mM respectively. This means that PEG 400 was less effective in displacing talinolol than Cremophor EL and Tween 80. Absorptive permeability of talinolol in Caco-2 cells was increased by 3.5 times while basolateral-to-apical permeability did not change significantly.

Johnson et al. [141] studied the potential of PEG 400 to enhance P-gp mediated transport of digoxin and metabolism of verapamil. They found that PEG 400 (5% w/v) inhibited basolateral-to-apical digoxin transport no matter if included on the apical or basolateral side or both. They suggested that changes in osmotic pressure at the apical membrane due to PEG 400 might result in decreased P-gp activity. Since PEG 400 also decreased basolateral-to-apical transport when added exclusively to the basolateral side and partitioning effects alone could not account for this effect they suggested that PEG 400 might also have an indirect effect on intracellular ATP levels as seen for Pluronic copolymers.

Furthermore, they demonstrated a decrease in verapamil metabolism when PEG400 was present indicating that PEG 400 might also act by inhibiting metabolism.

Hugger et al. [179] studied the effect of PEG 300 on ^{3}H-taxol and ^{3}H-doxorubicin transport across Caco-2 cell monolayers. PEG 300 was evaluated in concentrations from 2.5% to 20%. Because of the high concentration of PEG 300 used it was added basolaterally and apically sumltaneously in order to exclude any effects due to differences between basolateral and apical osmolarity. The b-to-a/a-to-b ratio was decreased for all concentrations and at the highest concentration of 20% PEG polarized transport was practically eliminated. No effect of PEG 300 was observed on testosterone and mannitol flux indicating that passive transcellular and paracellular transport is not enhanced. Therefore it was concluded that PEG 300 could inhibit P-gp and/or MRP mediated transport in Caco-2 cells. As a probable mechanism changes in membrane fluidity were proposed , since PEG300 at 20% significantly decreased fluorescence anisotropy of TMA-DPH (though not of DPH) which means that it decreases the fluidity of the polar head group region of the bilayer. This is different from the surfactants in that they rather decreased DPH anisotropy which monitors fluidity of the hydrophobic core part of the bilayer.

Interestingly , Hugger et al. [137] also showed that PEG300 inhibited transport in MDR1-MDCK cells while Cremophor EL and Tween 80 did not. Furthermore, Tween 80 decreased DPH anisotropy in Caco-2 cells while no such effect was seen in MDR1-MDCK cells. This supports the notion that inhibition of transporters also depends on their proximate environment since the membrane composition in these cells might differ.

Compared to the other surfactants PEGs seem to exert their effects at comparatively high concentrations (5-20%) while they had no effect at low concentrations (0.05-1.5%) (Table 3).

To our knowledge no in vivo studies investigating the effects of low molecular weight PEG on drug carrier activity in vivo have been published yet.

3g. Solutol HS 15

Solutol HS 15 contains mainly polyethylene glycol-15-hydroxystearate. It is used as a solubilizer for vitamin A, D, E and K and for lipophilic active pharmaceutical ingredients such as nifedipine, piroxicam, miconazole and alfadolone [180].

Solutol HS 15 was studied by Dudeja et al. [181] in the MDR (multi drug resistant) cell line KB 8-5-11 (human epidermoid carcinoma cell line). They showed that at a Solutol HS 15 concentration of 10 μg/ml (0.001%) multi-drug resistance of the KB 8-5-11 cells was reversed to a great extent as measured by rhodamine 123 uptake. Due to the fact that Solutol HS 15 is composed of several molecular entities a wide range is specified for the CMC of this product (0.005 – 0,02%).Thus, the concentration used in this study was above the CMC. Membrane fluidity studies with different probes including DPH and TMA-DPH were performed and it was concluded that Solutol HS 15 decreased membrane fluidity as measured by DPH and TMA-DPH.

Solutol HS 15 at concentrations ranging from 0.05% - 0.5% was effective in increasing digoxin transfer across rat everted intestinal tissue by about twofold [135]. LDH release by the tissue used as a marker of cellular toxicity was higher than control but less than 200% of control which was the limit regarded as not yet toxic by the investigators.

Bittner et al. [162] also showed that AUC of colchicine following oral administration was enhanced 4-fold by coadministration of Solutol HS 15 as compared to control. Since solubility of colchicine, a highly soluble drug, could not be enhanced by Solutol HS 15, other factors like P-gp inhibition or inhibition of CYP3A4 metabolism need to account for the improvement in colchicine bioavailability.

In conclusion, Solutol HS 15 was shown to enhance digoxin and rhodamine transport in vitro and colchicine bioavailability in rats in vivo, probably by P-gp inhibition or inhibition of metabolism and not by increasing drug solubility.

3h. Labrasol

Labrasol (caprylocaproyl macrogolglycerides EP/caprylocaproyl polyoxylglycerides USP/NF) is composed of a well-defined mixture of mono-, di- and triglycerides and mono- and di-fatty acid esters of polyethylene glycol. It is used as solubilizing agent, bioavailability enhancer of poorly soluble drugs, as surfactant in microemulsions and as permeation enhancer in topical preparations [182].

Effects of Labrasol on cephalexin a PEPT1 substrate were studied in vitro and in situ with rat intestine by Koga et al. [183]. It was found that permeability was enhanced by 10% when Labrasol (0.5%) was co-administerd under ATP-depleted conditions. Only about 50% of the enhancement was accounted for by active transport i.e. only 5% of the overall transport enhancement was due to modulation of active transport. Labrasol did not change the transepithelial electrical resistance of the tissue, though the short circuit current (I_{sc}), a measure of flow of electrogenic ions, was reduced. The authors concluded that the membrane barrier was maintained. Gelucire 44/14 (PEG-32 glyceryl laurate) did not affect transport at the same concentrations. The result would suggest an enhancement of absorptive transport since cephalexin is known as PEPT1 substrate. However, if it were a substrate of MRP or P-gp too, the result could as well be due to efflux inhibition.

Cornaire et al. [135] found a 5-fold increase of digoxin transport through everted rat intestinal tissue by 0.5% Labrasol, which indeed would suggest inhibition of P-gp. In these experiments, Labrasol also liberated LDH in significant amounts, which might indicate a potential toxic effect on the tissue, so that decreased cell viability might have been the reason for increased permeability.

Labrasol contained in a self microemulsifying drug delivery system was shown to increase paracellular transport across Caco-2 cell monolayers as measured by mannitol transport [184].

The sensitivity of cell viability and tight junctions towards Labrasol might be higher in Caco-2 cells than in living tissue because the latter shows inherent heterogeneity and superior protective mechanisms. A toxic effect on a monoculture cell line must not necessarily entail a toxic effect under in vivo conditions. To which extend LDH release can be correlated with cellular toxicity remains unresolved.

Hu et al. [185] studied bioavailability of gentamicin in a Labrasol containing and a non-Labrasol formulation. Though no polarized transport was observed for gentamicin alone, verapamil significantly enhanced apical-to-basolateral transport and decreased basolateral-to-apical transport of gentamicin in rat intestinal tissue. Gentamicin shows high solubility, is not metabolised and it is not well absorbed. In vivo bioavailability in rats was significantly enhanced when gentamicin was administered directly to the colon together with Labrasol. An implication of active transport systems has not been shown, but could also not be excluded.

For the moment data is too scarce to judge whether Labrasol can significantly enhance drug transport by modulation of drug carrier activity. It might as well enhance passive transcellular or paracellular transport. Nevertheless, it has been shown that to be effective in enhancing bioavailability of some low-bioavailability drugs [185].

3i. Others (Softigen 767, Imwitor 742, Methoxypolyethylene Glycol-block-polycaprolactone Diblock Copolymer Eudragit L100-55)

Softigen 767 (PEG-6 Caprylic/Capric Glycerides) and Imwitor 742 (caprylic/capric glycerides) were studied by Cornaire et al. [135]. Both increased digoxin and celiprolol absorption across rat gut tissue and AUCs for digoxin following oral administration in rats. Softigen 767 additionally increased AUC of celiprolol in the rat. Both increased LDH release of rat intestinal tissue less than twofold, which was set as an absolute toxicity boundary by the authors. I.e. any compound increasing LDH release above 200% was regarded as exerting substantial toxicity, those below as possibly but not necessarily toxic. The authors further state that Softigen 767 also increased mannitol transport suggesting that increased paracellular transport might contribute to the overall effect but that this route is not a common pathway for rather lipophilic substrates as digoxin and celiprolol.

A special aspect observed with these compounds in the in vivo experiments was that not only AUC increased but that the pharmacokinetic profile changed in that a second C_{max} appeared i.e. that the curves showed two peaks. The additional peak (as compared to control) appeared in the early stage of absorption. It was suggested that the compounds might have been more effective in the upper GI tract where P-gp expression is lower than in the lower parts of the GI tract [23]. Inversely, the concentration of the surfactants would be highest in the upper GI tract and due to dilution it would decrease in the lower GI tract.

Zastré et al. [186, 187] studied the effects of a methoxypolyethylene glycol-block-polycaprolactone diblock copolymer on rhodamine 123 uptake. Unlike shown for other surfactants rhodamine 123 accumulation in Caco-2 cells continued to increase even at concentrations 10 times higher than the CMC of the diblock copolymer. Partitioning into cell membranes might be a possible explanation. However, the CMC of Cremophor EL is 0.0095% [w/v] in water but 0.03 % [w/v] in the presence of cells and buffer [145] which only is about a threefold difference. The diblock copolymer was as effective in decreasing basolateral-to-apical flux as verapamil and enhanced apical-to-basolateral transport of rhodamine 123 at concentrations of 0.25 % while verapamil (50 μM) did not. Transport was also enhanced under ATP-depleted conditions so that probably both passive diffusion of rhodamine across the membrane and inhibition of active secretion by P-gp contributed to the effect.

The absorption of the antibiotics cefixim and cefadroxil, PEPT1 substrates, could be enhanced in an in situ study in rats by increasing the H^+-gradient in the rat ileum using a proton-releasing polymer (Eudragit L100-55) [188]. This complies with the idea of an H^+-dependent absorptive transporter. It is an example of actually enhancing absorptive transport in contrast to inhibiting efflux.

4. Possible Mechanism for Inhibition of Drug-carriers by Excipients

P-gp as well as MRP are saturable and ATP-dependent enzymes. Therefore their activity can be affected by substrate concentration or ATP depletion.

Saturable transport means that at high substrate concentrations V_{max} is reached and no further increase in active transport or secretion. V_{max} can be reduced by uncompetitive inhibition or noncompetitive inhibition. A change in membrane fluidity could trigger conformational changes of the transport protein into inactive, less active or even more active states which would be reflected in changes of V_{max} or K_m. Surfactants might interact with hydrophobic parts of the transmembrane domains of the transporter or might hinder access to putative binding sites sterically.

Transport of substrates by P-gp is coupled to ATP-hydrolysis. In fact P-gp contains two nucleotide binding sites with ATPase activity [189]. Any changes in binding affinity of ATP or availability of ATP (ATP depletion), any change in stability of intermediate states of ATP and the binding sites and changes in the release of ADP or P_i can affect the overall activity of P-gp. Such changes can be brought about by alterations of the three dimensional structure of the transporter by binding of a substrate or modulator or by changing the proximate environment of the protein i.e. membrane perturbations.

Depletion of intracellular ATP can inhibit P-gp mediated transport as was discussed for Pluronic P85. A proposed mechanism for ATP-depletion involves reduced mitochondria function [168] e.g. by uncoupling of oxidative phosphorylation [190] or inhibition of the NADH dehydrogenase complex [191].

Similarly, for secondary active transporters of the solute carrier type, as PEPT1, attenuation of the pH- gradient can lead to decreased activity.

Regev et al. [192] hypothesized that P-glycoprotein might be more sensitive to changes in membrane fluidization than other proteins. Most of the surfactants were able to alter membrane fluidity in one way or the other (e.g. TPGS decreased membrane fluidity, Polysorbate 80 increased membrane fluidity) at concentrations which had effects on transport, too. The question arises as to whether changes in membrane fluidity alone can cause inhibition of transporters. Rege et al [136] studied the effects of benzyl alcohol, a membrane fluidizer, and cholesterol, a membrane rigidizer on rhodamine 123 transport. Benzyl alcohol was shown to increase membrane fluidity but not transport of rhodamine 123 across Caco-2 cell monolayers and cholesterol pretreatment decreased membrane fluidity but did not significantly affect the rhodamine 123 transport. Therefore, alterations in membrane fluidity alone might not be sufficient to elicit changes in transport activity or might just reflect partitioning of surfactants into the membrane.

P-gp has been shown to be a substrate of protein kinase A and C which might change transporter conformation and activity by phosphorylation of certain residues. However, P-gp mutants, where the putative phosphorylation sites have been eliminated, showed normal transport function and generated drug resistance in formerly sensitive cells [193]. Furthermore, Rege et al. [136] showed that the PKC inhibitors staurosporine and chelerythrine chloride were not able to increase rhodamine 123 transport across Caco-2 cell monolayers. Therefore, it was regarded as unlikely that PKA or PKC play an important role in regulation of P-gp activity.

5. Conclusion

Excipients have been regarded as pharmacological inert substances formerly. However, the above cited works disclosed interactions between surfactants and polymers with members of at least four different transport protein types (P-gp, MRP, MCT and PEPT1). Though the mechanisms of inhibition have not been fully unravelled yet, it has been shown that transport activity of the mentioned transporters in the intestine can be altered, especially by surfactants, on a functional level.

Nevertheless, more clinical studies would be necessary to determine the in vivo relevance of the findings.

The review includes a row of excipients that seem to be safe with regard to acute and probably long-term toxicity, since these excipients have been used for years in pharmaceutical formulations and have been admitted to use by the responsible governmental bodies.

However, concomitant intake of two or more drug formulations, one containing the modulatory excipient the other a transporter substrate, might alter pharmacokinetics of the drug and may lead to toxicity for drugs with low therapeutic index.

Interestingly, most of the drugs formulated with surfactants (e.g. HIV-Protease inhibitors, Cyclosporine, Paclitaxel) are themselves transporter substrates or inhibitors (especially P-gp substrates), so that one would not normally co-administer them with other P-gp substrates in the first place. It might however be more than a coincidence that the formulations containing the surfactants with modulatory potential turned out most effective in formulation studies with P-gp substrates.

The cited works illustrate the importance of characterizing excipients not only by their physical but also by their biological properties. This would not only contribute to their safe use but could also lead to new ideas in drug delivery.

6. References

[1] Chan LM, Lowes S, Hirst BH. The ABCs of drug transport in intestine and liver: efflux proteins limiting drug absorption and bioavailability. *Eur J Pharm Sci.* 2004 Jan;21(1):25-51.

[2] Borst P. ER, Kool M., Wijnholds J. The multidrug resistance protein family. *Biochim Biophys Acta.* 1999 Dec 6;1461(2):347-57.

[3] Liang R, Fei YJ, Prasad PD, Ramamoorthy S, Han H, Yang-Feng TL, et al. Human intestinal H+/peptide cotransporter. Cloning, functional expression, and chromosomal localization. *J Biol Chem.* 1995 Mar 24;270(12):6456-63.

[4] Daniel H. GK. The proton oligopeptide cotransporter family SLC15 in physiology and pharmacology. *Pflügers Archiv European Journal of Physiology.* 2004 February;447(5):610 - 8.

[5] Koepsell H, Schmitt BM, Gorboulev V. Organic cation transporters. *Rev Physiol Biochem Pharmacol.* 2003;150:36-90.

[6] Takanaga H. TI, Inaba S., Sai Y., Higashida H., Yamamoto H., Tsuji A. cDNA cloning and functional characterization of rat intestinal monocarboxylate transporter. *Biochem Biophys Res Commun.* 1995 Dec 5;217(1):370-7.

[7] Halestrap AP, Price NT. The proton-linked monocarboxylate transporter (MCT) family: structure, function and regulation. *Biochem J.* 1999 Oct 15;343 Pt 2:281-99.

[8] Karlsson J, Kuo SM, Ziemniak J, Artursson P. Transport of celiprolol across human intestinal epithelial (Caco-2) cells: mediation of secretion by multiple transporters including P-glycoprotein. *Br J Pharmacol.* 1993 Nov;110(3):1009-16.

[9] Cavet ME, West M, Simmons NL. Transport and epithelial secretion of the cardiac glycoside, digoxin, by human intestinal epithelial (Caco-2) cells. *Br J Pharmacol.* 1996 Jul;118(6):1389-96.

[10] Collett A, Higgs NB, Sims E, Rowland M, Warhurst G. Modulation of the permeability of H2 receptor antagonists cimetidine and ranitidine by P-glycoprotein in rat intestine and the human colonic cell line Caco-2. *J Pharmacol Exp Ther.* 1999 Jan;288(1):171-8.

[11] Kim RB. Drugs as P-glycoprotein substrates, inhibitors, and inducers. *Drug Metab Rev.* 2002 Feb-May;34(1-2):47-54.

[12] Lowes S, Simmons NL. Multiple pathways for fluoroquinolone secretion by human intestinal epithelial (Caco-2) cells. *Br J Pharmacol.* 2002 Mar;135(5):1263-75.

[13] Friedman DI, Amidon GL. Passive and carrier-mediated intestinal absorption components of two angiotensin converting enzyme (ACE) inhibitor prodrugs in rats: enalapril and fosinopril. *Pharm Res.* 1989 Dec;6(12):1043-7.

[14] de Vrueh RLA, Smith, P.L., Lee, C.-P. Transport of L-valine aciclovir via the oligopeptide transporter in the human intestinal cell line , Caco-2. *J Pharmacol Exp Ther.* 1998;286:1166-70.

[15] Drescher S, Glaeser H, Murdter T, Hitzl M, Eichelbaum M, Fromm MF. P-glycoprotein-mediated intestinal and biliary digoxin transport in humans. *Clin Pharmacol Ther.* 2003 Mar;73(3):223-31.

[16] Anderle P, Niederer E, Rubas W, Hilgendorf C, Spahn-Langguth H, Wunderli-Allenspach H, et al. P-Glycoprotein (P-gp) mediated efflux in Caco-2 cell monolayers: the influence of culturing conditions and drug exposure on P-gp expression levels. *J Pharm Sci.* 1998 Jun;87(6):757-62.

[17] Hanafy A, Langguth P, Spahn-Langguth H. Pretreatment with potent P-glycoprotein ligands may increase intestinal secretion in rats. *Eur J Pharm Sci.* 2001 Feb;12(4):405-15.

[18] Collett A. T-HJ, Warhurst G. Rapid induction of P-glycoprotein expression by high permeability compounds in colonic cells in vitro: a possible source of transporter mediated drug interactions? *Biochem Pharmacol.* 2004 Aug 15;68((4)):783-90.

[19] Marzolini C PE, Buclin T, Kim RB. Polymorphisms in human MDR1 (P-glycoprotein): recent advances and clinical relevance. *Clin Pharmacol Ther.* 2004 Jan;75.(1):13-33.

[20] Westphal K, Weinbrenner A, Zschiesche M, Franke G, Knoke M, Oertel R, et al. Induction of P-glycoprotein by rifampin increases intestinal secretion of talinolol in human beings: a new type of drug/drug interaction. *Clin Pharmacol Ther.* 2000 Oct;68(4):345-55.

[21] Tsuji A. TI. Carrier-Mediated Intestinal Transport of Drugs. *Pharmaceutical Research.* 1996 July; 13(7):963 - 77.

[22] Steffansen B. NCU, Brodin B., Eriksson A.H., Andersen R., Frokjaer S. Intestinal solute carriers: an overview of trends and strategies for improving oral drug absorption. *Eur J Pharm Sci.* 2004 Jan;21(1):3-16.

[23] Mouly S, Paine MF. P-glycoprotein increases from proximal to distal regions of human small intestine. *Pharm Res.* 2003 Oct;20(10):1595-9.

[24] Benet LZ, Cummins CL, Wu CY. Unmasking the dynamic interplay between efflux transporters and metabolic enzymes. *Int J Pharm.* 2004 Jun 11;277(1-2):3-9.

[25] Zhang Y, Benet LZ. The gut as a barrier to drug absorption: combined role of cytochrome P450 3A and P-glycoprotein. *Clin Pharmacokinet.* 2001;40(3):159-68.

[26] Sparreboom A, van Asperen J, Mayer U, Schinkel AH, Smit JW, Meijer DK, et al. Limited oral bioavailability and active epithelial excretion of paclitaxel (Taxol) caused by P-glycoprotein in the intestine. *Proc Natl Acad Sci U S A.* 1997 Mar 4;94(5):2031-5.

[27] Kartner N, Shales M, Riordan JR, Ling V. Daunorubicin-resistant Chinese hamster ovary cells expressing multidrug resistance and a cell-surface P-glycoprotein. *Cancer Res.* 1983 Sep;43(9):4413-9.

[28] Tamai I, Yamashita J, Kido Y, Ohnari A, Sai Y, Shima Y, et al. Limited distribution of new quinolone antibacterial agents into brain caused by multiple efflux transporters at the blood-brain barrier. *J Pharmacol Exp Ther.* 2000 Oct;295(1):146-52.

[29] Jones K, Hoggard PG, Sales SD, Khoo S, Davey R, Back DJ. Differences in the intracellular accumulation of HIV protease inhibitors in vitro and the effect of active transport. *Aids.* 2001 Apr 13;15(6):675-81.

[30] Kim AE, Dintaman JM, Waddell DS, Silverman JA. Saquinavir, an HIV protease inhibitor, is transported by P-glycoprotein. *J Pharmacol Exp Ther.* 1998 Sep;286(3):1439-45.

[31] Kim RB, Fromm MF, Wandel C, Leake B, Wood AJ, Roden DM, et al. The drug transporter P-glycoprotein limits oral absorption and brain entry of HIV-1 protease inhibitors. *J Clin Invest.* 1998 Jan 15;101(2):289-94.

[32] Saeki T, Ueda K, Tanigawara Y, Hori R, Komano T. Human P-glycoprotein transports cyclosporin A and FK506. *J Biol Chem.* 1993 Mar 25;268(9):6077-80.

[33] Gramatte T, Oertel R. Intestinal secretion of intravenous talinolol is inhibited by luminal R-verapamil. *Clin Pharmacol Ther.* 1999 Sep;66(3):239-45.

[34] Tanigawara Y, Okamura N, Hirai M, Yasuhara M, Ueda K, Kioka N, et al. Transport of digoxin by human P-glycoprotein expressed in a porcine kidney epithelial cell line (LLC-PK1). *J Pharmacol Exp Ther.* 1992 Nov;263(2):840-5.

[35] Leier I, Jedlitschky G, Buchholz U, Cole SP, Deeley RG, Keppler D. The MRP gene encodes an ATP-dependent export pump for leukotriene C4 and structurally related conjugates. *J Biol Chem.* 1994 Nov 11;269(45):27807-10.

[36] Madon J, Eckhardt U, Gerloff T, Stieger B, Meier PJ. Functional expression of the rat liver canalicular isoform of the multidrug resistance-associated protein. *FEBS Lett.* 1997 Apr 7;406(1-2):75-8.

[37] Zelcer N, Saeki T, Reid G, Beijnen JH, Borst P. Characterization of drug transport by the human multidrug resistance protein 3 (ABCC3). *J Biol Chem.* 2001 Dec 7;276(49):46400-7.

[38] Suzuki M, Suzuki H, Sugimoto Y, Sugiyama Y. ABCG2 transports sulfated conjugates of steroids and xenobiotics. *J Biol Chem.* 2003 Jun 20;278(25):22644-9.

[39] Miller DS. Nucleoside phosphonate interactions with multiple organic anion transporters in renal proximal tubule. *J Pharmacol Exp Ther.* 2001 Nov;299(2):567-74.

[40] Ueda K, Okamura N, Hirai M, Tanigawara Y, Saeki T, Kioka N, et al. Human P-glycoprotein transports cortisol, aldosterone, and dexamethasone, but not progesterone. *J Biol Chem.* 1992 Dec 5;267(34):24248-52.

[41] Kakumoto M, Takara K, Sakaeda T, Tanigawara Y, Kita T, Okumura K. MDR1-mediated interaction of digoxin with antiarrhythmic or antianginal drugs. *Biol Pharm Bull.* 2002 Dec;25(12):1604-7.

[42] Uhr M, Steckler T, Yassouridis A, Holsboer F. Penetration of amitriptyline, but not of fluoxetine, into brain is enhanced in mice with blood-brain barrier deficiency due to mdr1a P-glycoprotein gene disruption. *Neuropsychopharmacology.* 2000 Apr;22(4):380-7.

[43] Polli JW, Jarrett JL, Studenberg SD, Humphreys JE, Dennis SW, Brouwer KR, et al. Role of P-glycoprotein on the CNS disposition of amprenavir (141W94), an HIV protease inhibitor. *Pharm Res.* 1999 Aug;16(8):1206-12.

[44] Perloff MD vML, Greenblatt DJ. Ritonavir and dexamethasone induce expression of CYP3A and P-glycoprotein in rats. *Xenobiotica.* 2004 Feb;34(2):133-50.

[45] Wu X, Whitfield LR, Stewart BH. Atorvastatin transport in the Caco-2 cell model: contributions of P-glycoprotein and the proton-monocarboxylic acid co-transporter. *Pharm Res.* 2000 Feb;17(2):209-15.

[46] Boyd RA, Stern RH, Stewart BH, Wu X, Reyner EL, Zegarac EA, et al. Atorvastatin coadministration may increase digoxin concentrations by inhibition of intestinal P-glycoprotein-mediated secretion. *J Clin Pharmacol.* 2000 Jan;40(1):91-8.

[47] Litman T, Brangi M, Hudson E, Fetsch P, Abati A, Ross DD, et al. The multidrug-resistant phenotype associated with overexpression of the new ABC half-transporter, MXR (ABCG2). *J Cell Sci.* 2000 Jun;113 (Pt 11):2011-21.

[48] Orlowski S, Valente D, Garrigos M, Ezan E. Bromocriptine modulates P-glycoprotein function. *Biochem Biophys Res Commun.* 1998 Mar 17;244(2):481-8.

[49] Kakumoto M, Sakaeda T, Takara K, Nakamura T, Kita T, Yagami T, et al. Effects of carvedilol on MDR1-mediated multidrug resistance: comparison with verapamil. *Cancer Sci.* 2003 Jan;94(1):81-6.

[50] Saitoh H, Aungst BJ. Possible involvement of multiple P-glycoprotein-mediated efflux systems in the transport of verapamil and other organic cations across rat intestine. *Pharm Res.* 1995 Sep;12(9):1304-10.

[51] Pan BF, Dutt A, Nelson JA. Enhanced transepithelial flux of cimetidine by Madin-Darby canine kidney cells overexpressing human P-glycoprotein. *J Pharmacol Exp Ther.* 1994 Jul;270(1):1-7.

[52] Pastan I, Gottesman MM, Ueda K, Lovelace E, Rutherford AV, Willingham MC. A retrovirus carrying an MDR1 cDNA confers multidrug resistance and polarized expression of P-glycoprotein in MDCK cells. *Proc Natl Acad Sci U S A.* 1988 Jun;85(12):4486-90.

[53] Sharp SY, Smith V, Hobbs S, Kelland LR. Lack of a role for MRP1 in platinum drug resistance in human ovarian cancer cell lines. *Br J Cancer.* 1998 Jul;78(2):175-80.

[54] Cui Y, Konig J, Buchholz JK, Spring H, Leier I, Keppler D. Drug resistance and ATP-dependent conjugate transport mediated by the apical multidrug resistance protein, MRP2, permanently expressed in human and canine cells. *Mol Pharmacol.* 1999 May;55(5):929-37.

[55] Wakasugi H, Yano I, Ito T, Hashida T, Futami T, Nohara R, et al. Effect of clarithromycin on renal excretion of digoxin: interaction with P-glycoprotein. *Clin Pharmacol Ther.* 1998 Jul;64(1):123-8.

[56] Lown KS, Mayo RR, Leichtman AB, Hsiao HL, Turgeon DK, Schmiedlin-Ren P, et al. Role of intestinal P-glycoprotein (mdr1) in interpatient variation in the oral bioavailability of cyclosporine. *Clin Pharmacol Ther.* 1997 Sep;62(3):248-60.

[57] Evers R, Kool M, Smith AJ, van Deemter L, de Haas M, Borst P. Inhibitory effect of the reversal agents V-104, GF120918 and Pluronic L61 on MDR1 Pgp-, MRP1- and MRP2-mediated transport. *Br J Cancer.* 2000 Aug;83(3):366-74.

[58] Zeng H, Bain LJ, Belinsky MG, Kruh GD. Expression of multidrug resistance protein-3 (multispecific organic anion transporter-D) in human embryonic kidney 293 cells confers resistance to anticancer agents. *Cancer Res.* 1999 Dec 1;59(23):5964-7.

[59] Doyle LA, Yang W, Abruzzo LV, Krogmann T, Gao Y, Rishi AK, et al. A multidrug resistance transporter from human MCF-7 breast cancer cells. *Proc Natl Acad Sci U S A.* 1998 Dec 22;95(26):15665-70.

[60] Zelcer N, Reid G, Wielinga P, Kuil A, van der Heijden I, Schuetz JD, et al. Steroid and bile acid conjugates are substrates of human multidrug-resistance protein (MRP) 4 (ATP-binding cassette C4). *Biochem J.* 2003 Apr 15;371(Pt 2):361-7.

[61] Lin JH, Chiba M, Chen IW, Nishime JA, deLuna FA, Yamazaki M, et al. Effect of dexamethasone on the intestinal first-pass metabolism of indinavir in rats: evidence of cytochrome P-450 3A [correction of P-450 A] and p-glycoprotein induction. *Drug Metab Dispos.* 1999 Oct;27(10):1187-93.

[62] Fardel O, Lecureur V, Guillouzo A. Regulation by dexamethasone of P-glycoprotein expression in cultured rat hepatocytes. *FEBS Lett.* 1993 Jul 26;327(2):189-93.

[63] Zhao JY, Ikeguchi M, Eckersberg T, Kuo MT. Modulation of multidrug resistance gene expression by dexamethasone in cultured hepatoma cells. *Endocrinology.* 1993 Aug;133(2):521-8.

[64] Sugimoto Y, Tsukahara S, Imai Y, Sugimoto Y, Ueda K, Tsuruo T. Reversal of breast cancer resistance protein-mediated drug resistance by estrogen antagonists and agonists. *Mol Cancer Ther.* 2003 Jan;2(1):105-12.

[65] de Lannoy IA, Silverman M. The MDR1 gene product, P-glycoprotein, mediates the transport of the cardiac glycoside, digoxin. *Biochem Biophys Res Commun.* 1992 Nov 30;189(1):551-7.

[66] Lowes S, Cavet ME, Simmons NL. Evidence for a non-MDR1 component in digoxin secretion by human intestinal Caco-2 epithelial layers. *Eur J Pharmacol.* 2003 Jan 1;458(1-2):49-56.

[67] Verstuyft C, Strabach S, El-Morabet H, Kerb R, Brinkmann U, Dubert L, et al. Dipyridamole enhances digoxin bioavailability via P-glycoprotein inhibition. *Clin Pharmacol Ther.* 2003 Jan;73(1):51-60.

[68] Wils P, Phung-Ba V, Warnery A, Lechardeur D, Raeissi S, Hidalgo IJ, et al. Polarized transport of docetaxel and vinblastine mediated by P-glycoprotein in human intestinal epithelial cell monolayers. *Biochem Pharmacol.* 1994 Oct 7;48(7):1528-30.

[69] Schinkel AH, Wagenaar E, Mol CA, van Deemter L. P-glycoprotein in the blood-brain barrier of mice influences the brain penetration and pharmacological activity of many drugs. *J Clin Invest.* 1996 Jun 1;97(11):2517-24.

[70] Fardel O, Lecureur V, Daval S, Corlu A, Guillouzo A. Up-regulation of P-glycoprotein expression in rat liver cells by acute doxorubicin treatment. *Eur J Biochem.* 1997 May 15;246(1):186-92.

[71] Brangi M, Litman T, Ciotti M, Nishiyama K, Kohlhagen G, Takimoto C, et al. Camptothecin resistance: role of the ATP-binding cassette (ABC), mitoxantrone-resistance half-transporter (MXR), and potential for glucuronidation in MXR-expressing cells. *Cancer Res.* 1999 Dec 1;59(23):5938-46.

[72] Takano M, Hasegawa R, Fukuda T, Yumoto R, Nagai J, Murakami T. Interaction with P-glycoprotein and transport of erythromycin, midazolam and ketoconazole in Caco-2 cells. *Eur J Pharmacol.* 1998 Oct 9;358(3):289-94.

[73] Huang L, Hoffman T, Vore M. Adenosine triphosphate-dependent transport of estradiol-17beta(beta-D-glucuronide) in membrane vesicles by MDR1 expressed in insect cells. *Hepatology.* 1998 Nov;28(5):1371-7.

[74] Loe DW, Almquist KC, Cole SP, Deeley RG. ATP-dependent 17 beta-estradiol 17-(beta-D-glucuronide) transport by multidrug resistance protein (MRP). Inhibition by cholestatic steroids. *J Biol Chem.* 1996 Apr 19;271(16):9683-9.

[75] Keppler D, Leier I, Jedlitschky G. Transport of glutathione conjugates and glucuronides by the multidrug resistance proteins MRP1 and MRP2. *Biol Chem.* 1997 Aug;378(8):787-91.

[76] Allen JD, Van Dort SC, Buitelaar M, van Tellingen O, Schinkel AH. Mouse breast cancer resistance protein (Bcrp1/Abcg2) mediates etoposide resistance and transport, but etoposide oral availability is limited primarily by P-glycoprotein. *Cancer Res.* 2003 Mar 15;63(6):1339-44.

[77] Cvetkovic M, Leake B, Fromm MF, Wilkinson GR, Kim RB. OATP and P-glycoprotein transporters mediate the cellular uptake and excretion of fexofenadine. *Drug Metab Dispos.* 1999 Aug;27(8):866-71.

[78] Robey RW, Medina-Perez WY, Nishiyama K, Lahusen T, Miyake K, Litman T, et al. Overexpression of the ATP-binding cassette half-transporter, ABCG2 (Mxr/BCrp/ABCP1), in flavopiridol-resistant human breast cancer cells. *Clin Cancer Res.* 2001 Jan;7(1):145-52.

[79] Pariante CM, Kim RB, Makoff A, Kerwin RW. Antidepressant fluoxetine enhances glucocorticoid receptor function in vitro by modulating membrane steroid transporters. *Br J Pharmacol.* 2003 Jul;139(6):1111-8.

[80] Bakos E, Evers R, Sinko E, Varadi A, Borst P, Sarkadi B. Interactions of the human multidrug resistance proteins MRP1 and MRP2 with organic anions. *Mol Pharmacol.* 2000 Apr;57(4):760-8.

[81] Payen L, Delugin L, Courtois A, Trinquart Y, Guillouzo A, Fardel O. The sulphonylurea glibenclamide inhibits multidrug resistance protein (MRP1) activity in human lung cancer cells. *Br J Pharmacol.* 2001 Feb;132(3):778-84.

[82] Yamaguchi H, Yano I, Hashimoto Y, Inui KI. Secretory mechanisms of grepafloxacin and levofloxacin in the human intestinal cell line caco-2. *J Pharmacol Exp Ther.* 2000 Oct;295(1):360-6.

[83] Perloff MD, von Moltke LL, Fahey JM, Daily JP, Greenblatt DJ. Induction of P-glycoprotein expression by HIV protease inhibitors in cell culture. *Aids*. 2000 Jun 16;14(9):1287-9.
[84] Huisman MT, Smit JW, Crommentuyn KM, Zelcer N, Wiltshire HR, Beijnen JH, et al. Multidrug resistance protein 2 (MRP2) transports HIV protease inhibitors, and transport can be enhanced by other drugs. *Aids*. 2002 Nov 22;16(17):2295-301.
[85] Miyama T, Takanaga H, Matsuo H, Yamano K, Yamamoto K, Iga T, et al. P-glycoprotein-mediated transport of itraconazole across the blood-brain barrier. *Antimicrob Agents Chemother*. 1998 Jul;42(7):1738-44.
[86] Kim RB, Wandel C, Leake B, Cvetkovic M, Fromm MF, Dempsey PJ, et al. Interrelationship between substrates and inhibitors of human CYP3A and P-glycoprotein. *Pharm Res*. 1999 Mar;16(3):408-14.
[87] Wang X, Furukawa T, Nitanda T, Okamoto M, Sugimoto Y, Akiyama S, et al. Breast cancer resistance protein (BCRP/ABCG2) induces cellular resistance to HIV-1 nucleoside reverse transcriptase inhibitors. *Mol Pharmacol*. 2003 Jan;63(1):65-72.
[88] Pauli-Magnus C, Rekersbrink S, Klotz U, Fromm MF. Interaction of omeprazole, lansoprazole and pantoprazole with P-glycoprotein. *Naunyn Schmiedebergs Arch Pharmacol*. 2001 Dec;364(6):551-7.
[89] Soldner A, Benet LZ, Mutschler E, Christians U. Active transport of the angiotensin-II antagonist losartan and its main metabolite EXP 3174 across MDCK-MDR1 and caco-2 cell monolayers. *Br J Pharmacol*. 2000 Mar;129(6):1235-43.
[90] Callaghan R, Riordan JR. Synthetic and natural opiates interact with P-glycoprotein in multidrug-resistant cells. *J Biol Chem*. 1993 Jul 25;268(21):16059-64.
[91] de Graaf D, Sharma RC, Mechetner EB, Schimke RT, Roninson IB. P-glycoprotein confers methotrexate resistance in 3T6 cells with deficient carrier-mediated methotrexate uptake. *Proc Natl Acad Sci U S A*. 1996 Feb 6;93(3):1238-42.
[92] Zeng H, Chen ZS, Belinsky MG, Rea PA, Kruh GD. Transport of methotrexate (MTX) and folates by multidrug resistance protein (MRP) 3 and MRP1: effect of polyglutamylation on MTX transport. *Cancer Res*. 2001 Oct 1;61(19):7225-32.
[93] Vlaming ML, Mohrmann K, Wagenaar E, de Waart DR, Elferink RP, Lagas JS, et al. Carcinogen and anticancer drug transport by Mrp2 in vivo: studies using Mrp2 (Abcc2) knockout mice. *J Pharmacol Exp Ther*. 2006 Jul;318(1):319-27.
[94] Chen C, Scott D, Hanson E, Franco J, Berryman E, Volberg M, et al. Impact of Mrp2 on the biliary excretion and intestinal absorption of furosemide, probenecid, and methotrexate using Eisai hyperbilirubinemic rats. *Pharm Res*. 2003 Jan;20(1):31-7.
[95] Kool M, van der Linden M, de Haas M, Scheffer GL, de Vree JM, Smith AJ, et al. MRP3, an organic anion transporter able to transport anti-cancer drugs. *Proc Natl Acad Sci U S A*. 1999 Jun 8;96(12):6914-9.
[96] Volk EL, Farley KM, Wu Y, Li F, Robey RW, Schneider E. Overexpression of wild-type breast cancer resistance protein mediates methotrexate resistance. *Cancer Res*. 2002 Sep 1;62(17):5035-40.
[97] Chen ZS, Robey RW, Belinsky MG, Shchaveleva I, Ren XQ, Sugimoto Y, et al. Transport of methotrexate, methotrexate polyglutamates, and 17beta-estradiol 17-(beta-D-glucuronide) by ABCG2: effects of acquired mutations at R482 on methotrexate transport. *Cancer Res*. 2003 Jul 15;63(14):4048-54.

[98] Consoli U, Van NT, Neamati N, Mahadevia R, Beran M, Zhao S, et al. Cellular pharmacology of mitoxantrone in p-glycoprotein-positive and -negative human myeloid leukemic cell lines. *Leukemia.* 1997 Dec;11(12):2066-74.

[99] Morrow CS, Peklak-Scott C, Bishwokarma B, Kute TE, Smitherman PK, Townsend AJ. Multidrug resistance protein 1 (MRP1, ABCC1) mediates resistance to mitoxantrone via glutathione-dependent drug efflux. *Mol Pharmacol.* 2006 Apr;69(4):1499-505.

[100] Aquilante CL, Letrent SP, Pollack GM, Brouwer KL. Increased brain P-glycoprotein in morphine tolerant rats. *Life Sci.* 2000;66(4):PL47-51.

[101] Gupta A, Zhang Y, Unadkat JD, Mao Q. HIV protease inhibitors are inhibitors but not substrates of the human breast cancer resistance protein (BCRP/ABCG2). *J Pharmacol Exp Ther.* 2004 Jul;310(1):334-41.

[102] Gutmann H, Miller DS, Droulle A, Drewe J, Fahr A, Fricker G. P-glycoprotein- and mrp2-mediated octreotide transport in renal proximal tubule. *Br J Pharmacol.* 2000 Jan;129(2):251-6.

[103] Breedveld P, Zelcer N, Pluim D, Sonmezer O, Tibben MM, Beijnen JH, et al. Mechanism of the pharmacokinetic interaction between methotrexate and benzimidazoles: potential role for breast cancer resistance protein in clinical drug-drug interactions. *Cancer Res.* 2004 Aug 15;64(16):5804-11.

[104] Kusuhara H, Suzuki H, Terasaki T, Kakee A, Lemaire M, Sugiyama Y. P-Glycoprotein mediates the efflux of quinidine across the blood-brain barrier. *J Pharmacol Exp Ther.* 1997 Nov;283(2):574-80.

[105] Wang E, Lew K, Barecki M, Casciano CN, Clement RP, Johnson WW. Quantitative distinctions of active site molecular recognition by P-glycoprotein and cytochrome P450 3A4. *Chem Res Toxicol.* 2001 Dec;14(12):1596-603.

[106] Schuetz EG, Beck WT, Schuetz JD. Modulators and substrates of P-glycoprotein and cytochrome P4503A coordinately up-regulate these proteins in human colon carcinoma cells. *Mol Pharmacol.* 1996 Feb;49(2):311-8.

[107] El Hafny B, Chappey O, Piciotti M, Debray M, Boval B, Roux F. Modulation of P-glycoprotein activity by glial factors and retinoic acid in an immortalized rat brain microvessel endothelial cell line. *Neurosci Lett.* 1997 Oct 31;236(2):107-11.

[108] Eytan GD, Regev R, Oren G, Hurwitz CD, Assaraf YG. Efficiency of P-glycoprotein-mediated exclusion of rhodamine dyes from multidrug-resistant cells is determined by their passive transmembrane movement rate. *Eur J Biochem.* 1997 Aug 15; 248(1): 104-12.

[109] Zaman GJ, Flens MJ, van Leusden MR, de Haas M, Mulder HS, Lankelma J, et al. The human multidrug resistance-associated protein MRP is a plasma membrane drug-efflux pump. *Proc Natl Acad Sci U S A.* 1994 Sep 13;91(19):8822-6.

[110] Schuetz EG, Schinkel AH, Relling MV, Schuetz JD. P-glycoprotein: a major determinant of rifampicin-inducible expression of cytochrome P4503A in mice and humans. *Proc Natl Acad Sci U S A.* 1996 Apr 30;93(9):4001-5.

[111] Cui Y, Konig J, Keppler D. Vectorial transport by double-transfected cells expressing the human uptake transporter SLC21A8 and the apical export pump ABCC2. *Mol Pharmacol.* 2001 Nov;60(5):934-43.

[112] Weiss J, Dormann SM, Martin-Facklam M, Kerpen CJ, Ketabi-Kiyanvash N, Haefeli WE. Inhibition of P-glycoprotein by newer antidepressants. *J Pharmacol Exp Ther.* 2003 Apr;305(1):197-204.

[113] Sakaeda T, Takara K, Kakumoto M, Ohmoto N, Nakamura T, Iwaki K, et al. Simvastatin and lovastatin, but not pravastatin, interact with MDR1. *J Pharm Pharmacol.* 2002 Mar;54(3):419-23.

[114] Nakamura T, Kakumoto M, Yamashita K, Takara K, Tanigawara Y, Sakaeda T, et al. Factors influencing the prediction of steady state concentrations of digoxin. *Biol Pharm Bull.* 2001 Apr;24(4):403-8.

[115] Durr D, Stieger B, Kullak-Ublick GA, Rentsch KM, Steinert HC, Meier PJ, et al. St John's Wort induces intestinal P-glycoprotein/MDR1 and intestinal and hepatic CYP3A4. *Clin Pharmacol Ther.* 2000 Dec;68(6):598-604.

[116] Kochi S, Takanaga H, Matsuo H, Naito M, Tsuruo T, Sawada Y. Effect of cyclosporin A or tacrolimus on the function of blood-brain barrier cells. *Eur J Pharmacol.* 1999 May 21;372(3):287-95.

[117] Akita H, Suzuki H, Ito K, Kinoshita S, Sato N, Takikawa H, et al. Characterization of bile acid transport mediated by multidrug resistance associated protein 2 and bile salt export pump. *Biochim Biophys Acta.* 2001 Mar 9;1511(1):7-16.

[118] Hirohashi T, Suzuki H, Takikawa H, Sugiyama Y. ATP-dependent transport of bile salts by rat multidrug resistance-associated protein 3 (Mrp3). *J Biol Chem.* 2000 Jan 28;275(4):2905-10.

[119] Kavallaris M, Madafiglio J, Norris MD, Haber M. Resistance to tetracycline, a hydrophilic antibiotic, is mediated by P-glycoprotein in human multidrug-resistant cells. *Biochem Biophys Res Commun.* 1993 Jan 15;190(1):79-85.

[120] Hendricks CB, Rowinsky EK, Grochow LB, Donehower RC, Kaufmann SH. Effect of P-glycoprotein expression on the accumulation and cytotoxicity of topotecan (SK&F 104864), a new camptothecin analogue. *Cancer Res.* 1992 Apr 15;52(8):2268-78.

[121] Evers R, Kool M, van Deemter L, Janssen H, Calafat J, Oomen LC, et al. Drug export activity of the human canalicular multispecific organic anion transporter in polarized kidney MDCK cells expressing cMOAT (MRP2) cDNA. *J Clin Invest.* 1998 Apr 1;101(7):1310-9.

[122] Broxterman HJ, Kuiper CM, Schuurhuis GJ, Tsuruo T, Pinedo HM, Lankelma J. Increase of daunorubicin and vincristine accumulation in multidrug resistant human ovarian carcinoma cells by a monoclonal antibody reacting with P-glycoprotein. *Biochem Pharmacol.* 1988 Jun 15;37(12):2389-93.

[123] Renes J, de Vries EG, Nienhuis EF, Jansen PL, Muller M. ATP- and glutathione-dependent transport of chemotherapeutic drugs by the multidrug resistance protein MRP1. *Br J Pharmacol.* 1999 Feb;126(3):681-8.

[124] Huang R, Murry DJ, Kolwankar D, Hall SD, Foster DR. Vincristine transcriptional regulation of efflux drug transporters in carcinoma cell lines. *Biochem Pharmacol.* 2006 Jun 14;71(12):1695-704.

[125] Fei YJ, Kanai Y, Nussberger S, Ganapathy V, Leibach FH, Romero MF, et al. Expression cloning of a mammalian proton-coupled oligopeptide transporter. *Nature.* 1994 Apr 7;368(6471):563-6.

[126] Bretschneider B, Brandsch M, Neubert R. Intestinal transport of beta-lactam antibiotics: analysis of the affinity at the H+/peptide symporter (PEPT1), the uptake

into Caco-2 cell monolayers and the transepithelial flux. *Pharm Res.* 1999 Jan;16(1):55-61.

[127] Ezra A, Hoffman A, Breuer E, Alferiev IS, Monkkonen J, El Hanany-Rozen N, et al. A peptide prodrug approach for improving bisphosphonate oral absorption. *J Med Chem.* 2000 Oct 5;43(20):3641-52.

[128] Tamai I, Takanaga H, Maeda H, Sai Y, Ogihara T, Higashida H, et al. Participation of a proton-cotransporter, MCT1, in the intestinal transport of monocarboxylic acids. *Biochem Biophys Res Commun.* 1995 Sep 14;214(2):482-9.

[129] Ritzhaupt A. WIS, Ellis A., Hosie K.B., Shirazi-Beechey S.P. Identification and characterization of a monocarboxylate transporter (MCT1) in pig and human colon: its potential to transport L-lactate as well as butyrate. *J Physiol.* 1998;513:719-32.

[130] Ritzhaupt A. WIS, Ellis A., Hosie K.B., Shirazi-Beechey S.P. Identification of monocarboxylate transporter isoform type 1 (MCT1) on the luminal membrane of human and pig colon. *Biochem Soc Trans.* 1998;26(S120).

[131] Woodcock DM, Jefferson S, Linsenmeyer ME, Crowther PJ, Chojnowski GM, Williams B, et al. Reversal of the multidrug resistance phenotype with cremophor EL, a common vehicle for water-insoluble vitamins and drugs. *Cancer Res.* 1990 Jul 15;50(14):4199-203.

[132] Nerurkar MM, Burton PS, Borchardt RT. The use of surfactants to enhance the permeability of peptides through Caco-2 cells by inhibition of an apically polarized efflux system. *Pharm Res.* 1996 Apr;13(4):528-34.

[133] Anderberg EK, Artursson P. Epithelial transport of drugs in cell culture. VIII: Effects of sodium dodecyl sulfate on cell membrane and tight junction permeability in human intestinal epithelial (Caco-2) cells. *J Pharm Sci.* 1993 Apr;82(4):392-8.

[134] Rege BD, Yu LX, Hussain AS, Polli JE. Effect of common excipients on Caco-2 transport of low-permeability drugs. *J Pharm Sci.* 2001 Nov;90(11):1776-86.

[135] Cornaire G, Woodley J, Hermann P, Cloarec A, Arellano C, Houin G. Impact of excipients on the absorption of P-glycoprotein substrates in vitro and in vivo. *Int J Pharm.* 2004 Jun 18;278(1):119-31.

[136] Rege BD, Kao JP, Polli JE. Effects of nonionic surfactants on membrane transporters in Caco-2 cell monolayers. *Eur J Pharm Sci.* 2002 Sep;16(4-5):237-46.

[137] Hugger ED, Novak BL, Burton PS, Audus KL, Borchardt RT. A comparison of commonly used polyethoxylated pharmaceutical excipients on their ability to inhibit P-glycoprotein activity in vitro. *J Pharm Sci.* 2002 Sep;91(9):1991-2002.

[138] Shono Y, Nishihara H, Matsuda Y, Furukawa S, Okada N, Fujita T, et al. Modulation of intestinal P-glycoprotein function by cremophor EL and other surfactants by an in vitro diffusion chamber method using the isolated rat intestinal membranes. *J Pharm Sci.* 2004 Apr;93(4):877-85.

[139] Koga K, Ohyashiki T, Murakami M, Kawashima S. Modification of ceftibuten transport by the addition of non-ionic surfactants. *Eur J Pharm Biopharm.* 2000 Jan;49(1):17-25.

[140] Hugger ED, Audus KL, Borchardt RT. Effects of poly(ethylene glycol) on efflux transporter activity in Caco-2 cell monolayers. *J Pharm Sci.* 2002 Sep;91(9):1980-90.

[141] Johnson BM, Charman WN, Porter CJ. An in vitro examination of the impact of polyethylene glycol 400, Pluronic P85, and vitamin E d-alpha-tocopheryl

polyethylene glycol 1000 succinate on P-glycoprotein efflux and enterocyte-based metabolism in excised rat intestine. *AAPS PharmSci.* 2002;4(4):E40.

[142] Batrakova E, Lee S, Li S, Venne A, Alakhov V, Kabanov A. Fundamental relationships between the composition of pluronic block copolymers and their hypersensitization effect in MDR cancer cells. *Pharm Res.* 1999 Sep;16(9):1373-9.

[143] Batrakova EV, Li S, Miller DW, Kabanov AV. Pluronic P85 increases permeability of a broad spectrum of drugs in polarized BBMEC and Caco-2 cell monolayers. *Pharm Res.* 1999 Sep;16(9):1366-72.

[144] Bogman K, Zysset Y, Degen L, Hopfgartner G, Gutmann H, Alsenz J, et al. P-glycoprotein and surfactants: effect on intestinal talinolol absorption. *Clin Pharmacol Ther.* 2005 Jan;77(1):24-32.

[145] Bogman K, Erne-Brand F, Alsenz J, Drewe J. The role of surfactants in the reversal of active transport mediated by multidrug resistance proteins. *J Pharm Sci.* 2003 Jun;92(6):1250-61.

[146] Nerurkar MM, Ho NF, Burton PS, Vidmar TJ, Borchardt RT. Mechanistic roles of neutral surfactants on concurrent polarized and passive membrane transport of a model peptide in Caco-2 cells. *J Pharm Sci.* 1997 Jul;86(7):813-21.

[147] Wagner D, Spahn-Langguth H, Hanafy A, Koggel A, Langguth P. Intestinal drug efflux: formulation and food effects. *Adv Drug Deliv Rev.* 2001 Oct 1;50 Suppl 1:S13-31.

[148] Miyamoto KI, Koga-Takeda K, Koga K, Ohshima T, Nomura M. Saturable function of P-glycoprotein as a drug-efflux pump in multidrug-resistant tumour cells. *J Pharm Pharmacol.* 1996 May;48(5):522-5.

[149] Martin-Facklam M, Burhenne J, Ding R, Fricker R, Mikus G, Walter-Sack I, et al. Dose-dependent increase of saquinavir bioavailability by the pharmaceutic aid cremophor EL. *Br J Clin Pharmacol.* 2002 Jun;53(6):576-81.

[150] Tayrouz Y, Ding R, Burhenne J, Riedel KD, Weiss J, Hoppe-Tichy T, et al. Pharmacokinetic and pharmaceutic interaction between digoxin and Cremophor RH40. *Clin Pharmacol Ther.* 2003 May;73(5):397-405.

[151] Bardelmeijer HA, Ouwehand M, Malingre MM, Schellens JH, Beijnen JH, van Tellingen O. Entrapment by Cremophor EL decreases the absorption of paclitaxel from the gut. *Cancer Chemother Pharmacol.* 2002 Feb;49(2):119-25.

[152] Malingre MM, Schellens JH, Van Tellingen O, Ouwehand M, Bardelmeijer HA, Rosing H, et al. The co-solvent Cremophor EL limits absorption of orally administered paclitaxel in cancer patients. *Br J Cancer.* 2001 Nov 16;85(10):1472-7.

[153] Chiu YY, Higaki K, Neudeck BL, Barnett JL, Welage LS, Amidon GL. Human jejunal permeability of cyclosporin A: influence of surfactants on P-glycoprotein efflux in Caco-2 cells. *Pharm Res.* 2003 May;20(5):749-56.

[154] Brouwers J, Tack J, Lammert F, Augustijns P. Intraluminal drug and formulation behavior and integration in in vitro permeability estimation: a case study with amprenavir. *J Pharm Sci.* 2006 Feb;95(2):372-83.

[155] Nakamura T, Sakaeda T, Ohmoto N, Tamura T, Aoyama N, Shirakawa T, et al. Real-time quantitative polymerase chain reaction for MDR1, MRP1, MRP2, and CYP3A-mRNA levels in Caco-2 cell lines, human duodenal enterocytes, normal colorectal tissues, and colorectal adenocarcinomas. *Drug Metab Dispos.* 2002 Jan;30(1):4-6.

[156] Taipalensuu J, Tornblom H, Lindberg G, Einarsson C, Sjoqvist F, Melhus H, et al. Correlation of gene expression of ten drug efflux proteins of the ATP-binding cassette transporter family in normal human jejunum and in human intestinal epithelial Caco-2 cell monolayers. *J Pharmacol Exp Ther.* 2001 Oct;299(1):164-70.

[157] Yu L, Bridgers A, Polli J, Vickers A, Long S, Roy A, et al. Vitamin E-TPGS increases absorption flux of an HIV protease inhibitor by enhancing its solubility and permeability. *Pharm Res.* 1999 Dec;16(12):1812-7.

[158] Chang T, Benet LZ, Hebert MF. The effect of water-soluble vitamin E on cyclosporine pharmacokinetics in healthy volunteers. *Clin Pharmacol Ther.* 1996 Mar;59(3):297-303.

[159] Argao EA, Heubi JE, Hollis BW, Tsang RC. d-Alpha-tocopheryl polyethylene glycol-1000 succinate enhances the absorption of vitamin D in chronic cholestatic liver disease of infancy and childhood. *Pediatr Res.* 1992 Feb;31(2):146-50.

[160] Dintaman JM, Silverman JA. Inhibition of P-glycoprotein by D-alpha-tocopheryl polyethylene glycol 1000 succinate (TPGS). *Pharm Res.* 1999 Oct;16(10):1550-6.

[161] Varma MV, Panchagnula R. Enhanced oral paclitaxel absorption with vitamin E-TPGS: effect on solubility and permeability in vitro, in situ and in vivo. *Eur J Pharm Sci.* 2005 Jul-Aug;25(4-5):445-53.

[162] Bittner B, Guenzi A, Fullhardt P, Zuercher G, Gonzalez RC, Mountfield RJ. Improvement of the bioavailability of colchicine in rats by co-administration of D-alpha-tocopherol polyethylene glycol 1000 succinate and a polyethoxylated derivative of 12-hydroxy-stearic acid. *Arzneimittelforschung.* 2002;52(9):684-8.

[163] Collnot EM, Baldes C, Wempe MF, Hyatt J, Navarro L, Edgar KJ, et al. Influence of vitamin E TPGS poly(ethylene glycol) chain length on apical efflux transporters in Caco-2 cell monolayers. *J Control Release.* 2006 Mar 10;111(1-2):35-40.

[164] Strickley RG. Solubilizing excipients in oral and injectable formulations. *Pharm Res.* 2004 Feb;21(2):201-30.

[165] Cornaire G, Woodley JF, Saivin S, Legendre JY, Decourt S, Cloarec A, et al. Effect of polyoxyl 35 castor oil and Polysorbate 80 on the intestinal absorption of digoxin in vitro. *Arzneimittelforschung.* 2000 Jun;50(6):576-9.

[166] Zhang H, Yao M, Morrison RA, Chong S. Commonly used surfactant, Tween 80, improves absorption of P-glycoprotein substrate, digoxin, in rats. *Arch Pharm Res.* 2003 Sep;26(9):768-72.

[167] Seeballuck F, Lawless E, Ashford MB, O'Driscoll CM. Stimulation of triglyceride-rich lipoprotein secretion by polysorbate 80: in vitro and in vivo correlation using Caco-2 cells and a cannulated rat intestinal lymphatic model. *Pharm Res.* 2004 Dec;21(12):2320-6.

[168] Kabanov AV, Batrakova EV, Alakhov VY. Pluronic block copolymers as novel polymer therapeutics for drug and gene delivery. *J Control Release.* 2002 Aug 21;82(2-3):189-212.

[169] Batrakova EV, Han HY, Miller DW, Kabanov AV. Effects of pluronic P85 unimers and micelles on drug permeability in polarized BBMEC and Caco-2 cells. *Pharm Res.* 1998 Oct;15(10):1525-32.

[170] Batrakova EV, Han HY, Alakhov V, Miller DW, Kabanov AV. Effects of pluronic block copolymers on drug absorption in Caco-2 cell monolayers. *Pharm Res.* 1998 Jun;15(6):850-5.

[171] Miller DW, Batrakova EV, Kabanov AV. Inhibition of multidrug resistance-associated protein (MRP) functional activity with pluronic block copolymers. *Pharm Res.* 1999 Mar;16(3):396-401.

[172] Huai-Yun H, Secrest DT, Mark KS, Carney D, Brandquist C, Elmquist WF, et al. Expression of multidrug resistance-associated protein (MRP) in brain microvessel endothelial cells. *Biochem Biophys Res Commun.* 1998 Feb 24;243(3):816-20.

[173] Draper MP, Martell RL, Levy SB. Indomethacin-mediated reversal of multidrug resistance and drug efflux in human and murine cell lines overexpressing MRP, but not P-glycoprotein. *Br J Cancer.* 1997;75(6):810-5.

[174] Batrakova EV, Li S, Alakhov VY, Elmquist WF, Miller DW, Kabanov AV. Sensitization of cells overexpressing multidrug-resistant proteins by pluronic P85. *Pharm Res.* 2003 Oct;20(10):1581-90.

[175] Batrakova EV, Li S, Elmquist WF, Miller DW, Alakhov VY, Kabanov AV. Mechanism of sensitization of MDR cancer cells by Pluronic block copolymers: Selective energy depletion. *Br J Cancer.* 2001 Dec 14;85(12):1987-97.

[176] Batrakova EV, Li S, Vinogradov SV, Alakhov VY, Miller DW, Kabanov AV. Mechanism of pluronic effect on P-glycoprotein efflux system in blood-brain barrier: contributions of energy depletion and membrane fluidization. *J Pharmacol Exp Ther.* 2001 Nov;299(2):483-93.

[177] Batrakova EV, Li S, Li Y, Alakhov VY, Kabanov AV. Effect of pluronic P85 on ATPase activity of drug efflux transporters. *Pharm Res.* 2004 Dec;21(12):2226-33.

[178] Batrakova EV, Zhang Y, Li Y, Li S, Vinogradov SV, Persidsky Y, et al. Effects of pluronic P85 on GLUT1 and MCT1 transporters in the blood-brain barrier. *Pharm Res.* 2004 Nov;21(11):1993-2000.

[179] Hugger ED CC, Raub TJ, Burton PS, Borchardt RT. Automated analysis of polyethylene glycol-induced inhibition of P-glycoprotein activity in vitro. *J Pharm Sci* 2003 Jan;92(1):21-6. 2003;92(1):21-6.

[180] Technical information Solutol HS15, *BASF ;* August 2004.

[181] Dudeja PK, Anderson KM, Harris JS, Buckingham L, Coon JS. Reversal of multidrug resistance phenotype by surfactants: relationship to membrane lipid fluidity. *Arch Biochem Biophys.* 1995 May 10;319(1):309-15.

[182] *Data sheet Labrasol,* Gattefossé ; specification number 3074/3 ; last update 07.12.04.

[183] Koga K, Kawashima S, Murakami M. In vitro and in situ evidence for the contribution of Labrasol and Gelucire 44/14 on transport of cephalexin and cefoperazone by rat intestine. *Eur J Pharm Biopharm.* 2002 Nov;54(3):311-8.

[184] Sha X, Yan G, Wu Y, Li J, Fang X. Effect of self-microemulsifying drug delivery systems containing Labrasol on tight junctions in Caco-2 cells. *Eur J Pharm Sci.* 2005 Apr;24(5):477-86.

[185] Hu Z, Tawa R, Konishi T, Shibata N, Takada K. A novel emulsifier, labrasol, enhances gastrointestinal absorption of gentamicin. *Life Sci.* 2001 Nov 2;69(24):2899-910.

[186] Zastre J, Jackson J, Bajwa M, Liggins R, Iqbal F, Burt H. Enhanced cellular accumulation of a P-glycoprotein substrate, rhodamine-123, by Caco-2 cells using low molecular weight methoxypolyethylene glycol-block-polycaprolactone diblock copolymers. *Eur J Pharm Biopharm.* 2002 Nov;54(3):299-309.

[187] Zastre J, Jackson J, Burt H. Evidence for modulation of P-glycoprotein-mediated efflux by methoxypolyethylene glycol-block-Polycaprolactone amphiphilic diblock copolymers. *Pharm Res.* 2004 Aug;21(8):1489-97.

[188] Nozawa T, Toyobuku H, Kobayashi D, Kuruma K, Tsuji A, Tamai I. Enhanced intestinal absorption of drugs by activation of peptide transporter PEPT1 using proton-releasing polymer. *J Pharm Sci.* 2003 Nov;92(11):2208-16.

[189] Ambudkar SV, Kimchi-Sarfaty C, Sauna ZE, Gottesman MM. P-glycoprotein: from genomics to mechanism. *Oncogene.* 2003 Oct 20;22(47):7468-85.

[190] Brustovetskii NN, Dedukhova VN, Egorova MV, Mokhova EN, Skulachev VP. [Uncoupling of oxidative phosphorylation by fatty acids and detergents suppressed by ATP/ADP antiporter inhibitors]. *Biokhimiia.* 1991 Jun;56(6):1042-8.

[191] Kirillova GP, Mokhova EN, Dedukhova VI, Tarakanova AN, Ivanova VP, Efremova NV, et al. The influence of pluronics and their conjugates with proteins on the rate of oxygen consumption by liver mitochondria and thymus lymphocytes. *Biotechnol Appl Biochem.* 1993 Dec;18 (Pt 3):329-39.

[192] Regev R, Assaraf YG, Eytan GD. Membrane fluidization by ether, other anesthetics, and certain agents abolishes P-glycoprotein ATPase activity and modulates efflux from multidrug-resistant cells. *Eur J Biochem.* 1999 Jan;259(1-2):18-24.

[193] Germann UA, Chambers TC, Ambudkar SV, Licht T, Cardarelli CO, Pastan I, et al. Characterization of phosphorylation-defective mutants of human P-glycoprotein expressed in mammalian cells. *J Biol Chem.* 1996 Jan 19;271(3):1708-16.

In: Drugs: Approval and Evaluation, Delivery and Control ISBN: 978-1-60456-533-1
Editors: A.O. Hartmann, L.K. Neumann

Chapter 4

VITAMIN B_6 AS LIVER-TARGETING GROUP IN DRUG DELIVERY

Guo-Ping Yan*, Xiao-Yan Wang and Li-Li Mei
School of Material Science and Engineering, Wuhan Instituite of Technology, Wuhan 430073, P. R. China

ABSTRACT

Vitamin B_6 includes a series of compounds containing the pyridoxal structure, such as pyridoxol, pyridoxamine, pyridoxaldehyde and their derivatives. The pyridoxal structure, the catalytically active form of vitamin B_6, possesses specific hepatocyte uptake by the pyridoxine transporter at the sinusoidal pole because the pyridoxine transporters that exist in hepatocytes can selectively recognize and bind to the pyridoxal structure, and transport it into the cells via a member transport system. Thus pyridoxine can be adopted as a liver-targeting group and be incorporated into the low molecular weight compounds and macromolecules for the use as magnetic resonance imaging (MRI) contrast agents and anticancer conjugates. The research progress of liver-targeting drug delivery system is discussed briefly. Previous researches have demonstrated that the incorporation of pyridoxine into these molecules can increase their uptake by the liver, and that these molecules containing pyridoxine groups exhibit liver-targeting properties.

Keywords: vitamin B6, liver-targeting, drug delivery, magnetic resonance imaging (MRI)

* Correspondence concerning this article should be addressed to: Guo-Ping Yan, School of Material Science and Engineering, Wuhan Instituite of Technology, Wuhan 430073, P. R. China. E-mail address: guopyan@ hotmail.com.

INTRODUCTION

Vitamin B_6, also known as pyridoxine, is water-soluble and is required for both mental and physical health. Vitamin B_6 includes a series of compounds containing the pyridoxal structure, such as pyridoxol, pyridoxamine, pyridoxaldehyde and their derivatives.

The liver has both a unique blood supply (arterial, venous and portal-venous) and specific cells that are capable of transporting/accumulating bulk amounts of both endo- and exobiotic substances [1-3]. The pyridoxine transporters that exist in hepatocytes at the sinusoidal pole can selectively recognize and bind to the pyridoxal structure, and transport it into the cells via a member transport system. The pyridoxal structure, the catalytically active form of vitamin B_6, possesses specific hepatocyte uptake by the pyridoxine transporter. Thus pyridoxine can be adopted as a liver-targeting group and be incorporated into the low molecular weight compounds and macromolecules for the use as magnetic resonance imaging (MRI) contrast agents and anticancer conjugates [4-7]. The research progress of liver-targeting drug delivery system is discussed briefly. Previous researches have demonstrated that the incorporation of pyridoxine into these molecules can increase their uptake by the liver, and that these molecules containing pyridoxine groups exhibited liver-targeting properties [8-19].

LIVER-TARGETING MRI CONTRAST AGENTS

Over the last three decades, nuclear magnetic resonance (NMR) has been perhaps the most powerful method for the non-invasive investigation of human anatomy, physiology and pathophysiology. Developed in 1973 by Paul Lauterbur [20], magnetic resonance imaging (MRI) has become widely used as the diagnosis and treatment of human diseases in hospitals around the world, since it received FDA approval for clinical use in 1985. It is a non-invasive clinical imaging modality, which relies on the detection of NMR signals emitted by hydrogen protons in the body placed in a magnetic field. In 2003, Paul C. Lauterbur and Sir Peter Mansfield won the Nobel Prize in physiology and medicine for their discoveries concerning MRI because it can be widely used for the diagnosis and treatment of human diseases, such as necrotic tissue, infarcted artery and malignant disease [21,22].

One important way to improve the contrast in MRI is to introduce contrast agents. MRI contrast agents are a unique class of pharmaceuticals that enhance the image contrast between normal and diseased tissue and indicate the status of organ function or blood flow after administration by increasing the relaxation rates of water protons in tissue in which the agent accumulates [8,9]. Paramagnetic substances, superparamagnetic and ferromagnetic materials have been used as MRI contrast agents because paramagnetic substances have a net positive magnetic susceptibility, having the ability to become magnetized in an external magnetic field. Some MRI exams include the use of contrast agents. The categorizations of currently available contrast agents have been described according to their effect on the image, magnetic behavior and biodistribution in the body, respectively [23].

Subsequently proper ligands have been designed and complexed with paramagnetic metal ions to form strong water-soluble chelates as the first generation MRI contrast agents, for example, gadolinium diethylenetriaminepentaacetic acid (Gd-DTPA, Magnevist®, Schering AG, Germany) (Figure 1) [24]. Some clinically used MRI contrast agents are small ionic molecules such as Gd-DTPA and gadolinium 1,4,7,10-tetraazacyclododecane-N, N', N'', N'''-tetraacetic acids (Gd-DTOA, Dotarem®, Guerbet SA, France) (Figure 2) [25,26] that can diffuse freely through the extracellular space and excreted rapidly by the kidney. Then their biodistribution are nonspecific although Gd-DTPA works well in organs such as the brain and spinal cord, where the normal brain parenchyma has a barrier to permeability of the contrast agent and pathologic conditions such as cancer do not. The injection of large quantities of the ionic complex will raise ion concentration *in vivo* and cause localized disturbances in osmolality, which, in turn leads to cellular and circulatory damage. Most commonly, Gd-DTPA and Gd-DOTA have been modified to form neutral molecules, which thus exhibited much lower osmolality and higher LD_{50}s in animals [27-31].

Nowadays ideal MRI contrast agent is focused on the neutral tissue- or organ-targeting materials with high relaxivity and specificity, low toxicity and side effect, suitable long intravascular duration and excretion times, high contrast enhancement with low doses *in vivo*, and minimal cost of procedure [8,9,27,28]. In general, tissue or organ-specific contrast agents consist of two components: a magnetic label capable of altering the signal intensity on MR images and a target-group molecule having a characteristic affinity for a specific type of cell or receptor. Some suitable residues have been incorporated into either the acetic side-arms or the diethylenetriamine backbone of Gd-DTPA and Gd-DOTA to obtain the tissue or organ-specific contrast agents. For example, liver-targeting agents such as gadobenate dimeglumine (Gd-BOPTA, Gadobenate, Multihance®, Bracco Imaging, Italy) and gadolinium ethoxybenzyltriamine pentaacetic acid (Gd-EOB-DTPA, Gadoxetate; Eovist®, Schering AG, Germany) have been developed, which can accumulate in the liver site, increasing contrast concentration, and producing greater signal in the MR images [32-42].

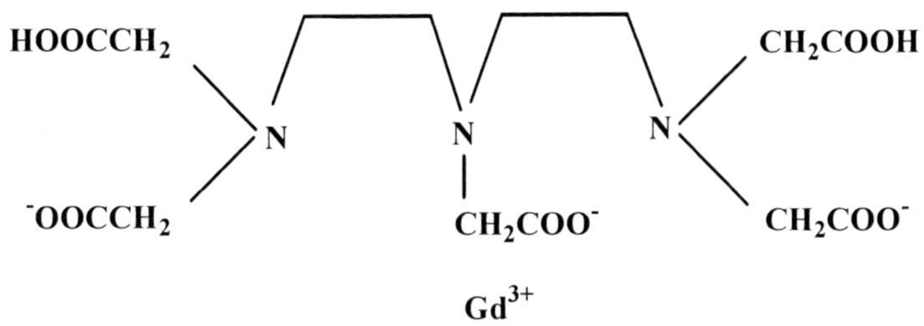

Figure 1. Structural formula of Gd-DTPA.

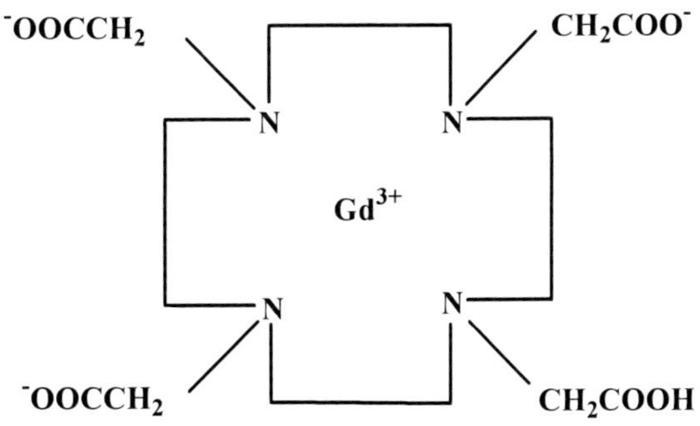

Figure 2. Structural formula of Gd-DOTA.

Low Molecular Weight Liver-Targeting MRI Contrast Agents

Manganese dipyridoxyl-diphosphate (mangafodipir, Mn-DPDP, Teslascan®, Nycomed Amersham Imaging, Princeton, NJ) is a contrast agent developed for imaging of the hepatobiliary system (Figure 3). Unlike Gd-DTPA, Mn-DPDP is an intracellular agent that is taken up specifically by hepatocytes and pancreas, and excreted in the bile since the ligand consists of two linked pyridoxal-5'-phosphate groups, the catalytically active form of vitamin B_6. Thus, it was thought that Mn-DPDP was a potential candidate for specific hepatocyte uptake by the pyridoxine transporter at the sinusoidal pole. However, it was reported that the complex dissociated both in the blood and in the liver and the uptake mechanism did not depend on the pyridoxine transporter [4-6].

Other liver-targeting DTPA derivates containing vitamin B_6 groups have also been prepared according to the liver-targeting property of Mn-DPDP. A series of DTPA derivatives ligands containing pyridoxol groups have been synthesized by the reaction of DTPA dianhydride with the pyridoxol derivatives with the different space groups. Compared with Gd-DTPA, their non-ionic bulky Gd^{3+} complexes have higher relaxivities, lower stability constants and the liver-targeting property. Moreover, Gd-DTPA and Gd-DOTA are modified to form neutral molecules, which thus exhibit much lower osmolality, while these neutral agents have been shown to have higher LD_{50}s in animals [7,43,44].

Macromolecular Liver-Targeting MRI Contrast Agents

Macromolecular MRI contrast agent can be prepared by the incorporation of a low molecular weight paramagnetic metal cheated complex such as Gd-DTDA or Gd-DOTA, to the backbone or the pendant chains of macromolecule. It usually exhibits more effective relaxation than that of the low molecular weight metal complex alone and improves the relaxivity of per gadolinium atom because of an increase in rotational correlation time. On the other hand, macromolecular MRI contrast agents may show prolonged intravascular retention due to its bulky molecular volume, it can be used clinically as a blood pool contrast agent. In addition, when an organ-targeting group, for example, PM is attached to this macromolecular metal complex, it can be endowed with liver-targeting property [45-58].

Macromolecular liver-targeting Gd(III) chelates have been developed by the incorporation of Gd-DTPA and pyridoxanine into polyasparamides, dendrimers and polyester. Relaxivity studies showed that the chelates possessed obviously higher relaxation effectiveness than that of Gd-DTPA. MR imaging of the liver in rats and experimental data of biodistribution in mice indicated that they exhibited liver-targeting properties and enhanced the contrast of MR images in the liver.

Polyester Liver-Targeting MRI Contrast Agents

Water-soluble polyester ligands were synthesized by the polycondensation of diethylenetriaminepentaacetic dianhydride (DTPAA) with protected polyalcohol 3-O-benzyl-sn-glycerol (3-O-Bz-GLYC), monobenzaldehyde-pentaerythritol (S-Bz-PETO) and N-benzyl-diethanolamine (N-Bz-DEA), respectively, and the protecting groups were then removed by hydrogenation to give polyesters P(DTPA-GLYC), P(DTPA-PETO) and P(DTPA-DEA). In the same manner, by adding ethylene glycol (EG) monomer into the polymerization system, polyesters P(DTPA-GLYC-EG), P(DTPA-PETO-EG) and P(DTPA-DEA-EG) were also synthesized (Table 1). Pyridoxamine as a liver-targeting group was first chlorocarbonylated and then incorporated into polyesters. The polyester ligands containing pyridoxamine group thus prepared were further reacted with $GdCl_3$ in water at room temperature to give the corresponding hepatic-targeting polyester gadolinium complexes (Figure 4) [11].

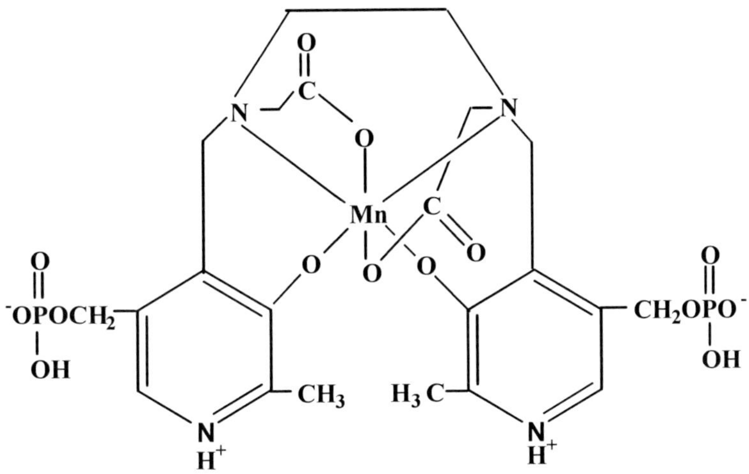

Figure 3. Structural formula of Mn-DPDP.

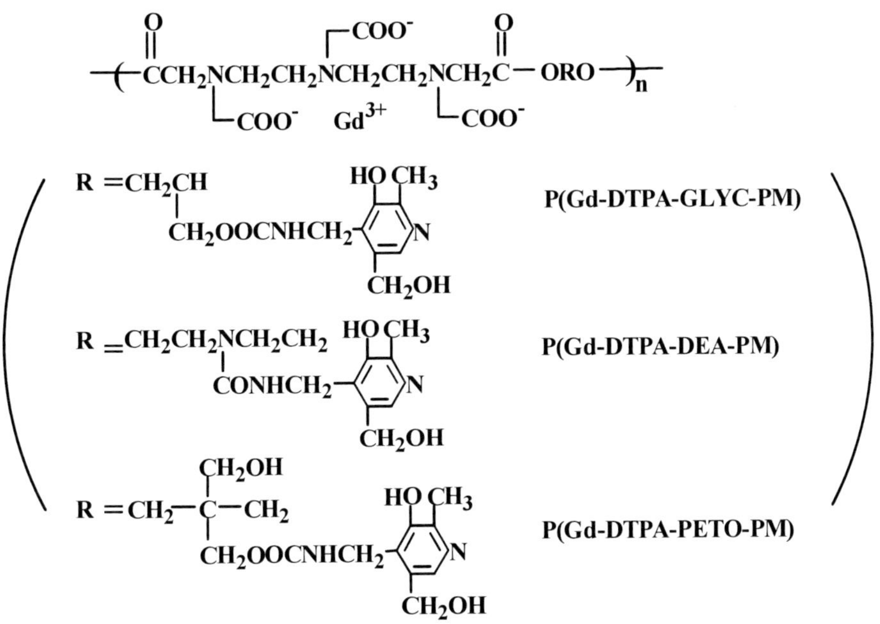

Figure 4. Structural formula of polyester gadolinium complexes.

Table 1. Molecular weight of polyesters

Polymer	*Mn (×10 ^{3})*	*Mw (×10 ^{3})*	*Polydispersity*
P(DTPA-GLYC)	7.51	9.08	1.21
P(DTPA-PETO)	10.9	11.4	1.04
P(DTPA-DEA)	8.33	10.6	1.27
P(DTPA-GLYC-EG)	8.73	16.8	1.92
P(DTPA-PETO-EG)	9.47	15.9	1.68
P(DTPA-DEA-EG)	19.7	37.6	1.95

Table 2. Experimental data of relaxivity

Gadolinium complexes	*$[Gd^{3+}]$(mmol· l^{-1})*	*T_1obsd (s)*	*R_1(mmol· l^{-1}·s)$^{-1}$*
Gd-DTPA	1.240	0.138±0.0071	5.6
P(Gd-DTPA-GLYC-PM)	1.3048	0.0631±0.0096	11.91
P(Gd-DTPA-PETO-PM)	1.6195	0.0577±0.0052	10.51
P(Gd-DTPA-DEA-PM)	1.5905	0.0531±0.0073	11.65
P(Gd-DTPA-GLYC-EG-PM)	1.8333	0.0441±0.0053	12.20
P(Gd-DTPA-PETO-EG-PM)	1.3643	0.0476±0.0063	15.17
P(Gd-DTPA-DEA-EG-PM)	1.3950	0.0575±0.0076	12.25

Temp: 25 °C; NMR Frequency: 80MHz; T_{1d} =3.23±0.021s.

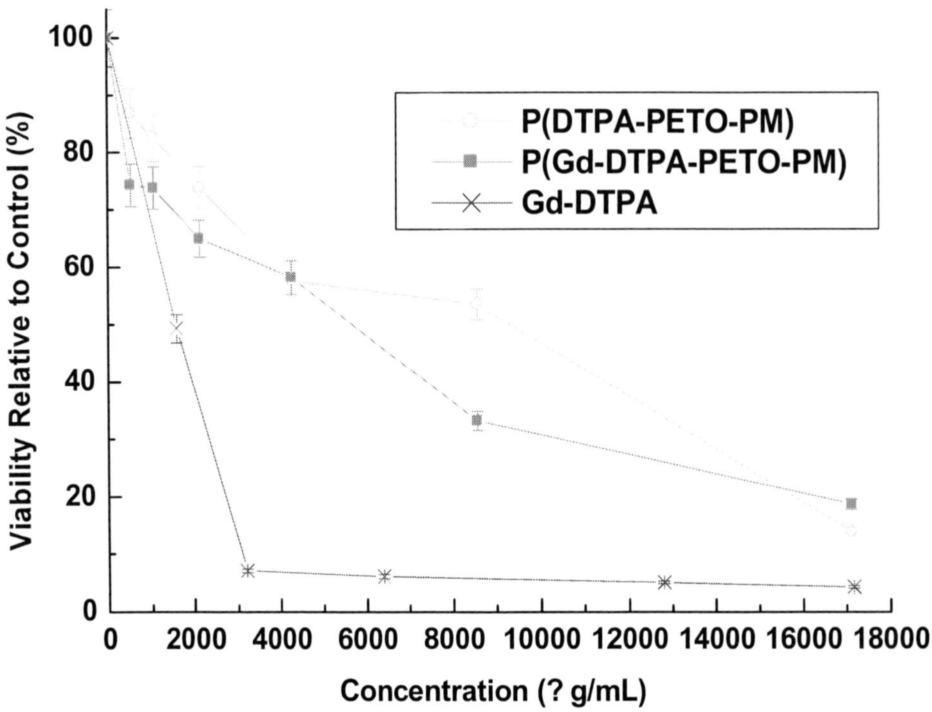

Figure 5. Cytotoxicity assay of anticancer drugs in L-02 cells.

Relaxivity studies showed that these polyester gadolinium complexes possess higher relaxation effectiveness than that of the clinically used small molecular gadolinium complex Gd-DTPA (Table 2). At the concentration (4280μg ml^{-1}) of polyester ligand and its gadolinium complex in the growth medium (RPMI-1640 media (10% foetal bovine serum (Gibco Co, USA), 100units ml^{-1} penicilium, 100μg ml^{-1} streptomycin)) , the viability of human normal liver cells (L-02) incubated with P(DTPA-PETO-PM) and P(Gd-DTPA-PETO-PM) retained 57.7% and 58.2%, respectively, relative to the control. It illustrated that possess low cytotoxicity to L-02 cells (Figure 5).

In comparison to the signal intensity (SI) of the liver in the rat injected of Gd-DTPA(0.1 mmol/kg) and P(Gd-DTPA-PETO) (0.1 mmol/kg) without the liver-targeting group PM, the signal intensity of the liver in the rat injected of P(Gd-DTPA-PETO-PM) (0.1mmol/kg) was obviously enhanced, the irradiated portion of the liver was brighter and the demarcation became clearer at the same time intervals during the detection time. This result illustrated that P(Gd-DTPA-PETO-PM) can greatly enhance the contrast of MR images of the liver after injection (Figures 6-8). Thirty minutes after injection of P(Gd-DTPA-PETO-PM), the signal enhancement of the liver (black cycle) is 176% (Table 3). It is better than that of Gd-DTPA (119%). On the other hand, P(Gd-DTPA-PETO-PM) has prolonged intravascular duration time for approximately one hour (127%). These results indicated that polyester gadonilium complexes containing pyridoxamine group can be targeted to the liver.

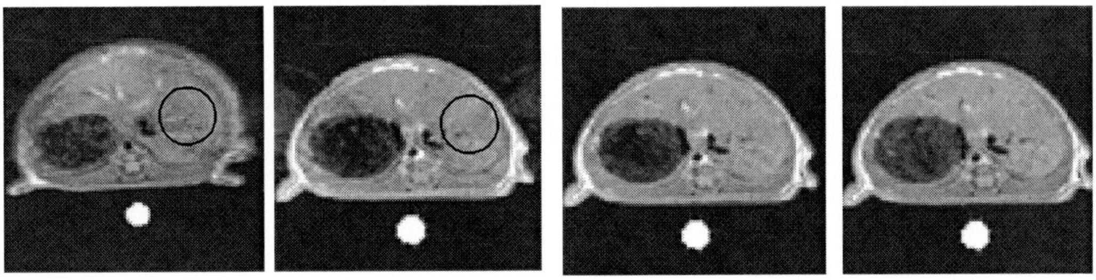

A_1 Control B_1 15 min C_1 30min D_1 45 min

Figure 6. A_1 is the T_1-weighted image of the rat received no injection of MRI contrast agent; B_1, C_1 and D_1 are the T_1-weighted images of the rat received injection of Gd-DTPA (0.1 mmol/kg, Magnevist) after 15 min, 30min and 45min.

Table 3. Enhancement (%) in the signal of the liver in different time after injection

Time after injection (min)	*Gd-DTPA*	*P(Gd-DTPA-PETO)*	*P(Gd-DTPA-PETO-PM)*
Control	100	100	100
5	107	107	111
15	114	112	160
30	119	114	176
45	115	115	154
60	114	116	127

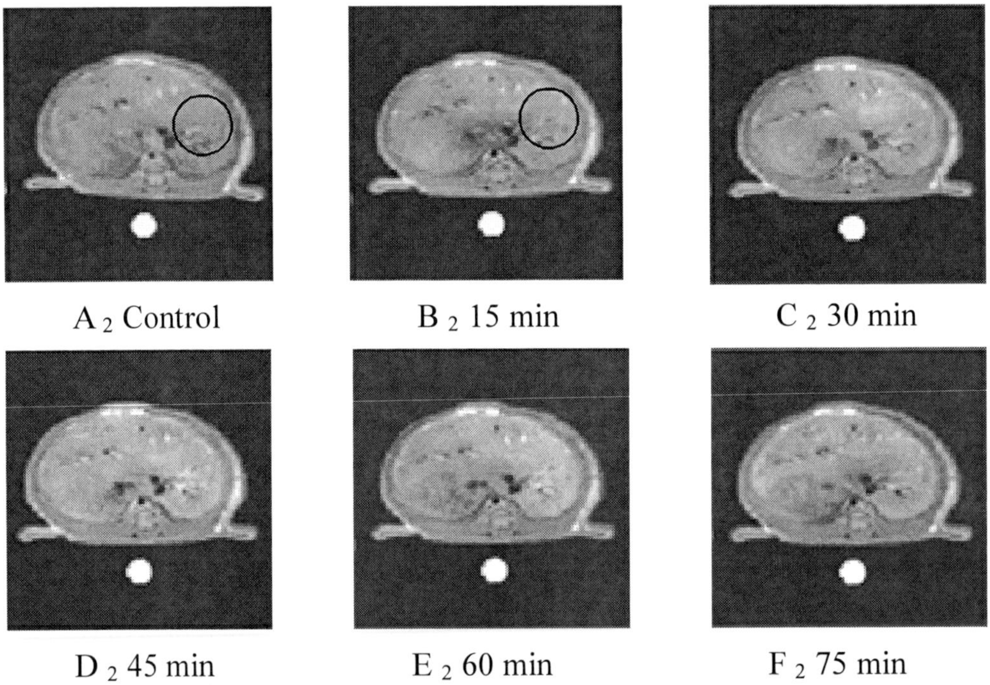

Figure 7. A_2 is the T_1-weighted image of the rat received no injection of MRI contrast agent; B_2, C_2 , D_2, E_2 and F_2 are the T_1-weighted images of the rat received injection of P(Gd-DTPA-PETO) (0.1 mmol/kg) without the liver-targeting groups PM after 15min, 30min, 45min, 60min and 75min.

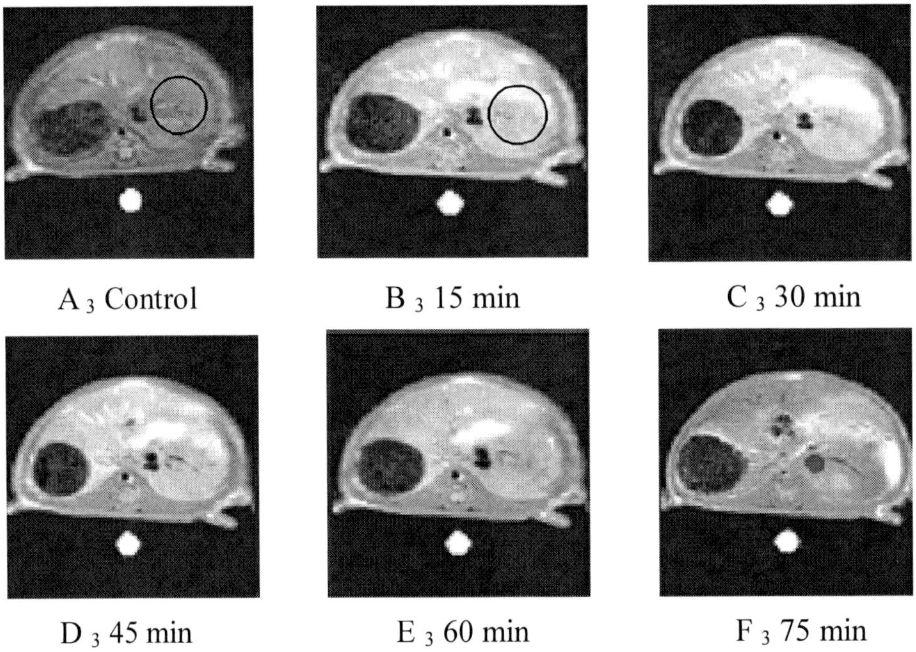

Figure 8. A_3 is the T_1-weighted image of the rat received no injection of MRI contrast agent; B_3, C_3 , D_3, E_3 and F_3 are the T_1-weighted images of the rat received injection of P(Gd-DTPA-PETO-PM) (0.1 mmol/kg) after 15min, 30min, 45min, 60min and 75min.

Polyaspartamide Liver-Targeting MRI Contrast Agents

Polyaspartamide is a biologically water-soluble synthetic polymer with a protein-like structure. It has been used as a plasma extender and a drug carrier and for some other biomedical applications because it is nontoxic, nonantigenic and degradable in living systems, and modified easily by reactions with the side chain. Antiviral drugs and anti-inflammatory agents have been covalently linked to (poly-α,β-[N-(2-hydroxyethyl)-D,L-aspartamide] (PHEA) forming drug-polymer conjugates capable of increasing drug stability and bioavailility [59-67].

The effects of PHEA and PAEA on cell growth and metabolism of HeLa cells *in vitro* were determined as a function of polymer concentration and compared to polylysine. The preliminary results show that over the concentration range tested, the cells incubated with PHEA and poly-α,β-[N-(2-amino ethy1)-L-aspartamide] (PAEA) retain 55.1% and 61.9% viabilities, while in the presence of polylysine (PLys), HeLa cells show no viability under the same concentration (100μg/mL). At a higher concentration (200μg/mL) of PHEA and PAEA, the cells still retain 62.4% and 49.8% viabilities respectively, relative to control (Figure 9). Thus polyaspartamides are the good polymeric carriers for MRI contrast agent and drug controlled release system [11].

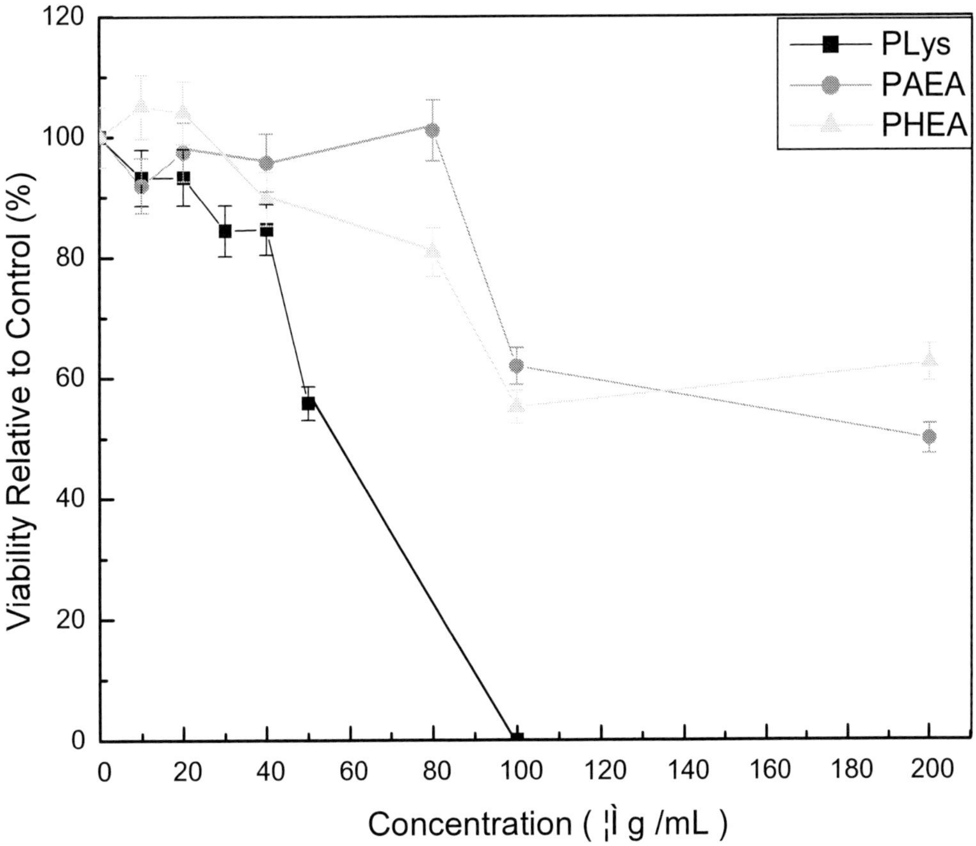

Figure 9. Cytotoxicity assay of PLys, PHEA and PAEA in HeLa cells.

Pyridoxamine (PM)-containing diethylenetriaminepentaacetic acid mono(N-hydroxysuccinimide) ester (SuO-DTPA-PM) was prepared by reacting PM with DTPA bis(N-hydroxysuccinimide) ester. The PM-containing DTPA active ester thus obtained was further incorporated into poly-α,β-[N-(2-hydroxyethy1)-L-aspartamide] (PHEA) and poly-α,β-[N-(2-amino ethy1)-L-aspartamide] (PAEA) to give liver-targeting macromolecular ligands PHEA-DTPA-PM and PAEA-DTPA-PM. Finally, by the metalation of the ligands with gadolinium Gd (III), two kinds of polyaspartamide gadolinium complexes were synthesized [11].

Relaxivity studies showed that these polyaspartamide gadolinium complexes possess higher relaxation effectiveness than that of Gd-DTPA. *In vitro* cytotoxicity assay showed that polyaspartamide gadolinium complexes have low cytotoxicity. Magnetic resonance imaging showed that the signal intensity (SI) of the liver in rat injected with PHEA-Gd-DTPA-PM (the average percent value of linked of polymeric repeat unit in gadolinium complexes (wt%): Gd 2.65) or PAEA-Gd-DTPA-PM (the average percent value of linked of polymeric repeat unit in gadolinium complexes (w%): Gd 11.04) was obviously enhanced. Experimental data of biodistribution in Kunming mice indicated that the rapid decrease of the polyaspartamide MRI contrast agent in blood, heart and spleen correlated with its increasing capture by the liver, indicating that these polyaspartamide MRI contrast agents containing pyridoxamine were taken up specifically by hepatcocytes.

DTPA and pyridoxamine (PM) as a liver-targeting group were both incorporated into polyaspartamides i. e. (poly-α,β-[N-(2-hydroxyethyl)-L-aspartamide] (PHEA), poly-α,β-[N-(3-hydroxypropyl)-L-aspartamide] (PHPA), poly-α,β-[N-(2-aminoethy1)-L-aspartamide] (PAEA) and poly-α,β-[N-(6-aminohexyl)-L- aspartamide] (PAHA) to obtain the polyaspartamide ligands. The polyaspartamide containing both DTPA ligands and pyridoxamine groups thus prepared were further reacted with gadolinium chloride to give the corresponding polyaspartamide gadolinium complexes with different amount of gadolinium ions PHEA-Gd-DTPA-PM, PHPA-Gd-DTPA-PM, PAEA-Gd-DTPA-PM and PAHA-Gd-DTPA-PM [12].

The polyaspartamide gadonilium complexes containing pyridoxamine groups possess obviously higher relaxation effectiveness than that of Gd-DTPA. PHEA-Gd-DTPA-PM (the average percent value of linked of polymeric repeat unit in gadolinium complexes (mol%): Gd-DTPA 5.30, PM 0.80) possesses the low intravenous acute toxicity and LD50/7days (intravenous, mouse) to IRC mice is 5.2g/kg±0.5g/kg.

MR imaging showed that the signal intensities (SI) of the liver in rat injected with low dosage of PHEA-Gd-DTPA-PM (0.1mmol/kg, 0.075mmol/kg, 0.05mmol/kg and 0.025 mmol/kg) were obviously enhanced in comparison to that of the liver in the rat injected with Gd-DTPA (0.1mmol/kg) (Figure 10). It greatly enhanced the contrast of MR image of the liver and provided prolonged intravascular duration in the liver (Table 4). These results indicated that the polyaspartamide gadonilium complex containing pyridoxamine groups could be used as the candidate of specific MRI contrast agent for the liver.

Table 4. Enhancement (%) in the signal from the liver at different times after injection

Time after injection (min)	*Gd-DTPA (0.1mmol/kg)*	*PHEA-Gd-DTPA-PM (M_2, 0.025 mmol/kg)*		*PHEA-Gd-DTPA-PM (M_2, 0.05 mmol/kg)*		*PHEA-Gd-DTPA-PM (M_2, 0.075 mmol/kg)*		*PHEA-Gd-DTPA-PM (M_2, 0.1 mmol/kg)*	
		Area 1	*Area 2*	*Area 1*	*Area 2*	*Area 1*	*Area 2*	*Area 1*	*Area 2*
Control	100	100	100	100	100	100	100	100	100
2	104	107	126	171	109	113	109	152	150
8	107	126	128	192	117	117	115	137	162
15	114	129	139	173	132	125	130	135	158
30	119	141	141	173	136	133	133	130	150
45	115	135	133	194	159	141	139	128	141
60	114	133	135	198	152	145	144	128	136
75		133	160	192	148	163	137	119	135
90		146	150	195	145	181	130	110	134
105		156	135	213	144	165	122	102	133
120		154	131	184	133	156	117	100	124

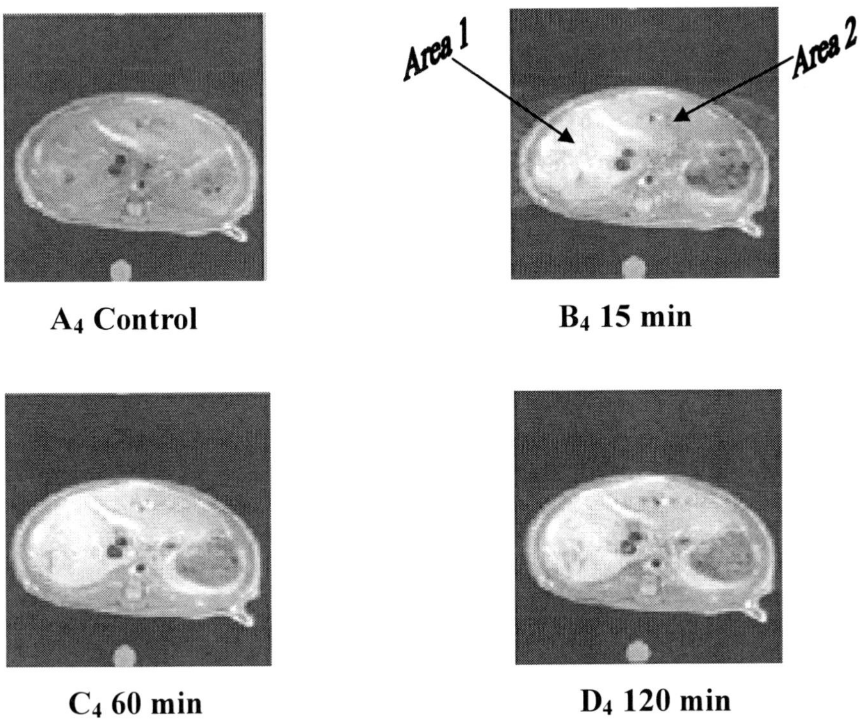

Figure 10. A_4 is the T_1-weighted image of the rats which received no MRI contrast agent; B_4, C_4 and D_4 are the T_1-weighted images of the rats which received injection with PHEA-Gd-DTPA-PM (the average percent value of linked of polymeric repeat unit in gadolinium complexes (mol%): Gd-DTPA 5.30, PM 0.80, 0.05mmol/kg) after 15min, 60min and 120min. Indicated areas 1 and 2 were used to calculate contrast enhancements listed in Table 4.

Dendritic Liver-Targeting MRI Contrast Agents

The conjugation of paramagnetic metal chelates to dendrimers is currently being explored as a new potential macromolecular MRI contrast agents because dendrimers have some advantages over other polymer carriers including the highly branched structure, low polydispersity molecule, uniform surface chemistry and high numbers of reactive functional groups per unit mass and volume for modification [68-80].

A series of liver-targeting dendritic gadolinium complexes were synthesized by conjugation of diethylenetriaminepentaacetic acid (DTPA) and pyridoxamine to the terminal amines of the dendrimers with 1,4,7,10-tetraazacyclododecane as the core (Generation: G1.0-5.0) and chelation with gadoliniumn chloride (Figure 11). These dendrimer-metal chelate conjugates have high ion relaxivities (of 13.0 - 23.5 $(mmol/L)^{-1}\cdot s^{-1}$ at 300MHz, 17℃, and pH of 7.4). MR imaging showed that the signal intensities (SI) of the liver in rats injected with low doses of G4.0-Gd-DTPA-PM (the average mole ratio of attached Gd-DTPA and PM to amine groups on the surface of the dendrimers (mol%): Gd-DTPA 10.84, PM 1.64) were significantly enhanced (Figure 12). G4.0-Gd-DTPA-PM greatly enhances the contrast of MR images of the liver, provides prolonged intravascular duration and produces highly contrasted visualization of blood vessels in the liver. These novel dendritic gadolinium complexes containing pyridoxamine groups demonstrate liver-targeting properties and show strong potential as new liver-targeting MRI contrast agents [13].

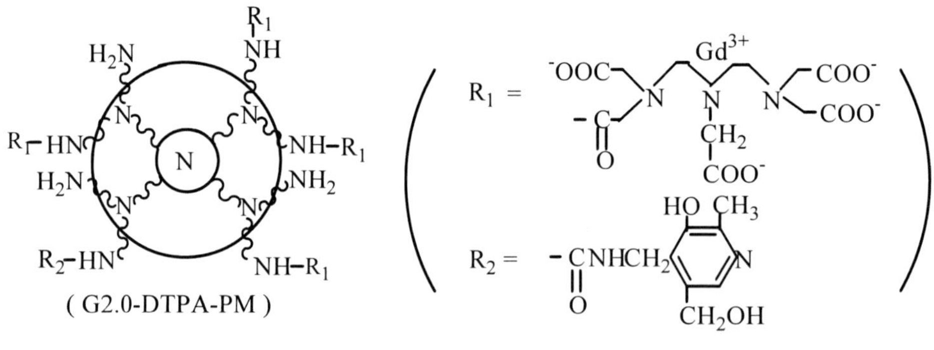

Figure 11. Structural formula of G2-Gd-DTPA-PM.

Table 5. Enhancement (%) in the signals from the liver at different times after injection

Time after injection (min)	*Gd-DTPA (0.1 mmol/kg)*	*G4.0-Gd-DTPA-PM (0.05 mmol/kg) Area 1 Area 2*	*G4.0-Gd-DTPA-PM (0.1 mmol/kg) Area 1 Area 2*
Control	100	100 100	100 100
8	107	137 107	131 135
15	114	147 118	145 152
30	119	154 126	148 179
45	115	160 131	153 176
60	114	165 148	169 172
75		159 147	166 169
93		155 144	162 166
105		149 128	145 165
120		148 127	137 164

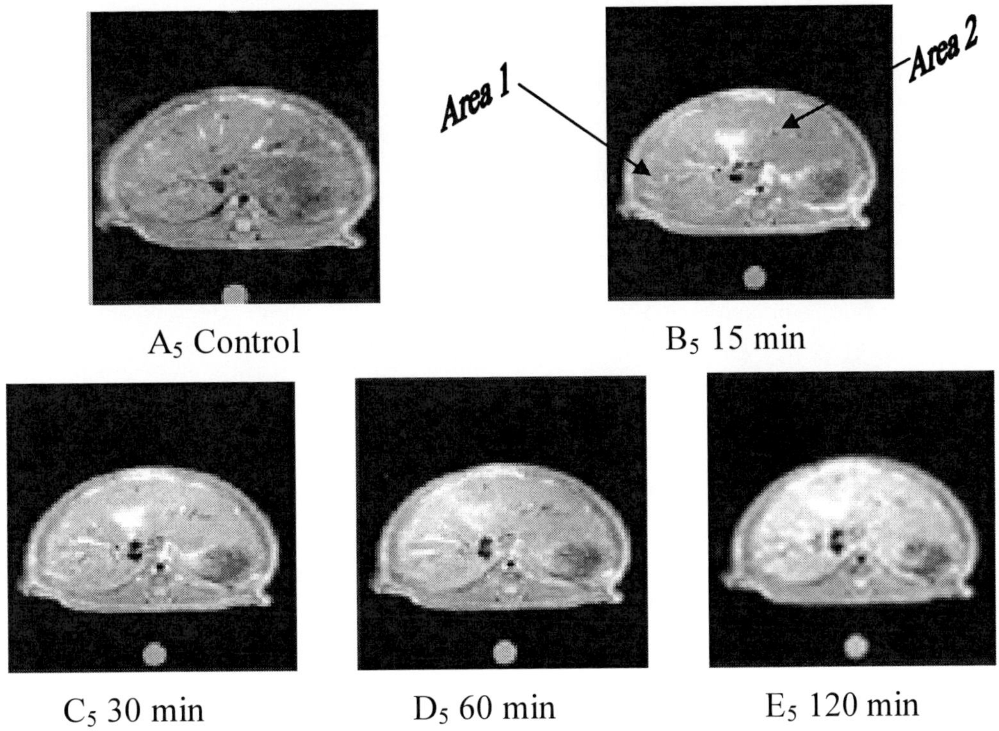

Figure 12. A_5 is the T_1-weighted image of the rat which received MRI contrast agent; B_5, C_5, D_2 and E_5 are the T_1-weighted images of the rat which received injections of dendritic G4-Gd-DTPA-PM (0.1 mmol/kg) after 15min, 30min, 60min and 120min. Indicated areas I and 2 were used to calculate contrast enhancements listed in Table 5.

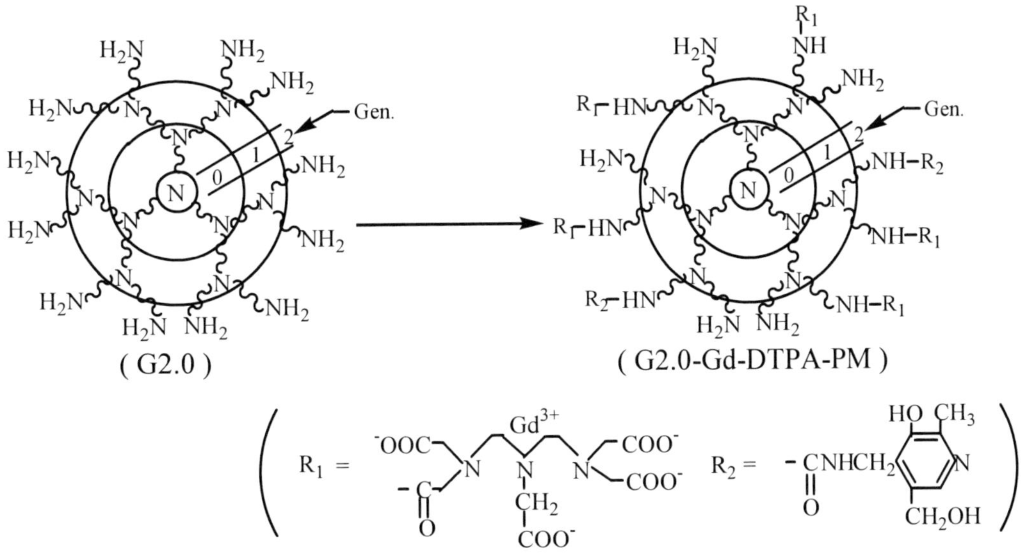

Figure 13. Structural formula of PAMAM-Gd-DTPA-PM.

In addition, diethylenetriaminepentaacetic acid (DTPA) and pyridoxamine (PM) were also both incorporated to the amine groups on the surface of the ammonia core poly(amidoamine) dendrimers (PAMAM, Generation 2.0-5.0) to obtain the dendritic ligands (Figure 13). These dendritic ligands were further reacted with gadolinium chloride to yield the corresponding dendritic gadolinium complexes. They also have high relaxivity and higher intravascular retention time, and greatly enhance the contrast of MR images of the liver. Animal tests showed that small doses of this dendrimer contrast agent could promise a highly resolved and contrasted visualization of blood vessels. So the results suggest that this new and powerful class of contrast agents have the potential for diverse and extensive application in MR imaging for the liver [14].

LIVER-TARGETING ANTICANCER CONJUGATES

Polymer-based drug delivery systems are used to optimize the therapeutic properties of drugs and render them safer, more effective and reliable. Moreover, polymeric drugs with macromolecules used as drug carriers can be easily synthesized at low cost, freely water-soluble, non-toxic, non-immunogenic and well characterized from the physico-chemical point of view. Now the development of biomedical polymers for drug controlled release was laid emphasis on the temporal control, distribution control and responsive drug delivery systems [81,82].

One important approach in drug delivery design is that the attached drugs can be targeted to specific organs, tissues or cells by the incorporation of a drug into a polymer containing organ or tissue-targeting group or moiety. By this method, the toxic side effects of the drugs can be suppressed and the distribution of drugs can be improved and reduce the drugs dose [83].

5-Fluorouracil (5-Fu) was chosen as a drug model because its structure and mode of action are well described and it is widely utilized in cancer chemotherapy. Anticancer conjugates of 5-fluorouracil and polyaspartamides containing pyridoxamine moiety were prepared by conjugating anticancer drug 5-fluorouracil and hepatocyte-targeting group pyridoxamine to the polyaspartamides with different side chains (poly-α,β-[N-(2-hydroxyethyl)-L-aspartamide] (PHEA), poly-α,β-[N-(2-aminoethy1)-L-aspartamide] (PAEA), poly-α,β-[N-(3- hydroxypropyl)-L-aspartamide] (PHPA) and poly-α,β-[N-(6- aminohexyl)-L-aspartamide] (PAHA). When the mole ratio of 5-Fu to the polymeric units in the feed of the reaction increased, the conversions of 5-Fu in polymeric drugs increased from 5.9wt% to 25.6wt%. Their properties i*n vitro* and *in vivo* were also evaluated [64].

In vitro drug release properties studies showed that these anticancer conjugates can sustain *in vitro* release rate 5-Fu in PBS. A steady release rate of the drug was maintained for more than 80h (Figure 14). 5-Fu-PHEA-PM and 5-Fu-PHPA-PM were released faster than 5-Fu-PAEA-PM and 5-Fu-PAHA-PM because the hydrolysis rate of –NCOO- from the side chains of 5-Fu-PHEA-PM and 5-Fu-PHPA-PM was faster than that of –NCONH- from the side chains of 5-Fu-PAEA-PM and 5-Fu-PAHA-PM.

In vitro cytotoxicity assay exhibited that polymeric drugs possess low cytotoxicity to the human liver cells (L-02) than Fluorofur and 5-fluorouracil (Figure 15). FT-207 is a derivative of 5-fluorouracil and possesses lower toxicity than 5-fluorouracil. At 225μg/ml of anticancer drugs in the growth medium, the L-02 cells incubated with FT-207 and 5-Fu-PAEA-PM, respectively, retained above 47.1% and 63.2% viabilities relative to control.

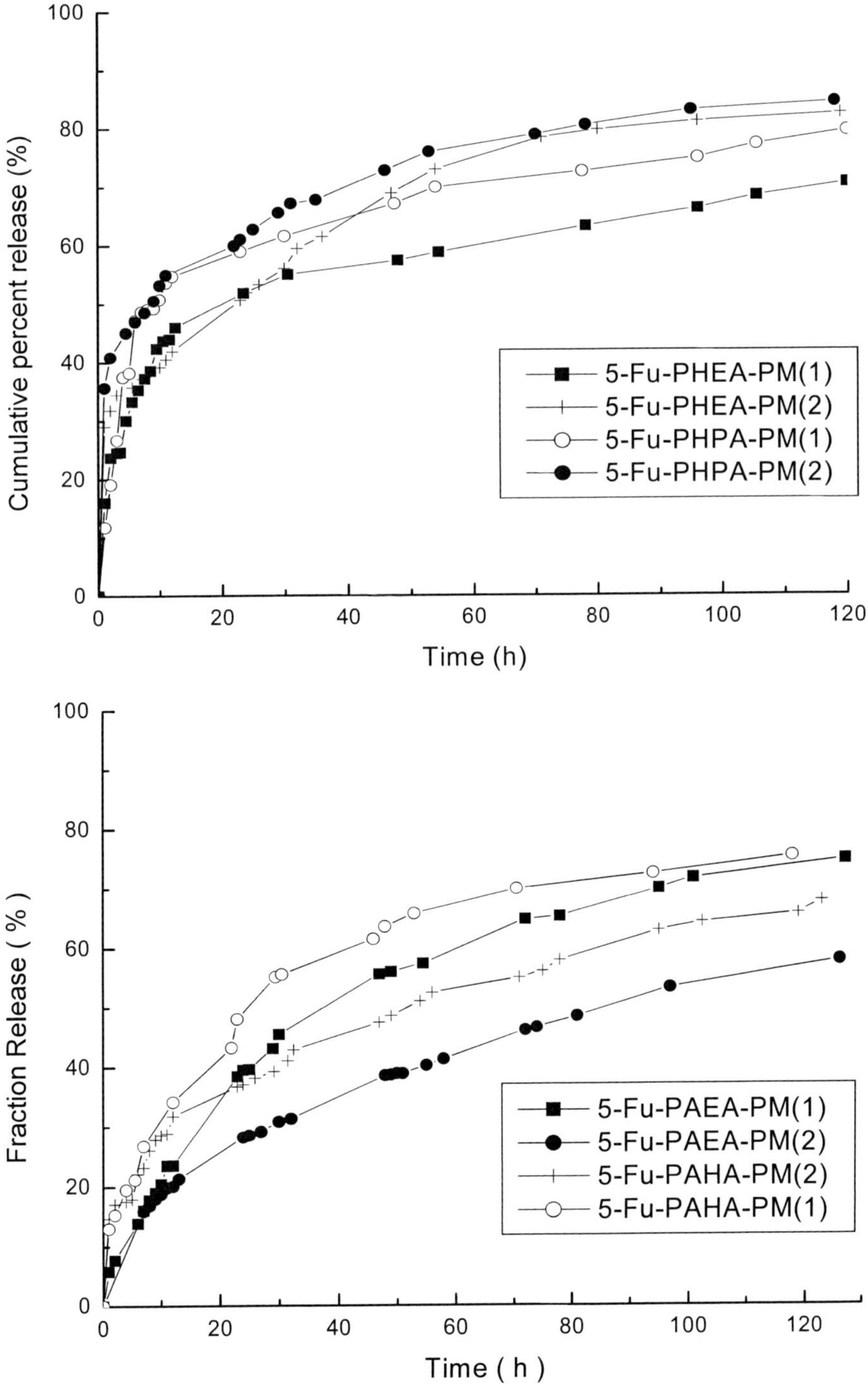

Figure 14. Release profiles 5-Fu of the polymeric drugs.

The distribution of PAEA-DTPA in mice tissues at various time points was shown that the agent was distributed to all the different tissues (such as the blood, liver, lung, heart and small intestine) showed no tissue-targeting property. It was rapidly cleared by the kidney, liver and small intestine, with the predominant excretion route of PAEA-DTPA is through kidney. The distribution of 5-Fu-PAEA-(DTPA)-PM in mice tissues at various time points was indicated that the majority of the polymeric drug was transferred from the blood into the liver within 20 min after injection. Very little amount of polymeric drug was found in the heart, spleen, lung, small intestine, muscle and bone at any time. This result shows the agent entered the liver from the blood and was excreted by kidneys later. A high content of 5-Fu-PAEA-(DTPA)-PM stayed in the liver for 90 min after injection. The incorporation of pyridoxamine in the polymers increased the pinocytic uptake by the liver.

The human hepatic tumor cells (Bel-7204) with different concentrations of 5-Fu-PAEA-PM (the content of polymeric drug (wt%): 5-Fu 25.6, PM 3.3) in the growth medium in culture were incubated for 24h in incubator (37℃, 5% CO_2). Induction of apoptosis was confirmed by formation of apoptotic bodies and fragmentation of cellular DNA (Figure 16). 5-Fu-PAEA-PM at 18μg/ml, 36μg/ml, 62.5μg/ml and 135μg/ml concentration induced apoptosis in about 27.6%, 43.1%, 50.7% and 62%, respectively, of human hepatic tumor cells after 48h incubation. When the concentration of 5-Fu-PAEA-PM (3) increased, the percentage of apoptosis in the human hepatic tumor cells became considerably larger. The apoptosis experiments showed the polymeric drugs could exhibit obviously high anticancer efficiencies and induce apoptosis in the human hepatic tumor cells (Bel-7204).

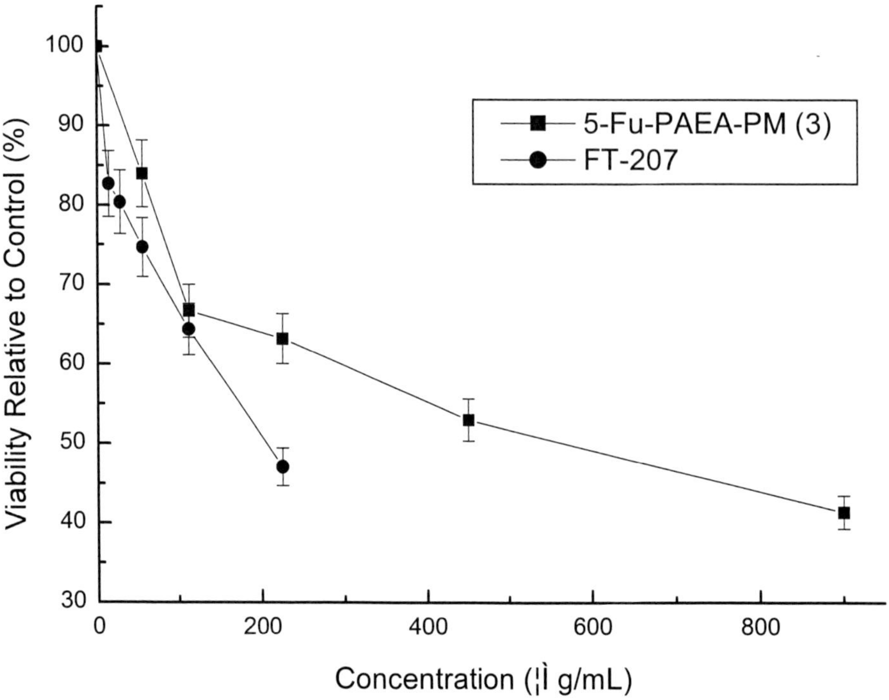

Figure 15. Cytotoxicity assay of anticancer drugs in L-02 cells.

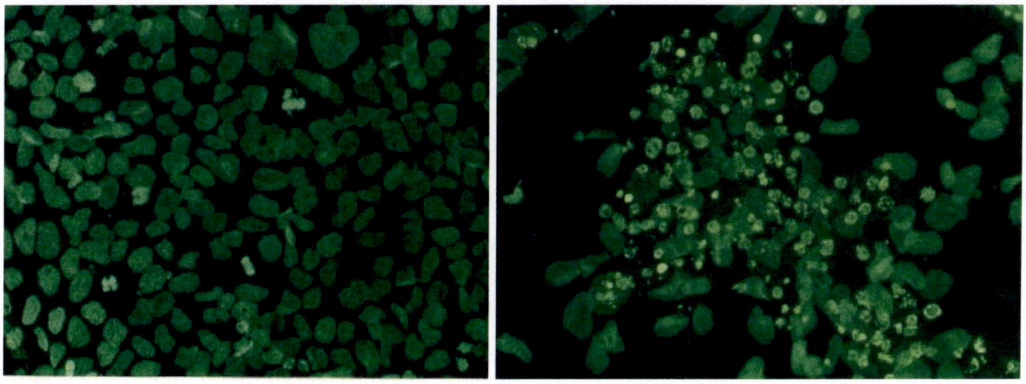

A B

Figure 16. Induced apoptosis photo of 5-Fu-PAEA-PM in the human hepatic tumor cells. A: control cells; B: 5-Fu-PAEA-PM (the content of polymeric drug (wt%): 5-Fu 25.6, PM 3.3) (135μg/mL).

SUMMARY

Although the liver-targeting mechanism and kinetic procedure of vitamin B_6 for MRI contrast agent and drug delivery have not described detailedly, previous researches have demonstrated that the incorporation of pyridoxine into MRI contrast agent and anticancer conjugates can increase their uptake by the liver, and that these molecules containing pyridoxine groups exhibit liver-targeting properties. Thus it is important to come to devote greater efforts to solving these problems.

One important approach in drug design for the disease in the liver is that the drugs can be targeted to the liver. By this method, the toxic side effects of the drugs can be suppressed and the distribution of drugs will be changed after administered, to improve the efficiency toward malignant cells and reduce the drugs dose. In future, the ideal drugs will be focused on the liver-targeting property with low toxicity and side effect, low doses *in vivo*, and minimal cost of procedure.

REFERENCES

[1] Van Beers, BE; Gallez, B; Pringot, J. Contrast-enhanced MR imaging of the liver. *Radiology*, 1997, 203: 297-306.

[2] Wen, J; Zhuo, RX; Wang, L. Aromatic DTPA-Bis(amide) gadolinium complexes as hepatobiliary contrast agents for magnetic resonance imaging. *Chin J Magn Reson* 1998, 15(3): 217-222.

[3] 3. Petre, C; Ni, Y; Marchal, G; Yu, J; Wevers, M; Lauffer, RB; Baert, AL. Detection and characterization of primary liver cancer in rats by MS-264-enhanced MRI. *Magn Reson Med* 1996, 35(4): 532-539.

[4] 4. Rocklage, SM; Cacheris, WP; Quay, SC; Hahn, FE; Raymond, KN. Magnanese (II) N, N'–dipyridoxyl ethylenediamine-N, N'-diactate-5, 5'-bis(phosphate): synthesis and

characterization of a paramagnetic chelate for magnetic resonance imaging enhancement. *Inorg Chem* 1989, 28: 477-485.

[5] Rummeny, E; Ehrenheim, C; Gehl, HB; Hamm, B; Laniado, M; Lodemann, KP; Schmiedel, E; Steudel, A; Vogl, TG. Manganese-DPDP as a hepatobiliary contrast agent in the magnetic resonance imaging of liver tumors: results of clinical phase II trials in Germany including 141 patients. *Invest Radiol* 1991, 26: S142-145.

[6] Mitchell, DG; Alam, F. Mangafodipir Trisodium: effects on T_2- and T_1- weighted MR cholangiography. *J Magn Reson Imaging* 1999, 9: 366-368.

[7] Wei, JF; Zhuo, RX. Studies on the novel liver-targeting MRI contrast agents containing vitamin B_6. *Chin Scien Bull* 1997, 42(14): 1519-1523.

[8] Yan, GP; Zhuo, RX. Research Progress of Magnetic Resonance Imaging Contrast Agents. *Chinese Science Bulletin* 2001, 46 (15): 1233-1237.

[9] Yan, GP; Robinsonand, L; Hogg, P. Magnetic Resonance Imaging Contrast Agents: overview and perspectives. *Radiography*, 2007 (In press).

[10] Yan, GP; Zhuo, RX; Xu, MY; Zhang, X; Li, LY; Liu, ML; Ye, CH. Hepatic targeting macromolecular MRI contrast agents. *Polym Int* 2002, 51: 892-898.

[11] Yan, GP; Zhuo, RX; Xu, MY; Li, LY; Tang, YF. Liver-targeting macromolecular MRI contrast agents. *Sci China, Ser B* 2001, 44 (4): 344-352.

[12] Yan, GP; Liu, ML; Li, LY. Studies on Polyaspartamide Gadolinium Complexes as potential Magnetic Resonance Imaging Contrast Agents. *Radiography*, 2005, 11: 117-122.

[13] Yan, GP; Bottle, SE; Zhuo, RX; Wei, L; Liu, ML; Li, LY. Evaluation on dendritic gadolinium complexes as MRI contrast agents. *J Bioact and Compatible Polym* 2004, 19(6): 453-465.

[14] Yan, GP; Hu, B; Liu, ML; Li, LY. Synthesis and Evaluation of Gadolinium Complexes Based on PAMAM as MRI Contrast Agents. *Journal of Pharmacy and Pharmacology*, 2005, 57(3): 351-357.

[15] Yan, GP; Bottle, SE; Zhuo, RX; Li, W; Liu, ML; Li, LY. Evaluation on Dendritic Gadolinium Complexes as MRI Contrast Agents. *Journal of Bioactive and Compatible Polymers*, 2004, 19(6): 453-465.

[16] Yan, GP; Zhuo, RX. Liver-targeting dendritic MRI contrast agents containing pyridoxamine group. *IUPAC World Polymer Congress 2002, Preprints, Part 2*: 946 (2002, Beijing, China)

[17] Yan, GP; Zhuo, RX; Xu, MY. Hepatic Targeting Macromolecular MRI Contrast Agents. *Polymer International, Polymers in the Third Millennium, Oral Abstracts*: Wednesday 5 September, Session A (2001, Montpellier, France).

[18] Yan, GP; Zhuo, RX; Xu, MY. Macromolecular MRI Contrast Agents Containing Hepatocyte-targeting Group. *Transactions of the Sixth World Biomaterials Congress Vol 3*: 1447 (2000, Kamuela, Hawaii, U.S.A)

[19] Yan, GP; Zhuo, RX; Xu, MY. Synthesis, Relaxivity, MR Imaging and Biodistribution of Macromolecular MRI Contrast Agents Containing Hepatocyte-targeting Group. *`2000 Cross-strait Polymer Learning Congress Summary*: 128-131 (2000, Gaoxiong, Taiwan).

[20] Lauterbur, PC. Image formation by induced local interactions: examples employing nuclear magnetic resonance. *Nature* 1973, 242: 190-191.

[21] Gallez, B; Swartz, HM. *In vivo* EPR: when, how and why? *NMR in Biomed* 2004, 17: 223-225.
[22] Lauffer, RB. Paramagnetic metal complexes as water proton relaxation agents for NMR imaging: theory and design. *Chem Rev* 1987, 87: 901-927.
[23] Nelson, KL; Runge, VM. Principles of MR contrast. In: Runge VM, editor. Contrast-enhanced clinical magnetic resonance imaging. USA: The University Press of Kentucky; 1996; 1-14.
[24] Weinmann, HJ; Brash, RC; Press, WR; Wesbey, GE. Characteristic of gadolinium-DTPA complex: a potential NMR contrast agent. *Am J Radiology* 1984, 142: 619-624.
[25] Mikei, K; Helm, L; Brucher, E; Merbach, A. ^{17}O NMR study of water exchange on $Gd(DTPA)(H_2O)^{2-}$ and $Gd(DOTA)(H_2O)^{2-}$ related to NMR imaging. *Inorg Chem* 1993, 32: 3844-3850.
[26] Zhuo, RX; Lu, ZR; Wei, JF; Yan, GP. The methods of synthesis of polyaminocarboxylates metal complexes. *Chinese Patent* 1995: 95 1 19302.3.
[27] Caravan, P; Ellison, JJ; Mcmurry, TJ; Lauffer, RB. Gadolinium (III) chelates as MRI contrast agents: structure, dynamics, and applications. *Chem Rev* 1999, 99: 2293-2352.
[28] Lowe, MP. MRI contrast agents: the next generation. *Aust J Chem* 2002, 55: 551-556.
[29] Aime, S; Dastrù, W; Crich, SG; Gianolio, E; Mainero, V. Innovative magnetic resonance imaging diagnostic agents based on paramagnetic Gd(III) complexes. *Biopolymers (Pept Sci)* 2002, 66: 419-428.
[30] Botta, M. Second coordination sphere water molecules and relaxivity of gadolinium(III) complexes: implication for MRI contrast agents. *Eur J Inorg Chem* 2000, 399-407.
[31] Wen, J; Zhuo, RX; Wang, L. Aromatic DTPA-Bis(amide) gadolinium complexes as hepatobiliary contrast agents for magnetic resonance imaging. *Chin J Magn Reson* 1998, 15(3): 217-222.
[32] Weinmann, HJ; Ebert, W; Misselwitz, B; Schmitt-Willich, H. Tissue-specific MR contrast agents. *Eur J Radio* 2003, 46: 33-44.
[33] Artemov, D. Molecular magnetic resonance imaging with targeted contrast agents. *J Cell Biochem* 2003, 90: 518-524.
[34] Enochs, WS; Weissleder, R. Organ- and Tissue-directed MRI contrast agents. In: Edelman RR, Hesselink JR, Zlatkin MB editors. Clinical magnetic resonance imaging. Pennsylvania, USA: WB Saunders Company; 1996; 192-219.
[35] Lorusso, V; Arbughi, T; Tirone, P; de Haen, C. Pharmacokinetics and tissue distribution in animals of gadobenate ion, the magnetic resonance imaging contrast enhancing component of gadobenate dimeglumine 0.5M solution for injection (MultiHance). *J Comput Assist Tomogr* 1999, 1(23): S181-194.
[36] Cavagna, F; Dapri, M; Maggioni, F; de Hahn, C; Felder, E. Gd-BOPTA/Dimeg: experimental disease imaging. *Magn Reson Med* 1991, 22: 329-333.
[37] Schuhmann-Giampieri, G; Schmitt-Willich, H; Press, WR; Negishi, C; Weinmann, HJ; Speak, U. Preclinical evaluation of Gd-EOB-DTPA as a contrast agent in MR imaging of the hepatobiliary system. *Radiology* 1993, 183(1): 59-64.
[38] Cynthia, R; Rogers, J; Arias, IM. Use of an asialoglycoprotein receptor-targeted magnetic resonance contrast agent to study changes in receptor biology during liver regeneration endoloxemia in rats. *Hepatology* 1996, 23(6): 1631-1638.

[39] Fu, YJ; Zhuo, RX. Studies on D-galactose-containing DTPA bisamide gadolinium complexes as liver-targeting MRI contrast agents. *Chem J Chin Univ* 1997, 18(7): 1072-1075.

[40] Moats, RA; Fraser, SE; Meade, TJ. A "smart" magnetic resonance contrast agent that reports on specific enzymatic activity. *Angew Chem Int Ed Engl* 1997, 36(7): 726-728.

[41] Leveille-Webster, C; Rogers, J; Arias, IM. Use of an asialoglycoprotein receptor-targeted magnetic resonance agent to study changes in receptor biology during liver regeneration and endotoxemia in rats. *Hepatology* 1996, 23: 1631-1641.

[42] Zhuo, RX; Fu, YJ; Liao, J. Synthesis, relaxivity and biodistribution of novel magnetic resonance imaging (MRI) contrast agents: polylysine (Gd-DTPA/DOTA) with pendent galactose moieties as hepatocyte-targeting groups. *Chin Chem Lett* 1997, 8 (2): 157-160.

[43] Ding, XJ; Zhuo, RX; Fu, GC. Studies on the synthesis, relaxivity and liver-targeting of DTPA-pyridoxol ester gadolinium and manganese complexes. *Chinese Science Bulletin* 2001, 46 (18): 1519-1523.

[44] Ding, XJ; Zhuo, RX; Fu, GC. Studies on the synthesis, relaxivity and liver-targeting of DTPA-pyridoxol ester gadolinium complexes. *Chemical Journal of Chinese Universities* 2002, 23 (1): 49-52.

[45] Duarte, MG; Gil, MH; Peters, JA; Colet, JM; Elst, LV; Muller, RN; Geraldes, CFGC. Synthesis, characterization, and relaxivity of two linear Gd(DTPA)-polymer conjugates. *Bioconjugate Chem* 2001, 12: 170-177.

[46] Tóth, E; Uffelen, IV; Helm, L; Merbach, AE; Ladd, D; Briley-SæbØ, K; Kellar, E. Gadolinium-based linear polymer with temperature-independent proton relaxivities: a unique interplay between the water exchange and rotational contributions. *Magn Reson Chem* 1998, 36: S125-134.

[47] Mohs, AM; Wang, XH; Goodrich, KC; Zong, YD; Parker, DL; Lu, ZR. PEG-*g*-poly(DTPA-*co*-L-cystine): a biodegradable macromolecular blood pool contrast agent for MR imaging. *Bioconjugate Chem* 2004, 15: 1424-1430.

[48] Lu, ZR; Parker, DL; Goodrich, KC; Wang, XH; Dalle, JG; Buswell, HR. Extracellular biodegradable macromolecular gadolinium(III) complexes for MRI. *Magn Reson Med* 2004, 51: 27-34.

[49] Ouyang, M; Zhuo, RX; Fu, GC. Study on synthesis and relaxivity of paramagnetic polyester metal complexes for MRI. *Ion Exchange and Adsorption* 1996, 12(4): 324-327.

[50] Bai, ZW; Zhuo, RX. The synthesis and relaxivity of polyester-amide MRI contrast agent. *Ion Exchange and Adsorption* 1996, 12(4): 332-335.

[51] Brasch, RC. Rationable and applications for macromolecular Gd-based contrast agents. *Magn Reson Med* 1991, 22: 282-287.

[52] Aime, S; Botta, M; Crich, SG; Giovenzana, GB; Pagliarin, R; Piccinini, M; Sisti, M; Terreno, E. Towards MRI contrast agent of improved efficacy NMR relaxometric investigations of the binding interaction HSA of a novel heptadentate macrocyclic triphosphonate Gd^{3+}-complex. *J Biol Inorg Chem* 1997, 2(4): 470-479.

[53] Schuhmann-Giampieri, G; Schmitt-Willich, H; Frenzel, T; Press, WR; Weinmann, HJ. *In vivo* and *in vitro* evaluation of Gd-DTPA-polylysine as a macromolecular contrast agent for magnetic resonance imaging. *Invest Radiol* 1991, 26: 969-974.

[54] Roberts, HC; Saeed, M; Roberts, TPL; Mühler, A; Brasch, RC. MRI of acute myocardial ischemia: comparing a new contrast agent, Gd-dtpa-24-cascade-polymer, with Gd-dtpa, *J magn Reson Imaging* 1999, 9: 204-208.

[55] Judd, RM; Reeder, SB; May-Newman, K. Effects of water exchange on the measurement of myocardial perfusion using paramagnetic contrast agents. *Magn Reson Med* 1999, 41: 334-342.

[56] Wen, XX; Jackson, EF; Price, RE; Kim, EE; Wu, QP; Wallace, S; Charnsangavej, C; Gelovani, JG; Li, C. Synthesis and characterization of poly(L-glutamic acid) gadolinium chelate: a new biodegradable MRI contrast agent. *Bioconjugate Chem* 2004, 15: 1408-1415.

[57] Lu, ZR; Wang, XH; Parker, DL; Goodrich, KC; Buswell, HR. Poly(L-glutamic acid) Gd(III)-DOTA conjugate with a degradable spacer for magnetic resonance imaging. *Bioconjugate Chem* 2003, 14: 715-719.

[58] Uzgiris, EE; Cline, H; Moasser, B; Grimmond, B; Amaratunga, M; Smith, JF; Goddard, G. Conformation and structure of polymeric contrast agents for medical imaging. *Biomacromolecules* 2004, 5: 54-61.

[59] Giammona, G; Carlisi, B; Palazzo, S. α,β-Poly (N-hydroxyethyl)- DL-aspartamide with derivatives of carboxylic acids. *J Polym Sci Polym Chem* 1987, 25: 2813-2818.

[60] Giammona, G; Carlisi, B; Cavallaro, G. Calorimetric investigation of the interaction betweenα,β-Poly (N-hydroxyethyl)-DL-aspartamide and surfactants. *Int J Pharm* 1990, 64: 239-242.

[61] Giammona, G; Carlisi, B; Pitarresi, G. Hydrophilic and hydropholic polymeric derivatives of antiinflammatory agents such as Alclofenac, Ketoprofen and Ibuprofen. *J Bioact Compatible polym* 1991, 6: 129-141.

[62] Giammona, G; Carlisi, B; Pitarresi, G. Water-soluble copolymers of an antiviral agent: synthesis and their interaction with a biomembrane model. *J Control Release* 1992, 22: 197-204.

[63] Giammona, G; Cavallaro, G; Fontana, G. Coupling of the antiviral agent zidovudine to polyaspartamide and in vitro drug release studies. *J Control Release* 1998, 54: 321-331.

[64] Yan, GP; Zhuo, RX; Zheng, CY. Study on the Anticancer Drug 5-Fluorouracil-conjugated Polyaspartamides Containing Hepatocyte-targeting Group. *Journal of Bioactive and Compatible Polymers* 2001, 16 (4): 277-293.

[65] Yan, GP; Liu, ML; Li, LY. Studies on Polyaspartamide Gadolinium Complexes Containing Sulfadiazine Groups as MRI Contrast Agents. *Bioconjugate Chemistry* 2005, 16: 967-971.

[66] Yan, GP; Zhuo, RX; Yang, YH; Xu, MY; Li, LY; Ye, ZH. Tumor-selective Macromolecular MRI Contrast Agents. *Journal of Bioactive and Compatible Polymers* 2002, 17 (2): 139-151.

[67] Esfand, R; Tomalia, DA. Poly(amidoamine) (PAMAM) dendrimers: from biomimicry to drug delivery and biomedical applications. *Drug Discovery Today* 2001, 6(8): 427-436.

[68] Kobayshi, H; Kawamoto, S; Jo, SK; Bryant, HL; Brechbiel, MW; Star, RA. Macromolecular MRI contrast agents with small dendrimers: pharmacokinetic differences between sizes and cores. *Bioconjugate Chem* 2003, 14: 388-394.

[69] Margerum, LD; Campion, BK; Koo, M; Shargill, N; Lai, JJ; Marumoto, A; Sontum, PC. Gadolinium (III) DO3A macrocycles and polyethylene glycol coupled to

dendrimers effect of molecular weight on physical and biological properties of macromolecular magnetic resonance imaging contrast agents. *Journal of Alloys and Compounds* 1997, 249:185-190.

[70] Yokoyama, M; Inoue, S. Preparation of adriamycin-conjugated poly(ethylene glycol)-poly(aspartic acid) block copolymer. *Macromol Chem Rapid Commun* 1987, 8: 431-435.

[71] Patri, AK; Majoros, IJ; Baker, JR. Dendritic polymer macromolecular carriers for drug delivery. *Current Opinion in Chemical Biology* 2002, 6: 466-471.

[72] Fischer, M; Vögtle, F. Dendrimers: from design to application—a progress report. *Angew Chem Int Ed* 1999, 38: 884-905.

[73] Wiener, EC; Brechbiel, MW; Brothers, H; Magin, RL; Gansow, OA; Tomalia, DA; Lauterbur, PC. Dendrimer-based metal chelates: a new class of magnetic resonance imaging contrast agents. *Magn Reson Med* 1994, 31: 1-8.

[74] Stiriba, SE; Frey, H; Haag, R. Dendritic polymers in biomedical applications: from potential to clinical use in diagnostics and therapy. *Angew Chem Int Ed* 2002, 41(8):1329-1334.

[75] Neerman, MF; Zhang, W; Parrish, AR; Simanek, EE. *In vitro* and *in vivo* evaluation of a melamine dendrimer as a vehicle for drug delivery. *Int J Pharmac* 2004, 281: 129-132.

[76] Wiener, EC; Auteri, FP; Chen, JW; Brechbiel, MW; Gansow, OA; Schneider, DS; Belford, RL; Clarkson, RB; Lauterbur, PC. Molecular dynamics of ion-chelate complexes attached to dendrimers. *J Am Chem Soc* 1996, 118: 7774-7782.

[77] Nicolle, GM; Toth, E; Schmitt-Willich, H; Raduchel, B; Merbach, AE. The Impact of Rigidity and Water Exchange on the Relaxivity of a Dendritic MRI Contrast Agent. *Chem Eur J* 2002, 8(5): 1040-1048.

[78] Bryant, LH; Brechbiel, MW; Wu, CC; Bulte, JWM; Herynek, V; Frank, JA. Synthesis and Relaxometry of High-Generation (G=5, 7, 9, and 10) PAMAM Dendrimer-DOTA-Gadolinium Chelates. *J Magn Reson Imaging* 1999, 9: 348-352.

[79] Stiriba, SE; Frey, H; Haag, R. Dendritic polymers in biomedical applications: from potential to clinical in diagnostics and therapy. *Angew Chem Int Ed*, 2002, 41(8): 1329-1334.

[80] Kobayashi, H; Jo, SK; Kawamoto, S; Yasuda, H; Hu, XZ; Knopp, MV; Brechbiel, MW; Choyke, PL; Star, RA. Polyamine dendrimer-based MRI contrast agents for functional kidney imaging to diagnose acute renal failure. *J Magn Reson Imaging* 2004, 20: 512-518.

[81] Langer, R. Polymer-controlled drug delivery systems. *Acc Chem Res* 1993, 26: 537-542.

[82] Nishikawa, M; Takakura, Y. Pharmacokinetic evalution of polymeric carriers. *Adv Drug Del Rev* 1996, 21: 135-155.

[83] Sezaki, H; Takakura, Y; Hashida, M. Souble macromolecular carriers for the delivery of antitumor drugs. *Adv Drug Del Rev* 1989, 3: 247-266.

In: Drugs: Approval and Evaluation, Delivery and Control ISBN: 978-1-60456-533-1
Editors: A.O. Hartmann, L.K. Neumann

Chapter 5

SHOULD THE EVALUATION AND PATENTING OF NOVEL MEDICINES FOLLOW A DISTINCTIVE TRACK?

Julio Sotelo*

National Institutes of Health of Mexico, Mexico

ABSTRACT

Biomedical research is the largest scientific enterprise; the twentieth century was its golden age. In that period, almost all therapeutic and preventive substances that participated in the doubling of life expectancy of humans were either discovered or synthesized. As natural consequence, the pharmaceutical industry grew immensely to become among the most successful of all economical investments. Human pathology moved from the acute infectious diseases, which were the principal causes of disease along the history, to the chronic degenerative and proliferative disorders, which have become nowadays the most frequent. The therapeutics of human disorders have also changed, from the preventive or curative, brief intervention (vaccines, antibiotics, vitamins, etc.), to the need for chronic, long-lasting ingestion of palliative remedies (antidepressants, antirheumatics, antihypertensives, lipid-lowering drugs, antiepileptics, etc.). This shift has produced an enormous and adverse impact on the economy of patients and medical institutions, together with a huge proliferation of innovative substances that attempt to participate in this lucrative market.

Evaluation by cost-benefit on the pertinence of new (generally expensive) vs. traditional (generally unexpensive) drugs, as well as fairness of new prices and propaganda strategies used by the pharmaceutical industry have become issues of paramount importance for the medical profession, as doctors are the necessary link between patients and drug-producers [1,2]. Nonetheless the ancestral codes of medical practice state undoubtedly that the moral and professional compromises of physicians are

* Correspondence to: Julio Sotelo, MD; Director, National Institutes of Health, Periferico Sur 4118, 01900 Mexico City, Mexico. Phone: (5255) 5652-8285; Fax: (5255) 5135-2229; e-mail: jsotelo@servidor.unam.mx

only with the patient [3]. Several peculiarities of research, testing and marketing of pharmaceutical substances indicate that novel and imaginative mechanisms of access to new substances must be found in the benefit of patients, particularly those with limited economical means, which are the great majority of humans, whether living in rich or in poor countries.

INTRODUCTION

While scientific advances in most fields of research remain stable and novelties accumulate over the basic discovery, advances in therapeutics produce new substances (many of them not entirely original) which, for the matter of patenting and commerce are taken as if the substance obtained was unique in its potential applications; therefore the price is set by the producers based entirely on marketing convenience, without any other consideration whatsoever [4]. In a recent communication I compared the way prices are set between two different goods, both based on modern research; cell phones and medicines [5]. If we have to define in brief terms our current times I would say that we live the times of "telecommunications and wonder drugs" they are among the finest products of human intellect and scientific talent, they have changed the world beyond the imagination of previous times and both have produced a dramatic impact in the every day life of most human beings. However, there have been dramatic differences in the commercial pathway that they have taken; particularly in the last twenty years. Telecommunication commodities are every year more accessible to more people all over the world, improving, in a wonderful convergence, the economical means of their clients extending their benefits to more groups of the less privileged economical strata. In contrast, the pharmaceutical advances are becoming every time less accessible to more and more people, so that nowadays, even in affluent countries, most novel treatments for severe disorders are beyond the means of a growing number of patients, the picture is pathetic in developing countries. In short, in regards to these two fields of scientific enquiries, as more scientific advances in telecommunications accumulate their goods and products become more and more accessible to the general public. In contrast, as more scientific advances in pharmaceutics accumulate their goods and products become more and more expensive and less accessible to the general public [6].

Scientific advances and their consequence, patenting and exploitation rights, are constantly applied to the products from the fields related above, however, at the end, the consumers are affected quite differently: Technological advances in communications facilitate life, improve economical potential, are a simple vehicle for entertainment or information and their costs to users have not changed sensibly from the past to the current models, which incorporate recently acquired scientific advances and bring enormous benefits to both, the producers and the consumers. In comparison, patenting and exploitation rights of pharmaceutical substances take quite a different tract; they also bring large benefits to the producers, but their potential benefit for consumers is usually hampered by the exorbitant prices of most novel pharmaceutical substances. The price of most recent medicines has no relation with their immediate predecessors used for the same clinical application.

The impact of scientific novelties on telecommunications (and there are many every year) is almost negligible for the every-day consumer. Just take as example the technological advances in television, instant information, computers, cell phones and so on, they are simply amazing; their prices are also amazing considering the wonders that the consumers enjoy, which augment every day, particularly the common citizen. We have to compare them with novel medicines, where the benefits reach less and less numbers of potential consumers, just because the skyrocketing of prices; although the practical benefits might continue being great for the producers. How this dichotomy became so? Why, contrary to the evolution of progress, in the case of pharmaceutical substances the benefits side unequivocally to one side?, the more scientific advances the more expensive they become. This lack of equilibrium might indicate that, although scientific research must continue, the commercial rules, in the case of pharmaceutical advances, should change towards an equilibrium that would favor both, consumers and producers.

When breakthrough scientific and technological advances are applied to the everyday life of the common citizen, the prices might be high at the beginning; however, once the novelty becomes a real gain in the public perception and its use is widespread two advantageous things occur, their cost lowers and the novel item joins the chain of progress in a mode that is difficult to predict, but it generates countless additional benefits which contribute to the progress of society. Lets consider as example the computer and its wonder companion, the internet, it would not be an exaggeration to affirm that they have changed almost every aspect of society; the enormous amount of research (and research money) employed in this field has generated countless patents, new pieces of information and amazing scientific findings. As consequence, it has brought large, enormous economical gains to producers, as compared with what could be seen in retrospective only as symbolic expenditures in research; these commodities have also been a fountain of richness for its consumers as well. In short, in the whole field of telecommunications scientific research, technological applications and marketing procedures have generated, on the side of investors and producers the biggest fortunes on earth and, on the side of consumers clear benefits that improve their life, economy and countless circumstances far beyond their immediate applications; very much as medicines used to be in former times.

Pharmaceutical Research

The impact of pharmaceutical research in the life of the common citizen has also been enormous, just see the history of the 20th century medicine, to mention only a few; the arrival of antibiotics, analgesics, antidepressants, antiparasitic drugs, hormones, vaccines, antihypertensives, tranquilizers, etc, have improved to an amazing degree both, the quality of life and the life expectancy of most humans. It is impossible to remain untouched by sight that followed the invention, or the discovery, of imaging studies, telemedicine and biochemical analysis as well as the advent of anesthetics; which made possible surgery, and transplants as its most elaborated craft. The products that medical and scientific research gave to modern society changed the life of most humans. It can be summarized in brief lines; biomedical research gave another life-span to humanity, in addition to the natural one of 35-40 years average that they lived throughout history (that is, before the 20th Century, the golden era of medical research) which was boosted to 70-80 years at the beginning of the 21st century, which is the new life expectancy of most children born today. So, modern humans, in contrast with their ancestors, live a life twice as long as their counterparts of all times. Most of this invaluable gain is due to biomedical research which paved the way for the understanding, prevention and treatment of most diseases that caused premature death through history. I believe that it is the most precious gift that scientific research has given to humanity in any field of knowledge.

For the fist time, in this contemporary age any subject has the logical expectation of living a very long life and die at an advanced age. In this notorious change for the wellbeing of society the pharmaceutical research played a protagonic role and, until recently, similarly to telecommunications and informatics, the gains had been shared by both sides: Hugh economical gains for the producers and drastic gains in health for the consumers.

PATHWAYS FOR DISCOVERY OF NEW MEDICINES

The inception of effective medicines led doctors to cure most diseases that were the principal causes of death and suffering along the history. For the sake of simplicity I will separate the origin of most human diseases in three groups: infectious, proliferative and degenerative (although some others like autoimmune or nutritional do not enter into this simplistic group). Scientific research of the past century was extraordinarily effective in the first one, infectious. The incomplete list of remedies include vaccines, antibiotics, antiparasitics, antiseptics, hormones, etc. In contrast, scientific gains in the last two groups, proliferative (cancer) and degenerative, have been rather modest. These disorders, have taken the first place in prevalence as causes of suffering and death while infectious disorders have receded. Thus, a new paradox has emerged in the spectrum of human diseases; the medical remedies for the most frequent diseases in the new epidemiological scenario go from palliative, to moderately effective to frankly inefficient. In any case, the cost of current treatments (even the ones of dubious efficacy) for most degenerative and proliferative diseases has blown up and became unaffordable for a very large number of patients from most countries, even the more affluent ones [7]. How came this paradox? Many old drugs that are highly effective and curative are inexpensive, whereas many other that are either palliative, or the ones that exert some degree of control over the progress of the disease but do not cure it, are more and more expensive as pharmaceutical research progresses.

Biomedical research, in contrast with most other branches of research is directed first to understand and then to modify the factors that affect the wellbeing of cells and systems within the human organism, its products can be separated in two main disciplines: one directed to the study and understanding of the biological process or its alterations (basic research) and another devoted to modify or mend the pathological process (clinical research) the latter is usually constructed upon the foundations settled by the former. Most biomedical advances follow the path first traced by basic research and then corrected or improved by applied research.

In general terms, basic biomedical research is organized and supported by federal funds or by non-lucrative agencies at universities and scientific centers, whereas applied research is usually supported by pharmaceutical companies. From basic research comes the discovery of the causes of diseases; from applied research comes the discovery of their pharmacological therapy. Both are a necessary chain for the progress of medicine, but their differences are large. Basic research represents a non-profit, hugh investment of society, it is very successful indeed for the generation of countless pieces of information to gain understanding of the biological and the pathological processes affecting human life. Once this knowledge is gained, the second step, which in the perception of the public is the spectacular one, is to find a substance that could intervene in the pathological process inducing either its reversal or the control of the abnormal function.

Marketing of Novel Drugs

There is a despairingly large inequality from the side of applied pharmaceutical research. Drug companies benefit from basic research without substantial expenditure on it, which usually is a non-patented public property. The information obtained by basic research leads unequivocally to the knowledge of the cellular, chemical and molecular disturbances associated to the pathological process. After this knowledge is obtained, the pharmaceutical industry sets the appropriate protocols to produce a substance aiming to intervene favorably or to interfere with the pathological process. There is nothing wrong with this sequence of events; it is the very foundation for the discovery of several wonder drugs that have changed the spectrum of diseases in the last hundred years (though the last fifty were the best). In my opinion the problem raises form the concept, which recently became highly deleterious for the ethical aims of medicine, that prices for new medicines, which were discovered throughout the above described track, can be settled by the pharmaceutical manufacturers without external contentions or any parameter other than their own economical calculations, which run according to their market studies and particular expectations. Although in legal terms the current internationally accepted scheme of patenting and marketing allows this unilateral conception, we must remember that the great majority of novel pharmaceutical substances are only improvements (many of them quite modest) upon current or former therapies. For instance any new anti-hypertensive synthesized today could be marginally better than a classical one in lowering the high pressure; but until now no anti-hypertensive cures hypertension, which would be the real breakthrough. In the same example, this hypothetical new anti-hypertensive, which might be 10% superior to the old one, is not 8 or 10 or even 20 percent more expensive than former ones, as it would be logically expected due to its marginal superiority. This increase would be sufficient to conquer the huge market of arterial hypertension and produce large and fair, economical gains for its producers. Contrary to the above lucubration, this hypothetical new anti-hypertensive becomes three or four times more expensive than the classical one. In the case of anticancer drugs this phenomenon has became outrageously wicked; several antineoplastics, whose benefits are meager, manifested only as minor (though statistically significant) increases in the length of survival after diagnosis, are sold at unbelievably high prices. Nothing to do with the traditional ways of medicine, particularly when the remedy is, at the end, rather inefficacious.

In former times, the most expensive materials in the world were the gems and precious metals, there is no need to explain the reasons, nobody argues against them, nor to their high price. Besides, they are only a personal option for supplemental luxury. As for substances, some edibles were also quite expensive (great wines, caviar, truffles, etc.) as scant and laborious products. Nowadays, the most expensive substances in the world are some pharmaceutical products elaborated by patented formulas, many of them quite inexpensive to produce. Their applications are singular for the lowering or tempering of human pain and suffering, they are used for the therapy of incurable diseases, which continue incurable even after their treatment. Some of these novel substances cost, by the milligram large amounts of money, reaching unprecedent amounts they are given as a single shot to the patient, to be repeated by a similar one few hours later. The medical profession can not allow this to happen, physicians should not participate candidly in the prescription of these medicines [8,9]. Moreover, governments must regulate this unfair market.

Pharmaceutical companies refer to "research costs" to justify whichever price they deem appropriate for novel, patented drugs. However, I believe that "research costs" in the pharmaceutical industry, as well as in other business are only part of the natural costs that any innovative industry has to spend in order to obtain large economical gains. Curiously, the pharmaceutical industry refer as "research costs" the whole enterprise of expenses in research, together with fees for doctors, travel expenses, publicity, lobbing, gifts and entertaining of professionals directed to the promotion of their medicines, inside a frequently naive medical profession [10,11].

Conclusion

As pharmaceutical research is only the final step in a long chain of costly research, mostly supported in its origin by federal grants and non lucrative agencies, the marketing of new medicines should be considered within a peculiar chapter of commerce in modern society [12]. Also, as any new medicine has to be prescribed by a third party (the doctor), I do propose that within the patenting and licensing processes of any substance intended for the therapy of human diseases an ethical commission, vigilant of the intended prices, must intervene mainly by setting the limits for economical gains of drug producers [5].

I have also proposed changes in the traditional regulation of clinical research of pharmaceutical substances which should care more for the integral benefit (in health, social and economical protection) of the patient than for the financial progress of the enormously successful pharmaceutical industry [13,14]. Currently, the testing of novel pharmaceutical substances is carried out in clinical research settings hired by the company that produces the substance. This peculiar relationship between the pharmaceutical industry and institutions of medical research is the source of countless biases, as it has mixed for the same enterprise scientific talent with commercial interest. Thus, in no few cases, the evaluation of new compounds does not cover entirely their long term toxicity, their limits of effectiveness or the margin of superiority of these substances as compared with traditional, inexpensive medicines in use for the same therapeutic goal. I think that a third party, called "collegiated research council" [13,14], integrated by distinguished scholars selected by leading universities and medical centers; should be included as an autonomous scientific board who would oversight the selection of investigators and institutions for the testing of new drugs and would intervene, representing the medical profession in the analysis of the intended pricing of the drug prior to their approval for commercialization by the regulatory agencies.

A big contention recently made by leading medical journals is the obscurity of information in regard to current schemes of financing clinical investigation of novel drugs indicating that in the case of the classical (and necessary) relationship pharmaceutical industry-medical profession [3,6] new mechanisms and rules have to be found in favor of the most important (and frequently forgotten) beneficiary of this relation, the patient.

REFERENCES

[1] Campbell EG, Gruen RL, Mountford J, Miller LG, Cleary PD, Blumenthal D. (2007). A national survey of physician-industry relationships. *N Engl J Med, 356*, 1742-1750.

[2] Angell M. (2005). *The truth about drug companies: How they deceive us and what to do about it.* New York: Random House.

[3] Moynihan R. (2003). Who pays for the pizza? Redefining the relationships between doctors and drug companies. 2: Disentanglement. *BMJ 326,* 1193-1196.

[4] Kassirer JP. *On the take: how medicine's complicity with big business can endanger your health.* New York: Oxford University Press; 2005.

[5] Sotelo J. (2007). How to make the prices of new drugs fairer. *BMJ, 334,* 369.

[6] Blumenthal D, Causino N, Campbell E, Louis KS. (1996). Relationships between academic institutions and industry in the life sciences--an industry survey. *N Engl J Med, 334,* 368-373.

[7] Tudor J. (2006). *The Political Economy of Health Care: A Clinical Perspective.* Bristol, UK: Policy Press.

[8] Brennan TA, Rothman DJ, Blank L, Blumenthal D, Chimonas SC, Cohen JJ, Goldman J, Kassirer JP, Kimball H, Naughton J, Smelser N. (2006). Health industry practices that create conflicts of interest: a policy proposal for academic medical centers. *JAMA, 295,* 429-433.

[9] Horton R. (Review) What's Wrong with Doctors. In: *How Doctors Think* by Jerome Groopman, Houghton Mifflin, 307 pp. The New York Review of Books, 54: May 31, 2007. http://www.nybooks.com/articles/20214

[10] Roehr B. (2007). More than 90% of US doctors receive favours from drug companies. *BMJ, 334,* 869. doi:10.1136/bmj.39196.342847.DB

[11] Hopkins J. (2007). US campaign aims to end industry gifts, speaking fees, and travel for doctors. *BMJ, 334,* 385. doi:10.1136/bmj.39132.345174.DB

[12] Studdert DM, Mello MM, Brennan TA. (2004). Financial conflicts of interest in physicians' relationships with the pharmaceutical industry--self-regulation in the shadow of federal prosecution. *N Engl J Med, 351,* 1891-1900.

[13] Sotelo J. (2006). Regulation of clinical research sponsored by pharmaceutical companies; a proposal. *Plos Medicine 3*, 945-947.

[14] Sotelo J. (2006). Industry-Sponsored Research: Author's Reply. *Plos Medicine, 3,* 464. http://medicine.plosjournals.org/perlserv/?request=get-document&doi=10.1371/journal.pmed.0030464.

In: Drugs: Approval and Evaluation, Delivery and Control ISBN: 978-1-60456-533-1
Editors: A.O. Hartmann, L.K. Neumann

Chapter 6

INVESTIGATION OF NEW MOLECULAR ENTITIES OF DRUGS APPROVED IN THREE REGIONS, JAPAN, US AND EU

Mitsuo Saito and Ryuichi Hasegawa
Division of Medicinal Safety Science, National Institute of Health Sciences, Tokyo, Japan

ABSTRACT

The number of new molecular entities (NMEs) approved in 2006 was 20 in Japan, 24 in US and 25 in EU, respectively. Among 70 NMEs approved in both Japan and US and/or EU during 2002 to 2006, 69 NMEs had been approved in US and 35 in EU by 2006, and there was only one common approval solely between Japan and EU. On the other hand, 39 NMEs were solely approved in US and EU during this period. Among 109 NMEs approved in either two or three regions, the number of preceding NMEs was 3 in Japan, 85 in US and 21 in EU.

1. INTRODUCTION

In order to promptly supply medicinal products that are needed in medical practice, measures for improving the efficiency of the drug approval review system have been undertaken. In the present study, in order to clarify the situation of drug approval, an investigation was conducted for the circumstances of approval of medicinal products containing a new molecular entity (NME) in 2006 in the three regions: Japan, the US and the EU; and comparative analyses were also conducted for NMEs that were approved between 2002 and 2006.

2. Methods of Investigating the Circumstances of Approvals in the Three Regions

For the approval situation in Japan, we investigated review reports obtained from the website of the Pharmaceuticals and Medical Devices Agency (http://www.info.pmda.go.jp/shinyaku/shinyaku_index.html). Regarding the US, we extracted brand names of NMEs from the FDA's CDER Drug and Biologic Approval Reports (http://www.fda.gov/cder/rdmt/). We also examined approval history obtained from Drugs@FDA (http://www.accessdata.fda.gov/scripts/cder/drugsatfda/index.cfm). For the EU, we extracted brand names of NMEs through the Centralized Approval Process from the Community Register of medicinal products (http://ec.europa.eu/enterprise/pharmaceuticals/register/index.htm) provided by the European Commission, and investigated product overview on target drugs from the EMEA's EPARs for authorized medicinal products for human use (http://www.emea.europa.eu/htms/human/epar/a.htm).

Table 1. NMEs approved in Japan, US and EU in 2006

Japan	US	EU
Aripiprazole	Sunitinib	Daptomycin
Silodosin	Ranolazine	Human normal Ig
Letrozole	Lubiprostone	Galsulfase
Clopidogrel	Anidulafungin	Fentanyl
Follitropin Alfa	Decitabine	Pegaptanib
Cetrorelix	Varenicline	Rotigotine
Tolterodine	Rasagiline	Alglucosidase alpha
Sertraline	Darunavir	Tigecycline
Solifenacin	Dasatinib	Timolol
Gabapentin	Avobenzone	Parathyroid hormone
Mozavaptane	Ecamsule	Clofarabine
Temozolomide	Octocrylene	Rimonabant
Interferon Beta-1a	Posaconazole	Entecavir
Entecavir	Biskalcitrate	Natalizumab
Bortezomib	Vorinostat	Sorafenib
Ropinirole	Sitagliptin	Sunitinib
Remifentanil	Ciclesonide	Dexrazoxane
Perflubutane	Telbivudine	Antithrombin alfa
Agalsidase Alfa	Kunecatechins	Sitaxentan
Laronidase	Paliperidone	Perflutren
	Alglucosidase alfa	Deferasirox
	Ranibizumab	Buprenorphine
	Idursulfase	Varenicline
	Panitumumab	Exenatide
		Dasatinib

In addition, regarding NMEs that have been approved in the last five years, we investigated the presence/absence of approvals and the times in the US and the EU, based on review reports of Japan. If the precedent approvals in other countries were described, we included those situations. Furthermore, we sought confirmation for UK medicines at the website of electronic Medicines Compendium Updates (http://www.medicines.org.uk/mcupdates/). In the tables, ingredients are presented using International Non-proprietary Names (INN).

3. NMEs that were Approved in 2006

The numbers of NMEs that were approved in 2006 in Japan, the US and the EU (EMEA) were 20, 24 and 25, respectively, showing no major differences (Table 1). Among them, there were no NMEs approved by all three regions in 2006; but entecavir was approved in both Japan and the EU, and 4 NMEs (sunitinib, varenicline, dasatinib and alglucosidase alfa) were approved in both the US and the EU.

4. Analysis of NMEs Approved in More than One Region and Precedent Approvals

Among the NMEs approved in Japan between 2002 and 2006 (including fixed combination drugs containing two NMEs), there were 70 ingredients that have been approved to date in the US or the EU; of which 69 were approved in the US, and 35 in the EU (Tables 2 and 3). On the other hand, there were 23 ingredients that were not approved in the EU but were approved in other countries including the UK. Of the 70 ingredients, only 3 received precedent approval in Japan: eletriptan, gefitinib and micafungin. The number of ingredients receiving precedent approval in the US was 57, and this included 42 ingredients that were approved before 2001. Inulin was approved in 1940 in the US and has been listed in the US Pharmacopeia, but is not sold in the US at present. Ten ingredients received precedent approval in the EU. Furthermore, there are 14 ingredients that were confirmed to have received precedent approval in countries other than the three regions: 6 ingredients in the UK, 2 each in France and Germany (among them, solifenacin was approved during the same period in both countries), and one each in Switzerland, New Zealand, Australia, the Netherlands, and Sweden.

On the other hand, there were 39 ingredients that were not approved in Japan but were approved in both the US and the EU between 2002 and 2006 (Tables 4 and 5). Of these 39 ingredients, those receiving precedent approvals numbered 28 in the US, and 11 in the EU.

Of the above 109 ingredients that were approved in two or three regions, those receiving precedent approval numbered 3 in Japan, 85 in the US, and 21 in the EU. If differences of 6 months or less in the timing of approval are regarded as simultaneous approvals, there were few simultaneously approved ingredients between Japan: 2 in 2003 in Japan and the US; and 1 in 2003, 2 in 2004, and 1 in 2006 in both Japan and the EU. On the other hand, for simultaneous approval in the US and the EU, the numbers were 6 before 2001, and then 2 in 2002, 5 in 2003, 6 in 2004, 1 in 2005, and 4 in 2006.

Table 2. NMEs approved in Japan and at least one other region (2002-2006)

NMEs	Japan	US	EU	Others*
Quinupristin/ Dalfopristin **	01/2002	09/1999	--	08/2002: UK
Infliximab	01/2002	08/1998	08/1999	--
Basiliximab	01/2002	05/1998	10/1998	--
Cladribine	01/2002	02/1993	04/2004	02/1995:UK
Risedronate	01/2002	03/1998	--	10/1999: UK
Palivizumab	01/2002	06/1998	08/1999	--
Gatifloxacin	04/2002	12/1999	--	--
Salmeterol	04/2002	02/1994	--	10/1996: UK
Eletriptan	04/2002	12/2002	--	02/2001:UK
Exemestane	07/2002	10/1999	--	12/1998: UK
Loratadine	07/2002	04/1993	--	09/2002: UK
Gefitinib	07/2002	05/2003	--	--
Esmolol	10/2002	12/1986	--	--
Ivermectin	10/2002	11/1996	--	--
Micafungin	10/2002	03/2005	--	--
Telmisartan	10/2002	11/1998	12/1998	--
Brinzolamide	10/2002	04/1998	03/2000	--
Sevelamer	01/2003	10/1998	01/2000	--
Leflunomide	04/2003	09/1998	--	07/1999: UK
Capecitabine	04/2003	04/1998	02/2001	--
Rizatriptan	07/2003	06/1998	--	06/1998: UK
Pramipexole	10/2003	07/1997	10/1997	--
Telithromycin	10/2003	04/2004	07/2001	--
Peginterferon Alfa-2a	10/2003	10/2002	6/2002	07/2001: Switzerland
Verteporfin	10/2003	04/2000	07/2000	--
Insulin glargine	10/2003	04/2000	06/2000	--
Atazanavir	12/2003	06/2003	03/2004	--
Dexmedetomidine	01/2004	12/1999	--	--
Raloxifene	01/2004	12/1997	--	07/2003: UK
Olmesartan	01/2004	04/2002	--	08/2002: Germany
Agalsidase Beta	01/2004	04/2003	--	--
Tenofovir	03/2004	10/2001	02/2002	--
Vardenafil	04/2004	08/2003	03/2003	--
Zoledronic Acid	10/2004	08/2001	04/2005	03/2003:UK
Tiotropium	10/2004	01/2004	--	05/2002:UK
Adefovir	10/2004	09/2002	03/2003	--
Peginterferon Alfa-2b	10/2004	01/2001	03/2000	--
Valganciclovir	11/2004	03/2001	--	04/2002: UK
Fosamprenavir	12/2004	10/2003	07/2004	--
Etanercept	01/2005	11/1998	02/2000	--
Rosuvastatin	01/2005	08/2003	--	03/2003:UK

NMEs	Japan	US	EU	Others*
Oxaliplatin	03/2005	08/2002	--	04/1998: France
Emtricitabine	03/2005	07/2003	10/2003	--
Bosentan	04/2005	11/2001	05/2002	--
Voriconazole	04/2005	05/2002	03/2002	--
Follitropin beta	04/2005	09/1997	05/1996	1995: New Zealand
Fludeoxyglucose(18F)	07/2005	1994	--	2002:UK
Gemtuzumab	07/2005	05/2000	--	--
Inulin	10/2005	1940	--	--
Finasteride	10/2005	06/1992	--	04/1992: Australia
Miglitol	10/2005	12/1996	--	07/1996: Netherland
Moxifloxacin	10/2005	12/1999	--	06/1999: Germany
Aripiprazole	01/2006	11/2002	06/2004	
Letrozole	01/2006	07/1997	--	11/1996:UK
Clopidogrel	01/2006	11/1997	07/1998	
Follitropin alpha	01/2006	09/1997	10/1995	
Cetrorelix	04/2006	08/2000	04/1999	
Tolterodine	04/2006	05/1998	--	09/1997: Sweden
Sertraline	04/2006	12/1991	--	
Solifenacin	04/2006	12/2004	--	12/2003: Germany, France
Gabapentin	07/2006	12/1993	--	11/2005: UK
Temozolomide	07/2006	08/1999	01/1999	
Interferon bera-1a	07/2006	05/1996	03/1997	
Entecavir	07/2006	03/2005	06/2006	
Bortezomib	10/2006	05/2003	04/2004	
Ropinirole	10/2006	09/1997	--	07/1996:UK
Remifentanil	10/2006	07/1996	--	10/1996:UK
Agalsidase alfa	10/2006	--	08/2001	
Laronidase	10/2006	04/2003	06/2003	

* Except for the drugs approved through EMEA centralized procedures.

** Combination drug.

Table 3. Number of approval and preceding drugs in Japan and other regions*

	Number of approval	Number of preceding drugs
Japan	70	3
US	69	57
EU	35	10

* Number of preceding drugs and NMEs approved in Japan and at least one other region in 2002 to 2006.

Table 4. NMEs approved solely in US and EU (2002-2006)

NMEs	US	EU
Nitisinone	01/2002	02/2005
Fulvestrant	04/2002	03/2004
Oxybate	07/2002	10/2005
Pegvisomant	03/2003	11/2002
Enfuvirtide	03/2003	05/2003
Aprepitant	03/2003	11/2003
Miglustat	07/2003	11/2002
Palonosetron	07/2003	03/2005
Daptomycin	09/2003	01/2006
Memantine	10/2003	05/2002
Tadalafil	11/2003	11/2002
Bevacizumab	02/2004	01/2005
Cetuximab	02/2004	06/2004
Pemetrexed	02/2004	09/2004
Cinacalcet	03/2004	10/2004
Insulin glulisine	04/2004	09/2004
Duloxetine	08/2004	12/2004
Erlotinib	11/2004	09/2005
Natalizumab	11/2004	06/2006
Iloprost	12/2004	09/2003
Pregabalin	12/2004	07/2004
Darifenacine	12/2004	10/2004
Ziconotide	12/2004	02/2005
Palifermin	12/2004	10/2005
Pegaptanib	12/2004	01/2006
Clofarabine	12/2004	05/2006
Exenatide	04/2005	11/2006
Galsulfase	05/2005	01/2006
Insulin Detemir	06/2005	06/2004
Tripranavir	06/2005	10/2005
Tigecycline	06/2005	04/2006
Deferasirox	11/2005	08/2006
Sorafenib	12/2005	07/2006
Sunitinib	01/2006	07/2006
Alglucosidase alpha	04/2006	03/2006
Rasagiline	05/2006	02/2005
Varenicline	05/2006	09/2006
Dasatinib	06/2006	11/2006
Posaconazole	09/2006	10/2005

Table 5. Number of approval and preceding drugs in US and EU*

Year of approval	Number of approval in US	US preceding	EU preceding
2002	3	3	0
2003	8	4	4
2004	15	12	3
2005	7	6	1
2006	6	3	3
Total	39	28	11

* Number of preceding drugs and NMEs approved solely in US and EU (2002-2006).

Conclusion

For the year 2006, there were no major differences in the number of approvals among the three regions. On the other hand, the analysis of NMEs approved in the three regions between 2002 and 2006 showed that the number judged to have been simultaneously approved in both Japan and the US or the EU was only 6, in contrast to 18 ingredients approved in both the US and the EU. In this study, the evaluation for the EU included only those ingredients approved by the Centralized Approval Process by the EMEA, and hence did not include individual ingredients approved by each country's government or by the Mutual Recognition Procedure in the EU region. As a consequence, the number of approved ingredients may have been reduced; though new ingredients that have already been used in the EU region but approved for the first time by the EMEA for brand new indications such as orphans may have been counted in the annual number of approvals. In the investigation performed previously to review the period between 2000 and August 2004 [1], it was shown that among 105 ingredients approved in the US, the average review periods for 21 ingredients approved in both Japan and the US were 18.2 months and 19.0 months, respectively, not significantly different, despite 82 ingredients were not approved in Japan at that time. This result may suggest that there are many cases in which a drug marketed in Western countries is introduced to Japan after effectiveness, safety have been confirmed. In the US, as the review system has been strengthened by the Prescription Drug User Fee Act, new drugs have received precedent approval, thereby allowing the public to benefit from the newest medical advances [2]. However, it has been pointed out that people are initially exposed to risks, and this analysis also confirmed that observation. In Japan, there is increasing concern about promptly providing necessary drugs to clinical practitioners in terms of enhancing both medical care and economy. Japan established the Pharmaceuticals and Medical Devices Agency in 2004 to strength the review system. Furthermore, numerous proposals have been made regarding strengthening of the review system and expediting the review process in the "New Health Frontier Strategy (Eminent Persons Meeting on New Health Frontier Strategy, April 18, 2007)," the "5-Year Strategy for Innovative Pharmaceuticals and Medical Devices Creation (Ministry of Education, Culture, Sports, Science and Technology; Ministry of Health, Labour and Welfare; and Ministry of Economy, Trade and Industry, April 26, 2007)", Innovation 25 (promulgated at a Cabinet meeting, June 01, 2007), the Basic Policies for Economic and Fiscal Reform 2007 (Council on Economic and Fiscal Policy, June 19, 2007),

The Report of the Study Group on promptly providing safe and effective drugs (Ministry of Health, Labor and Welfare, July 27, 2007) , etc. However, we must consider not only the review time, but also the necessity of striving for promotion of development stages leading up to the approval application that involves improving the environments of clinical studies designed to promote participation and competition in simultaneous global developments.

References

[1] Saito M, Hirata-Koizumi M, Miyake S, Hasegawa R. Comparison of approval times for new prescription drugs in Japan and USA. *Proceedings of the 125th Annual Meeting of the Pharmaceutical Society of Japan,* 4,218 (2005).

[2] Berndt ER, Gottschalk AH, Philipson TJ, Strobeck MW., Industry funding of the FDA: effects of PDUFA on approval times and withdrawal rates. *Nat Rev Drug Discov.*, 4, 545-554 (2005).

In: Drugs: Approval and Evaluation, Delivery and Control
Editors: A.O. Hartmann, L.K. Neumann
ISBN: 978-1-60456-533-1

Chapter 7

GLOBAL CONTROL OF TUBERCULOSIS AND NEW DRUGS: PUBLIC HEALTH ASPECTS OF NEW DRUG DEVELOPMENT FOR TUBERCULOSIS

Donald A. Enarson
International Union Against Tuberculosis and Lung Disease, Paris, France

The public health strategy to conquer tuberculosis is focused on primary prevention. Normally with an infectious disease, this would entail the use of a vaccine but, in the case of tuberculosis, the vaccine currently available acts as secondary prevention: it does not prevent infection but rather, prevents progress from infection to disease during the phase of dissemination following primary infection. Consequently, the approach to primary prevention differs for tuberculosis as compared with other infectious diseases; focus on the 'control' of the patients who are the most potent sources of transmission of the contagion. In order to understand this focus, and its difference from other infectious diseases, it would be important to understand the sequence of events that leads to disease with tuberculosis and to transmission of its causative organism, *Mycobacterium tuberculosis* and the role of various interventions in cutting this 'chain of transmission'.

To describe this 'chain of transmission', a transition model has been outlined [1], based on previous mathematical modeling exercises [2] identifying the priorities in the fight against tuberculosis. The role of drugs in this fight is clear from this model. The transitions of relevance to primary prevention are those that occur prior to infection. This includes the transition from susceptibility to exposure and the transition from exposure to infection. Normally, a vaccine functions to prevent the latter transition, from exposure to infection. With respect to the current vaccine, it acts on the transition from infection to illness, limiting the dissemination of bacilli from the primary site of infection, and preventing secondary foci (from which most adult-type cases arise) from developing. Incidentally, it also prevents those severe forms of tuberculosis associated with this phase of the pathogenesis, disseminated tuberculosis and tuberculous meningitis, forms that are particularly common in the young infant whose immunity is not yet well developed.

In the absence of a vaccine that provides primary prevention, the focus shifts to avoidance / reduction in exposure to the causative organism, *Mycobacterium tuberculosis*. This aims at

- Diminishing the number of cases in the community, thus reducing the probability of contact;
- Reducing the duration of infectiousness of the individual case, thus reducing the total 'vector' of contagion.

Thus, the transition upon which this primary prevention acts is that between susceptibility and exposure. Effective drug treatment of tuberculosis accomplishes both of these aims. When the treatment is applied systematically and carefully, the prevalence of cases declines, followed by a decline in infection of susceptible members of the population (in most communities, composed of young children) [3 4 5] This, in turn, leads to the objective of tuberculosis control, a generation free of tuberculous infection.

Drug treatment also reduces the duration of infectiousness of the individual case by rapidly reducing the viable population of bacilli in the most highly infectious cases of tuberculosis [6]. The most potent transmitter among all cases is the case of tuberculosis that is sputum smear positive [7] and particularly the case with a high bacterial count (often accompanied with cavities in the lungs). For this reason, the case of pulmonary tuberculosis that is smear positive is the case that has the highest priority in tuberculosis control. Consequently, every effort must be made to ensure that the treatment given is effective the first time it is given as, should the patient remain, or become again, sputum smear positive, not only does this increase the prevalence of the most contagious cases [8] but it also renders the case more difficult to cure and promotes transmission of the disease in the community [9].

Do we Need New Drugs?

The promise of new drugs, just over the horizon, is something that the professional community has been living with for decades. In 1985, O'Brien and Snider [10] editorialized that the demonstration of the ability of a new drug, ofloxacin, to act against tuberculosis augured well for the immediate development of new tools for the treatment of tuberculosis. Thirteen years later, in 1998, O'Brien and Vernon [11] reflected on this misplaced 'optimism' and identified a series of technical issues that required attention in moving forward with new tools development. This analysis, by focusing on relatively straightforward technical issues that could be rather easily addressed if there was great momentum in the community for development of new drugs, side stepped the larger issues facing the progress in developing new treatment for tuberculosis. This chapter will try to identify some of these larger issues.

The Limited Options Presently Available

It has often been stated that 'we have all the tools we need to control tuberculosis; what we need now is to apply them'. There are many aspects of this statement that are true and it emphasizes that much more could be done than is being done at present to reduce avoidable suffering and death due to tuberculosis. In another sense, this is not a true statement.

While we have a group of drugs (principally six drugs – isoniazid, rifampin, pyrazinamide, ethambutol, streptomycin and thioacetazone) that, used in correct combinations and applied according to standardized principals, can cure the vast majority of tuberculosis patients, this group of drugs will not be sufficient in future to fully control, and eventually eliminate, tuberculosis. Each of these drugs has been available for over twenty-five years and all have been widely used. No new drug of equal potency has been introduced into general use over this period of time. Moreover, at least one of these drugs (thioacetazone) is disappearing from the market and is no longer widely used. Another (streptomycin) is often avoided and was, for a time, very difficult to obtain in the private market. This steady erosion of available armaments developed in the third quarter of the twentieth century is a cause of major concern when viewed in light of the progress in developments of new drugs over the recent past.

The Threat of Drug Resistance

One of the most important limitations of a treatment-based strategy for control and prevention of an illness is the virtual inevitability of the development of drug resistance. The emergence of clinically significant drug resistance was noted since the first drugs were used in the treatment of tuberculosis [3]. This led many to believe that drug treatment would probably never be successful in the total eradication of the bacilli, even in the individual patient. It was only after the demonstration of the effectiveness of multidrug treatment that emphasis was placed on treatment as a means to permanently cure the individual patient. Indeed, many investigators from the United States of America (principally among them, Edith Lincoln, a physician caring for children with tuberculosis) viewed the major role of drug treatment as that for secondary prevention (preventing the development of disease once the individual was infected) [12].This led to a programme of research into 'preventive chemotherapy' [13] that has been a remarkably productive line of research in the United States to the present day and explains the particular focus of investigators from that country on the utility of this approach in the fight against tuberculosis.

Resistance to the drugs used for the treatment of tuberculosis is a natural phenomenon and is present in all large populations of *Mycobacterium tuberculosis*. It is due to natural mutations in the genes of the bacillus that occur at a well-defined rate. Thus, for example, in any population of 10^6 bacilli, there will be one bacillus naturally resistant to one of the medications commonly used for the treatment of tuberculosis. The population of bacilli in a case of cavitary pulmonary tuberculosis is estimated to be between 10^6 and 10^{12}. Consequently, in any case of this nature, there will be naturally resistant bacilli. This is one of the reasons why such cases are a particular priority in tuberculosis control because, if they are not treated carefully, this natural resistance will become clinically significant.

What is clinically significant drug resistance and how does it appear? Clinically significant drug resistance is that in which a high proportion of a bacterial population is resistant to at least one of the drugs routinely used for the treatment of tuberculosis. This occurs when, due to incorrect treatment, the bacteria that are susceptible to the drug are killed and those resistant are preserved, expanding to occupy the biological space left by the drug-sensitive population. This results in the high proportion of the bacterial population resistant to this drug. When such a drug-resistant population predominates, it becomes the 'engine' of the disease and carries its drug-resistance characteristic when it is transmitted to cause infection (and subsequent disease) in another individual. The patient developing a population of bacilli resistant to the medication improperly used is said to harbor 'acquired' drug resistance. When those drug-resistant organisms infect another individual who then goes on to develop disease, the patient with the resultant disease is said to harbor 'primary' drug resistance.

Acquired drug resistance, therefore, is the first step in the process of development of primary drug resistance. This frequently results when treatment is given without standardization, i.e. is individualized, based on the choice of the caregiver or the patient, and it is not carefully followed. Emergence of acquired drug resistance followed, in many locations, some years after the introduction and extensive use of isoniazid throughout the world; this was followed by the appearance of primary drug resistance in these locations [14]. Although inadequate treatment has been clearly seen, since the very first period of its use, to lead to acquired drug resistance in a very short period (within one month) in individual patients [15], its documentation as acquired drug resistance in a group of patients takes much longer and as primary drug resistance even longer. For example, while isoniazid was introduced into routine practice in the late 1950s and early 1960s, it was not until the mid 1970s that extensive primary isoniazid resistance was widely recognized. Similarly, rifampin was routinely used in many locations starting in the mid 1970s. It was not until the late 1980s that the problem posed by resistance to both isoniazid and rifampin was generally recognized. Thus, the period of time from initial misuse of medications until the recognition of the resulting primary resistance to these same medications is typically a decade and a half. What we are measuring today, as primary drug resistance, is due to the mistakes we have made several decades ago.

In spite of the presence of drug resistance to any one of these drugs, some clinical trials experts have suggested that patients can still be successfully treated in most instances [16]. Why, then, should we have any concern about this issue? Multidrug-resistance is said to be present when the organisms causing tuberculosis in an individual patient are resistant to at least both isoniazid and rifampin. When a patient has disease due to multidrug-resistant organisms, such a patient is very difficult to treat. The treatment must be prolonged from so-called 'short-course' treatment of a minimum of six months to prolonged treatment of a minimum of eighteen months [17]. Moreover, many of the drugs used in this treatment are notoriously difficult for the patient to tolerate, with the consequence that the treatment regimen may be frequently changed or the patient may refuse to continue the medication. Even when the medication is tolerated and taken, the outcome of treatment is disappointing.

Scientific evaluation of the outcome of treatment of multidrug-resistant tuberculosis remains very limited. Clinical trials are widely accepted as the 'gold standard' for the scientific evaluation of drug treatment for any disease. Up to the present moment, there are no published reports of any clinical trials for the evaluation of treatment of multidrug-resistant tuberculosis. Secondary evidence has been published and this is the only information currently available for evaluation. This consists of two types of evidence: routine evaluation of series of patients treated in selected institutions (clinical series) and systematic evaluation of all cases in a given location (community series). For the evaluation of the outcome of treatment in either a clinical series or in a community series, the generally accepted approach is to undertake evaluation of treatment by 'cohort evaluation'. The principle behind cohort evaluation is that all cases entered into a series (whether 'clinical' or 'community') must be accounted for and that the proportions presented as 'outcomes' are calculated based on the total 'population at risk'. Using this principle, the outcome of treatment of multidrug-resistant tuberculosis is substantially less satisfactory as compared with the outcome of treatment of patients with drug-susceptible tuberculosis [18]. This is common knowledge to all those who care for such patients.

In spite of this, the majority of all patients in all locations at the present time are not multidrug-resistant cases, even in the 'hot spots' of multidrug-resistance. How, then, does this pose a risk to the control of tuberculosis? We need only remind ourselves that what we are measuring today is what has occurred in the past and that to understand what is happening currently will take some years, using current methods of analysis.

Do we need new drugs? I would suggest that the answer to this question is yes! If we do not have new drugs in the next few years, we will begin to lose the battle against tuberculosis.

The Limitations of Current Treatment

A major challenge to successful treatment is the fact that current treatment is not 'user friendly'. It is neither friendly to the 'consumer' (the patient) nor to the 'merchant' (the health care provider). The current standard regimens recommended for the treatment of drug-susceptible tuberculosis is termed 'short-course' chemotherapy. This treatment requires a minimum of six months of treatment. This can, by no stretch of the imagination, be seriously termed 'short'.

The prolonged duration of treatment has several negative aspects. The first negative aspect is the cost this implies. Many have the impression that tuberculosis treatment is free-of-charge. This is a misconception. While the drugs may be provided without cost to the patient, the treatment requires major financial and social investment from the patient, the family and the community. In addition, the prolonged duration of commitment to attendance and pill taking behavior is a major obstacle to successful treatment and represents an inordinate demand on an individual (and community) that is already stressed by the impact of ill health and its environment of poverty. The impact of these constraints on adherence among patients is well understood by behavioral scientists.

What is less well understood is what are the constraints this imposes on the health care provider? Health services are focused more on the provision of direct, time-limited and incident-responsive activities. Their ability to provide services that require prolonged commitment to, often repetitive, activities is less successful. Tuberculosis, along with asthma, diabetes mellitus and other similar 'chronic' disease are prime examples. Maintaining adherence to such a prolonged commitment requires a rather intensive investment in quality assurance activities, prime among which is treatment support, supervision and monitoring. Ensuring that these activities continue over months and years is exceedingly complex. As political commitment wanes and as constraints are imposed on financial and human resources, the first casualty is usually these quality assurance activities. While these components have been at the core of the reform of tuberculosis services represented by the current global strategy, these are the components that are currently at greatest risk. These complex requirements are, to a large extent, mandated by the need for prolonged treatment required by the medications presently used for treatment of tuberculosis. Thus, if we are to make major strides in the care of tuberculosis patients and in the prevention of transmission of the causative organism, we will need drugs that allow treatment that is truly 'short-course' (not more than ten days in duration). Will this be possible?

Current Strengths we Can Harness in our Fight to Conquer Tuberculosis

The main strength we have historically enjoyed in the fight against tuberculosis has been the nature of the bacillus and its interaction with the human host.

Mycobacterium tuberculosis could be termed 'the lazy bacillus'. What is the background to this rather odd description? In order for a contagious disease to maintain equilibrium in the ecological niche in which it finds itself, each contagious case of the disease must produce, at a minimum, one other contagious case. Failure to do this will result in the natural decline and eventual disappearance of the pathogen. This observation lies at the base of the observed trends of tuberculosis in human populations over the centuries in which the disease has been tracked.

'Natural' Trend in Tuberculosis

It is clear that tuberculosis has been declining in Western Europe at least since the middle of the eighteenth century [19]. Generally reliable records from several major cities in Europe (London, Stockholm, Hamburg) have demonstrated a steady decline in deaths from tuberculosis since that time. These data have been supplemented with many others from all over Europe, North America and some places in Asia, showing a steady and progressive decline in the disease before there was any specific intervention available against the disease. This decline was more recently documented, using estimates of disease trend derived from tuberculin surveys, in multiple locations around the globe, including many low-income countries. This steady decline has been explained by a general improvement in nutrition, hygiene and standard of living [20] said to have occurred globally over the past century. This, however, is unlikely because similar trends have been observed in many different places, including places with very different socioeconomic characteristics. What is much more likely is that the transmission of tuberculosis has changed because of societal changes related to predictors of exposure.

This is best illustrated by examining two factors. The first is the size of the family. The number of individuals sharing the same living space has changed considerably in many locations and this change has been greatest in relation to intergenerational interaction. Secondly, the size of the dwelling, particularly in those locations where people are most likely to be enclosed in a poorly ventilated space, has changed a great deal. This is especially true of temperate and sub-arctic locations where people might be likely to spend long periods of time in an enclosed and poorly ventilated space. This is much less likely to have any effect in subtropical and tropical locations where people are more likely to spend more time out-of-doors or where doors and windows might be more likely to be left open, encouraging ventilation.

The 'natural' tendency for tuberculosis to decline has been one of the most important aspects to encourage a move toward control of the disease.

'Vector' of Transmission

A second factor in favor of actions to control and eliminate tuberculosis is the low degree of infectiousness of tuberculosis. Some infectious agents (measles, for example) are highly infectious. If a susceptible host is exposed to the agent, virtually one hundred per cent of such hosts will become infected by the agent and will develop disease as a result of this infection. This is not the case with respect to tuberculosis. Several large studies [7 21] have demonstrated clearly that, given exposure to *Mycobacterium tuberculosis*, only a minority of individuals become infected. Thus, for example, in the large study of contacts of cases of active pulmonary tuberculosis in Canada, even among those with prolonged and intensive contact with cases of pulmonary tuberculosis with high bacterial loads (sputum smear-positive cases) only a minority of individuals became infected by this contact. Moreover, among those who become infected with *M. tuberculosis*, when they have intact immune systems, only a minority go on to develop disease at some point in their life time [22 23]. From these large studies, an estimate can be made of the probability of transition from exposure to infection (approximately one in six individuals) and from infection to disease (approximately one in six individuals). This represents a combined probability of one in thirty-six individuals who makes the full transition from exposure to disease. Possibly as many as three-quarters of these individuals, in situations where no specific interventions are applied, might be the most highly infectious, sputum smear-positive cases, which means that overall, the transition from exposure to contagious disease is one in forty-eight. The consequence of this is that it is necessary to infect as many as forty-eight individuals in order to maintain the same burden of disease.

This 'transition probability' explains why the bacillus can be considered 'lazy' and why it requires more than simply the host and the agent to maintain the disease in the community. Components of the 'more' that are required include the conditions of poverty (principally overcrowding) and factors that impair immunity (most notably infection with the human immunodeficiency virus). Other factors that are undoubtedly important are long delays in diagnosis (where access to health services is limited or diagnostic suspicion is low [24]), large numbers of susceptible individuals exposed (as in residential care facilities) and where cases are very difficult to cure (as with multidrug-resistant tuberculosis).

Political Mobilization

Another strength that has emerged in recent years is an increasing awareness and commitment to the global fight against tuberculosis. Interest in this subject steadily waned after the introduction of effective therapy in the 1960s until the disease had virtually disappeared from the international agenda by the end of the 1980s, when the staff of the World Health Organization (WHO) dedicated to this work was a single individual. Since 1990, increasing attention has been given to tuberculosis, due to efforts of the WHO, the World Bank and then other structures of the international community, such as the G8 group of industrialized nations. This has led to a conclusion that efforts to address key diseases (HIV / AIDS, tuberculosis and malaria) are an important component of fighting poverty. This has led to mobilization of substantial resources that need to be directed strategically and should be focused on 'new tools'.

Gaps / Challenges where Novel Strategies May Be Desirable / Required to Enable Elimination

While we have certain advantages in the fight against tuberculosis, there are also many challenges that call for new approaches and new tools. These are not presently addressed by either the current strategy or available tools and constitute a serious block to further progress in the fight against tuberculosis.

Latency

Unlike many other infectious diseases, the pathogenesis of tuberculosis comprises a concept of latency. That is to say, as we have previously described, only a small minority of individuals infected with *M. tuberculosis* under usual circumstances ever develop the disease in their lifetime. However, they continue to experience a risk of disease for many years and even decades after having become infected [24] and often carry this risk throughout their entire lifetime. The full characteristics and mechanisms by which this occurs are not well understood. Indeed, while innovative studies had been undertaken in the 1920s to investigate the phenomenon [26], the unequivocal demonstration of these 'latent' bacilli is a relatively recent phenomenon [27], while the mechanism whereby they retain their dormant state is not understood at all. This phenomenon is the most likely explanation for why treatment duration remains so long (in spite of the use of the term 'short-course' chemotherapy for treatment requiring a minimum of six months) and why there is a need for the 'continuation' phase of treatment. Moreover, when treatment is given to individuals to treat latent infection (where the bacilli targeted are these 'dormant' microbes), the optimal duration of treatment is even longer (estimated to be nine months [28]). To achieve significant advances in the treatment of tuberculosis will require an approach that directly confronts the issue of 'latency' or 'dormancy'. Clearly six- or nine-month treatment is totally impractical and unacceptable as a final approach to the elimination of tuberculosis. Improvements will necessitate either 'awakening' these dormant bacilli to enable the drugs to attack the metabolically active processes of the microbes, or finding mechanisms to kill them without targeting metabolic processes. This is a major challenge and calls for entirely new paradigms in therapeutics.

Limitations in Efficiency of Clinical Trials

This issue must also be addressed in the evaluation of treatment of tuberculosis. A key challenge in demonstrating advances in treatment of tuberculosis is the prolonged period required for assessing new treatments in clinical trials. The 'usual' period for evaluating a proposed new treatment is a minimum of five years from conception of the new approach until its demonstration. A large proportion of the time required is the duration of the treatment and the need for prolonged follow up to detect relapse (a minimum of two years which, if added to the duration of treatment – at least six months to compare with the current gold standard – and the recruitment period – often at least another six months – amounts to a total of a minimum of three years). The poor progress that has been made in identifying 'surrogate markers' is a major challenge to any progress.

Challenge of HIV

All of these issues are present in the absence of the human immunodeficiency virus (HIV). There is mounting evidence [29 30] that all issues related to the treatment of tuberculosis change in the presence of HIV. It is clear that the timetable and process of pathogenesis is dramatically altered. Instead of a long period of time and a low probability of progression in the transitions in the pathogenesis of tuberculosis, the period from and probability of transition from infection to disease is dramatically altered [31]. This alteration, in turn and by definition, shortens the timeline for the appearance of drug resistance, if by no other means, by the rapid progression from infection to disease, thereby increasing the proportion of cases of tuberculosis that are due to recent infection/reinfection. The introduction of anti-retroviral treatments may go a long way to addressing the impact of HIV by reconstituting the immune function and thereby reducing the risk / rate of progression of disease. However, implementing this treatment in a whole community and to all the persons who need it will be a major challenge. Moreover, even if this treatment is widely given, eventually it will fail as it does not cure but only prolongs / suppresses the disease.

Evolving Genotype

The evolving genotype profile of the tuberculosis epidemic must also be considered as we reflect on the development of new tools for the elimination of tuberculosis. The changing pattern of tuberculosis observed in a variety of populations has been putatively explained by selection of the genetic characteristics of the human host [32], although evidence supporting this hypothesis is non-existent. That it can occur has been demonstrated in other infectious diseases. What is clear is that the genotype profile of the parasite (*M. tuberculosis*) is changing. The identification of the W-Beijing strain associated with outbreaks of tuberculosis in the United States [33] has been documented in other locations [34] where the association of large clusters with drug-resistant organisms has suggested an ecological advantage of the genetic mutations and a change in the characteristics of pathogenesis associated with this genotype. This variant profile is further illustrated by poorer vaccination protection in individuals exposed to the W-Beijing strain [35]. Its strong association with drug resistance further promotes its spread in the community [36]. Will this shift in genetic profile of the tuberculosis epidemic be accompanied by other changes in the pathogenesis of the disease and, thus in the responses to interventions? This question needs to be seriously addressed as we move forward in developing new approaches to treatment and control.

The challenge posed by drug resistance in the treatment of tuberculosis has already been discussed. What has not been discussed is the need to develop innovative approaches to treatment that avoid the (inevitable and inherent) problem of drug resistance. Current treatment methods, as noted above, are all associated with selection of inherent, genetic modifications that render the microbes naturally resistant to the chemicals used for treatment. Are there treatment modalities that can avoid this entirely? This is a key question and one that, if answered affirmatively, would represent a major step forward in the treatment of tuberculosis and its eventual elimination. Clearly the answer to this question does not lie in the current base of knowledge and research that is available. Are there clues from other disciplines / domains? If so, they need to be exploited as a matter of urgency.

Hurdles to Overcome in Development and Application of New Therapy

Even if it is recognized that there is a need for new tools for treatment of tuberculosis and that new strategies are required, developing them and applying them will not be straightforward. A number of issues need to be addressed in carrying innovation to implementation.

Economic Hurdles

Current approaches to the development of new treatments for any disease depend on a demonstrable economic benefit for those engaged in these developments. The preferred approach to advance new therapy is the engagement of the private sector in developing the new tools that are needed. The risks and costs inherent in such activities are enormous. Careful planning is necessary to maintain market advantage of a private concern. Thus, priorities for new developments must be market-driven. The fact that tuberculosis is a disease mainly of the economically marginalized is an important factor in maintaining a low priority for new tools development to deal with it. Even in wealthy communities, those most likely to be affected are those with the least access to resources. Moreover, it is entirely possible that the policy of services free-of-charge for tuberculosis patients, which has been the tradition for many decades, may actually impede efforts to mainstream tuberculosis services and to develop new tools to deal with it. Because this is such a 'sacred cow' within the community committed to the fight against tuberculosis, it has not been sufficiently critically analyzed.

Dependence on Service Provision

Another hurdle or obstacle to advances in the fight against tuberculosis is the constraints of a strategy for disease control / elimination that is highly dependent on service provision. Where elimination strategies have been most successful [37], they have been based on actions that do not require the long-term commitments to maintaining, in perpetuity, general services in all communities of the world. The successful fight against smallpox was dependent on a highly efficient, but relatively short-term and focused, provision of vaccination services. The fight against tuberculosis is highly dependent on the quality and sustainability of routine health services in increasingly more inaccessible, marginalized and unstable areas of the globe. Establishing and maintaining high quality services in all locations is difficult, if not impossible. That is why, even with new medications, it will be difficult to maintain diagnostic and treatment services for at least a whole generation. Even in rich countries, this has been a major challenge where decline in the quality of the services to the poor and marginalized is associated with a rise in burden of disease [38]. Moreover, political instability and conflict is also a major factor mitigating against advances in the fight against tuberculosis when this is dependent on long-term service provision [39].

Necessity of Long-Term Political Engagement

Stimulating action for control of tuberculosis is essential but not easy. One of the greatest challenges, but one of the essential components in successful action, is political commitment on the part of decision-makers and community leaders. That is why this is one of the first planks in the currently recommended global strategy to fight tuberculosis [40]. Recent emphasis on fighting disease as a means of fighting poverty (most clearly demonstrated by the Global Fund for AIDS, Tuberculosis and Malaria) is encouraging. However, it is not clear if this kind of commitment can be sustained. A major argument for investment in the fight against tuberculosis has been the proposal that tuberculosis has a major economic impact due to the fact that those affected are primarily in the economically-productive age group and that investment in such services is among the most cost-efficient of any investment in health [41]. Added to this is the argument that even short-term but effective investment could 'ratchet down' the burden of disease. However, these arguments are being eroded by the reversals associated with the epidemic of HIV / AIDS. In addition, as the 'easy returns' on investment are realized, it will take increasing investment with lower returns to make further progress and this may be difficult to sustain.

Professional Conservatism

In addition to the other hurdles that need to be addressed, there is one that is somewhat unexpected: professional conservatism. Tuberculosis has traditionally been recognized as a public health challenge. The medical care provided for a disease within a public health context virtually always includes a package of 'standard case management'. In respect to tuberculosis, standardization of care has been a key to quality improvement and to achieving the goals associated with a disease control and elimination strategy. The harm caused to the fight against tuberculosis by anarchic, individualized approaches to treatment have been clearly demonstrated [8] and the systematization of care recommended for tuberculosis patients has been a key to virtually all advances made against the disease, from the very start of the organized campaigns [42]. The systematic development and definition of standard treatment regimens for tuberculosis has been a key to modern care [43]. While individual clinicians are often quick to pick up and adopt new tools for the management of their patients, the adoption of new developments into packages of standard case management takes a great deal longer. For example, while the efficacy of 6-month regimens for the treatment of tuberculosis was demonstrated in 1972 [44], they were not formally adopted as standard treatment until many years later in most countries. For example, in British Columbia in Canada, they were only accepted as standard treatment ten years later. This is a common occurrence in definition of standard case management for public health practice. The development and demonstration of efficacy of new drugs and therapies for tuberculosis will need to be picked up and adopted as standard practice within public health definitions of standard case management. The history of doing so for past innovations illustrates the need for clearly defined mechanisms whereby this can be achieved more efficiently.

Conclusion

It is clear that we need new drugs: not ten years from now, but tomorrow. The drugs available to us for routine treatment of new patients are actually fewer than they were twenty-five years ago, and we are having an increasing number of patients whose disease is very difficult, if not impossible to cure. There is no question that, for the immediate future, the number of tuberculosis patients and the number multidrug-resistant will increase rather than decline.

The new drugs we need cannot be like the old ones that we have had. They must be more efficient, being recommended for much shorter periods (preferably days rather than months). Moreover, we must immediately embark on a systematic evaluation, through a program of clinical trials, of drugs being currently used, and those going to be introduced for the treatment of multidrug-resistant tuberculosis. We have to, as a matter of high priority, improve the efficiency of our methods of evaluation of efficacy of drugs through clinical trials.

In parallel to the program of new drugs development, we must also evaluate and improve our methods of assessing evidence and introducing it into policy. Finally, we must, as a matter of the highest priority, and for the security of the whole world, commit ourselves fully and wholeheartedly to the implementation of what we know and of what we newly develop.

References

[1] Enarson DA, Ait-Khaled N. Tuberculosis. In: Annesi-Maesano I, Gulsvik A, Viegi G, ed. Respiratory Epidemiology in Europe. *Eur Respir Mon* 2000; 15: 67-91.

[2] Waaler HT, Piot MA. The use of an epidemiological model for estimating the effectiveness for tuberculosis control measures. Sensitivity of the effectiveness of tuberculosis control measures to the coverage of the population. *Bull Wld Health Org* 1969; 41: 75-93.

[3] Crofton J. The contribution of treatment to the prevention of tuberculosis. *Bull Int Union Tuberc* 1962; 32: 6.43-653.

[4] Zhang L-X, Tu D-H, He G-X, Ma Z-Q, Nagelkerke NJ, Borgdorff MW, Enarson DA, Broekmans JF. Risk of Tuberculosis Infection and Tuberculous Meningitis after

Discontinuation of Bacillus Calmette-Guerin in Beijing. *Am J Respir Crit Care Med* 2000; 162; 1314-1317.
[5] Zhang L-X, Tu D-H, Enarson DA. The impact of directly-observed treatment on the epidemiology of tuberculosis in Beijing. *Int J Tuberc Lung Dis* 2000; 4: 904-910.
[6] Jindani A, Aber VR, Edwards EA, Mitchison DA. The early bactericidal activity of drugs in patients with pulmonary tuberculosis. *Am Rev Respir Dis* 1980; 121: 939-949.
[7] Grzybowski S Barnet GD, Styblo K. Contacts of cases of active pulmonary tuberculosis. *Bull Int Union Tuberc* 1975; 50: 90-106.
[8] Grzybowski S, Enarson DA. The fate of cases of pulmonary tuberculosis under various treatment programmes. *Bull Int Union Tuberc* 1978; 53: 70-75.
[9] Schulzer M, Enarson DA, Grzybowski S, Hong JP, Kim SJ, Lin TP. An analysis of tuberculosis data in Taiwan and Korea. *Int J Epidemiol* 1987; 16: 584-589.
[10] O'Brien RJ, Vernon AA. New tuberculosis drug development: how can we do better? *Am J Respir Crit Care Med* 1998; 157: 1705-1707.
[11] O'Brien RJ, Snider DE. Tuberculosis drugs – old and new. *Am Rev Respir Dis* 1985; 131: 309-311.
[12] Lincoln EM. The effect of antimicrobial therapy on the prognosis of primary tuberculosis in children. *Am Rev Tuberc* 1954; 69: 682-689.
[13] Ferebee SH. Controlled chemoprophylaxis trials in tuberculosis. a general review. *Adv Tuberc Res* 1969; 17: 28-106.
[14] Kleeberg HH, Olivier MS. *A World Atlas of Initial Drug Resistance.* 2nd ed. Pretoria: Tuberculosis Research Institute of South African Medical Research Council. 1984.
[15] British Medical Research Council. Streptomycin treatment of pulmonary tuberculosis. A Medical Research Council Investigation. *Brit Med J* 1948; 2: 769-783.
[16] Mitchison DA, Nunn AJ. Influence of initial drug resistance on the response to short-course chemotherapy of pulmonary tuberculosis. *Am Rev Respir Dis* 1986; 133: 423-430.
[17] World Health Organization. Guidelines for the Management of Drug-Resistant Tuberculosis. *WHO-TB*-96.210. 1997: pp48.
[18] Schaaf HS, Botha P, Beyers N, Gie RP, Vermeulen HAS, Groenewald P, Coetzee GJ, Donald PR. The 5-year outcome of multidrug resistant tuberculosis patients in Cape Province of South Africa. *Trop Med Int Health* 1996; 1: 718-722.
[19] Grigg ERN. The arcana of tuberculosis. With a brief epidemiologic history of the disease in the USA. *Am Rev Tuberc* 1958; 78: 426-453.
[20] McKeown T, Record RG. Reasons for the decline of mortality in England and Wales during the nineteenth century. *Popul Studies* 1962; 16: 94-122.
[21] Shaw JB, Wynn-Williams N. Infectivity of pulmonary tuberculosis in relation to sputum status. *Am Rev Tuberc* 1954; 69: 724-732.
[22] D'Arcy Hart P, Sutherland I. Final report of the Medical Research Council by its Tuberculosis Vaccines Clinical Trials Committee. BCG and vole bacillus vaccines in the prevention of tuberculosis in adolescence and early adult life. *Brit Med J.* 1977; ii: 293-295.
[23] Ferebee SH, Mount FW. Tuberculosis morbidity in a controlled trial of the prophylactic use of isoniazid among household contacts. *Am Rev Respir Dis* 1962; 85: 490-521.
[24] Xie HJ, Enarson DA, Chao CW, Allen EA, Grzybowski S. Deaths in tuberculosis patients in British Columbia, 1980-1984. *Tuber Lung Dis* 1992; 73: 77-82.

[25] Enarson DA, Sjogren I, Grzybowski S. Incidence of tuberculosis among Scandinavian immigrants in Canada. *Eur J Respir Dis* 1980; 61: 139-14.

[26] Opie EL, Aronson JD. Tubercle bacilli in latent tuberculous lesions and in lung tissue without tuberculous lesions. *Arch Pathol Lab Med* 1927; 4: 1-21.

[27] Hernandez-Pando R, Jeyanathan M, Mengistu G, Aguilar D, Orozoco H, Harboe, M, Rook GAW, Bjune G. Persistence of DNA from *Mycobacterium tuberculosis* in superficially normal lung tissue during latent infection. *Lancet* 2000; 356: 2133-2137.

[28] Comstock GW. How much isoniazid is needed for prevention of tuberculosis among immunocompetent adults? (Counterpoint). *Int J Tuberc Lung Dis* 1999; 3: 847-850.

[29] Vernon A, Burman W, Benator D, Khan A, Bozeman L. Acquired rifamycin monoresistance in patients with HIV-related tuberculosis treated with once-weekly rifapentine and isoniazid. *Lancet* 1999; 353: 1843-1847.

[30] Jindani A, Nunn AJ, Enarson DA. Two 8-month regimens of chemotherapy for treatment of newly diagnosed pulmonary tuberculosis: international multicentre randomised trial. *Lancet* 2004; 364: 1244-1252.

[31] Selwyn PA, Hartel D, Lewis VA, et al. A prospective study of the risk of tuberculosis among intravenous drug users with human immunodeficiency virus infection. *N Engl J Med* 1989; 320: 545-550.

[32] Grzybowski S, Enarson D. Tuberculosis. In: Current Pulmonology. Simmons DH, ed. *Chicago: Year Book Medical Publishers*, 1985: 73-96. ISBN 0 163 7800.

[33] Centers for Disease Control and Prevention. Outbreak of multidrug-resistant tuberculosis at a hospital – New York City, 1991. *MMWR Morb Mortal Wkly Rep* 1993; 42: 427-433.

[34] Toungoussova OS, Caugant DA, Sandven P, Mariandyshev AO, Bjune G. Impact of drug resistance on fitness of *Mycobacterium tuberculosis* strains of the W-Beijing genotype. *FEMS Immunol Clin Mocrobiol* 2004; 42: 281-290.

[35] Lopez B, Aguilar D, Orozco H, Burger M, Espitia C, Ritacco V, et al. A marked difference in pathogenesis and immune response induced by different *Mycobacterium tuberculosis* genotypes. *Clin Exp Immunol* 2003; 133: 30-37.

[36] Drobniewski F, Balabanova J, Ruddy M, Weldon L, Jeltkova K, Brown T, et al. Rifampin and multidrug-resistant tuberculosis in Russian civilians and prison inmates: dominance of the Beijing strain family. *Emerg Infect Dis* 2002; 8: 1320-1326.

[37] Henderson DA. The challenge of eradication: lessons from past eradication campaigns. *Int J Tuberc Lung Dis* 1998; 2: S4-S58.

[38] Brudney K, Dobkin J. Resurgent tuberculosis in New York City: Human immunodeficiency virus, homelessness and the decline of tuberculosis control programs. *Am Rev Respir Dis* 1991; 144: 745-749.

[39] Barr RG, Menzies R. The effect of war on tuberculosis: results of a tuberculin survey among displaced persons in El Salvador and a review of the literature. *Tuber Lung Dis* 1994; 75: 251-259.

[40] Enarson DA. Principles of IUATLD Collaborative Tuberculosis Programmes. *Bull Int Union Tuberc Lung Dis* 1991; 66: 195-200.

[41] Murray CJL, Styblo K, Rouillon A. Tuberculosis in developing countries: burden, intervention and cost. *Bull Int Union Tuberc Lung Dis* 1990; 65: 2-20.

[42] World Health Organization. WHO Expert Committee on Tuberculosis, Ninth Report. *WHO Technical Report Series* 552, Geneva: 1974: pp16.

[43] Fox W, Ellard GA, Mitchison DA. Studies on the treatment of tuberculosis undertaken by the British Medical Research Council Tuberculosis Units, 1946-1986, with relevant subsequent publications. *Int J Tuberc Lung Dis* 1999; 3: S231-S279.

[44] East African / British Medical Research Council. Controlled clinical trial of four 6-month regimens of chemotherapy for pulmonary tuberculosis. Second report. *Am Rev Respir Dis* 1976; 114: 471-475.

In: Drugs: Approval and Evaluation, Delivery and Control ISBN: 978-1-60456-533-1
Editors: A.O. Hartmann, L.K. Neumann

Chapter 8

Reliability and Pitfalls of Anesthetic Depth Measurement

Axel Heller
Critical Care Meeicine, University Hospital Carl Custav Carus,
University of Technology, Dresden, Germany

For more than 160 years anesthetic techniques are being carried out, in order to facilitate surgical procedures without pain sensation. Sufficient, reliable and reproducible control of anesthetic depth is of essential importance in modern anesthetic practice. Unnecessary deep anesthesia may lead to hemodynamic deterioration or prolonged emergence in case of high dose administration of anesthetic agents. Inadequate low anesthetic depth may lead to intraoperative awareness and recall, a frightening event for patients. Some of them may develop a posttraumatic stress disorder (PTSD) and need psychotherapeutic support for several years.

Schwender at al. in the 90´s distinguished 5 different stages of intraoperative awareness: (1) conscious awareness with explicit recall and with severe pain; (2) conscious awareness with explicit recall but no complaints of pain; (3) conscious awareness without explicit recall and possible implicit recall; (4) subconscious awareness without explicit recall and possible implicit recall; (5) no awareness. [1]. Sandin and colleagues published 2,000 a study of intraoperative awareness among 11,785 patients and detected an incidence of 0.18% when patients received neuromuscular blocking agents, whereas the incidence of awareness was 0.1% in the absence of neuromuscular blocking drugs [2].

Despite the low incidence of awareness as described by Sandin, with or without neuromuscular blocking agents, Osterman et al. estimated that in the US every year 30,000 patients experience intraoperative awareness, which only rarely leads to claims [3].

Patients scheduled for cardiothoracic procedures, polytraumatized patients or parturients for caesarean section under general anesthesia, are of higher risk for intraoperative awareness due to reduced myocardial performance and circulating blood volume, or to the required anesthetic technique not allowing the use of opioids until the section of the umbilical cord, respectively.

Furthermore, new anesthetic techniques, which actually are concerned to be beneficial for the patients regarding perioperative superior quality of pain relief, intraoperative organ protection and faster emergence from anesthesia, may increase the risk of intraoperative awareness. In Particular, the combination of neuraxial analgesia (thoracic epidural analgesia) and general anesthesia has been shown to reduce the amount of required inhaled and intravenous anesthetic agents for maintenance of an accurate anesthetic depth [4-6]. At present, the practice of anesthesia is based on the concept of components of anesthesia resulting from separate pharcological actions of multiple agent administration. Many anesthesiologists rely on somatic signs (motor responses, changes in respiratory pattern) and autonomic signs (tachycardia, hypertension, lacrimation, diaphoresis) to guide the dosage of anesthetic agents in order to achieve the basic goals of anesthetic management, that is unconsciousness, (hypnotic effects), blockade of somatic motor responses and suppression of autonomic responses to noxious stimuli. However, these clinical signs are not reliable measures of the conscious state of anesthetized patients [7]. The use of these clinical signs in judging dosage of anesthetic agents can lead to either overdosage or underdosage, especially in the presence of hypotensive episodes and bradycardia due to blockade of the pain stimuli at spinal level and sympathicolysis due to thoracic epidural analgesia.

An individual adjustment of the anesthetic depth to its actual demand can be achieved by the use of electroencephalographic devices which can process the encephalogram (EEG), processed EEG (p-EEG) monitors, simultaneously and transform it to an index of anesthetic depth. The precise definition of the term anesthetic depth and consecutively its assessment have been an important objective for over than 150 years and were almost developed in an equal manner like the anesthetic techniques and became more and more well described. John Snow, in 1847, first described five degrees of "narcotism" for ether anesthesia [8]. Guedel refined these terms in 1937 into four stages basing on somatic muscle tone, respiratory parameters and ocular signs [9] and in the same year Loomis described electroencephalographic pattern changes during human sleep and was the first who brought the EEG in relation with the term anesthesia [10]. Woodbridge in 1957 defined anesthesia as a combination of 4 components: Sensory blockade, motor blockade, blockade of autonomic reflexes and loss of consciousness [11].

Bispectral Index (BIS)

In the early 1990s the Bispectral Index- monitor (BIS), Aspect Medical Systems, monitor received Food and Drug Administration approval and since then it has been established in the daily anesthetic practice as a monitor of anesthetic depth and several studies have evaluated his contribution to the assessment of anesthetic depth, patients´ outcome and its limitations.

BIS is a dimensionless number scaled from 100-0, with 100 represanting an awake EEG and 0 representing complete electrical silence (burst suppression). The BIS integrates various EEG descriptors into a single variable. The mixture of subparameters of EEG activity was derived empirically from a prospectively collected database of anesthetized volunteers with measures of clinically relevant sedative endpoints and hypnotic drug concentrations. The EEG was recorded onto a computer and was time-matched with clinical endpoints and, where available, drug concentrations. The raw EEG data were inspected, sections containing artifacts were rejected and spectral calculations were then performed to produce both bispectral and power spectral variables. Bispectral analysis is a statistical technique allowing study of phenomena with nonlinear character, such as wave breaking. Bispectral analysis provides a description to a continuous pseudo-randomly varying signal (EEG) that is an alternative to other conventional power spectral analysis techniques derived from fast Fourier transformation. Conventional analysis of the EEG using fast Fourier transformation produces information regarding the power, frequency, and the phase of the EEG signal. Bispectral analysis represents a different description of the EEG in that interfrequency phase relations are measured, i.e. the bispectrum quantifies relations among the underlying sinusoidal components of the EEG [12].

The BIS algorithm includes 3 EEG subparameters, depending on the depth of anesthesia: "Burst suppression", the "SynchFastSlow" and the "BetaRatio". Burst suppression has a greater weight in the calculation of BIS values during general anesthesia when compared to sedation. The SynchFastSlow is defined as the logarithm of the following ratio: the sum of bispectrum peaks in the 0.5-47 Hz range divided by the sum of the bispectrum peaks in the 40-47 Hz range. The weight of SynchFastSlow in the BIS index calculation relates to the degree of EEG activity during general anaesthesia. The weight of BetaRatio is greatest at light sedation. The BetaRatio is calculated as the log of the ratio of power in two empirically derived frequency bands: log (P30-40 Hz / P11-20 Hz) [13].

Several studies have been conducted in order to assess the effects of BIS monitoring on the utilization of currently available anesthetic agents, such as propofol, desflurane and sevoflurane during general and combined anesthesia. BIS guided titration of propofol led to significant reduction in propofol requirement at about 1.30 mg/kg/hr [14] as well as to a decrease in the consumption of volatile anesthetics (desflurane, isoflurane and sevoflurane) with an overall decrease of 0.17 MAC equivalents [15-18].

Early recovery times were studied, described as time to eye opening, time to response to command, time to extubation and time to orientation. The effect of BIS guided anesthesia was a reduction in early recovery times. The time to eye opening was reduced by 2.34 minutes, the time for response to command was reduced by 2.28 minutes, time to extubation was reduced by 3.05 minutes and the time to orientation was reduced by 2.46 minutes [19].

The intraoperative advantages of BIS monitoring led to significant effect regarding postanesthesia care unit (PACU) with an overall reduction of 6.83 minutes. Nevertheless, intraoperative monitoring failed to reduce significantly a reduction in time of home readiness, although, it should be kept in mind that this endpoint depends on many factors beside anesthetic regimen [15]. Since late discharge home is the main cost driving factor in diagnoses related reimbursement systems, cost effectiveness of BIS- monitoring will be hard to detect. Even taking into account slightly shorter stay in cost intensive units (e.g. PACU).

Patients receiving individual adjusted anesthesia, were less in danger of intraoperative awareness and recall when compared with patients without BIS monitoring. BIS guided anesthesia among patients with an increased risk of intraoperative awareness (cardiac surgery) led to a significant decrease in the incidence of awareness [20].

However, an increasing number of studies, case reports and letters to the editor points out some limitations of the BIS monitoring during anesthesia [21-27]. Electromyographic activity influences the BIS monitor in a manner that adequate anesthetized patients suddenly appear to be in a very low level of anesthesia when neuromuscular blockade diminishes. This may mislead the anesthesiologists to increase the dosage of anesthetics in an attempt to re- adjust the anesthetic depth, resulting in a possible hemodynamic deterioration or a prolonged recovery due to inadequate deep anesthesia and unnecessary additional muscular paralysis. In case that, anesthesiologists who are eventually familiar with this interaction between the muscular activity and the BIS, ignore the elevated BIS levels, then awareness and intraoperative recall may occur, in case of an actual increased demand on anesthetic agents, or malfunction of the anesthetic equipment.

A possible explanation for the influence of increased electromyographic activity on the accuracy of the BIS is the fact that BIS algorithm includes frequencies between 0.5 and 47 Hz to compute the raw EEG into a narcotic stage. EMG activity creates frequencies from 25 to 300 Hz and this overlapping of frequencies might be the reason of elevated BIS levels in the absence of neuromuscular blocking drugs. The new BIS XP platform contains an EMG activity bar, which indicates the muscle activity throughout the measure and the manufacturers point out the improvements in the software of the BIS in combination with the new BIS Quattro® electrode regarding indicating and filtering artifacts, like electromyographic activity. However, the results of an investigation of Panousis et al. did not confirm the expectations of these improvements [28]. Vasoactive substances with high lipid solubility and thus fast passage through the blood brain barrier as well as warming devices using hot air in order to increase patients′ body temperature have been found to cause sporadical elevations of BIS values during general anesthesia as described by Ishiyama and Hemmerling, respectively.

Narcotrend

Another monitor of anesthetic depth, the Narcotrend (MonitorTechnik, Bad Bramstedt, Germany), has been commercially available in Europe since 2000 and 2006 received Food and Drug Administration approval. It has been developed by anesthesiologists and bioengineers from the University Medical school of Hannover, Germany and includes, similar to the BIS, a computerized analysis of the raw EEG. The raw EEG signal can be recorded by standard electrocardiogram electrodes for single- and double-channel registration. After an automatic artifact analysis, the raw EEG signal is processed by the Narcotrend using a multivariate analysis algorithm and is then assigned to defined EEG stages. The Narcotrend algorithm is in part based on the classification of the sleep EEG and differentiates six EEG stages from A (awake) to F (burst suppression to down cortical silence), with 15 substages. Additionally, a Narcotrend index is displayed with a range from 100 (awake) to 0. The methods for automatic classification were developed on the basis of a visual assessment of the EEG, which, in its origins, is related to sleep classification. In 1937, Loomis et al. described systematic changes of the EEG during human sleep and defined five stages, A-E to distinguish different EEG patterns. The scale was subsequently extended, refined by the definition of substages and applied to the classification of EEGs recorded during anesthesia. Schultz and colleagues used a scale with the substages A, $B_{0\text{-}2}$, $C_{0\text{-}2}$, $D_{0\text{-}2}$, $E_{0\text{-}1}$ and $F_{o\text{-}1}$ for visually characterizing and classifying EEG patterns observed during anesthesia with different volatile and intravenous agents.

The signals are sampled at 128 samples per second with a 12-bit resolution, and are bandpass filtered to 0.5-45 Hz. During recording, impedances and electrode potentials are tested at defined time intervals to ensure a constantly high quality of the EEG signal. Trace segments with a length of 20 seconds, the so called epochs, are the units of classification. In order to provide a smooth and continuous assessment of the EEG signal, the preceding 20 seconds period is classified every 5 seconds, yielding an overlap of 75% of the recorded data at every time point. "Background" parameters are calculated and updated during the course of an EEG recording. These parameters are sensitive to EEG patterns atypical of general anesthesia, for example distinct epileptiform activity, and are used for plausibility checks of the classification results. Finally, a smoothed value of the Narcotrend classification is calculated as a weighted mean.

Several clinical and validation studies have been conducted in order to evaluate the impact of a Narcotrend guided anesthesia on the requirement of volatile and anesthetic agents, as well as recovery and ambulation times. An early study comparing BIS and Narcotrend showed that change of Narcotrend stages was accompanied by significant changes in BIS values [29]. EEG changes during propofol-remifentanil anesthesia appear to be recorded and interpreted in a similar manner by both monitors. Various clinical studies involving the Narcotrend are available. Kraus et al. examined the extubation times in patients undergoing carotid artery surgery with propofol-remifentanil anesthesia controlled either by clinical assessment or by Narcotrend monitoring. Patients in the Narcotrend group required significantly less propofol and were extubated earlier [30]. The influence of Narcotrend monitoring on recovery time after total intravenous anesthesia with propofol was examined in a multicenter study including 46 institutions. A total of 521 patients were assessed using clinical criteria, whereas, in 4109 patients the depth of anesthesia was assessed by the Narcotrend aiming a narcotic stage between D and E. Recovery times were significantly shorter under continuous Narcotrend monitoring. Furthermore, the number of patients who were orientated after surgical procedure was also significantly higher in the Narcotrend group [31].

However, there are also several limitations regarding the use of the Narcotrend as a reliable tool for assessment of anesthetic depth: Schneider and colleagues presented challenging data about the ability of the Narcotrend to measure accurately the anesthetic depth under dynamic conditions during transition between anesthesia and wakefulness: After induction of general anesthesia, the authors allowed a certain time of stabilization of the Narcotrend values. After that they discontinued the administration of the anesthetic agents and as patients became awake the authors compared the clinical signs with the Narcotrend index. Patients were then anesthetized for a second time and the authors compared once more the clinical signs with the Narcotrend values. In both scenarios the Narcotrend failed to adequately detect the anesthetic depth, i.e. the monitor indicated sufficient anesthetic depth while patients were regaining consciousness and in the second case the Narcotrend indicated beginning consciousness [32]. Russell et al. used the isolated forearm technique in order to evaluate the ability of the Narcotrend to assess adequately the anesthetic depth and and concluded that the Narcotrend is unable to detect consciousness during general anesthesia due to the fact that patients responded to verbal commands [33].

It is important to mention that Russell intended a Narcotrend stage of C, which in most cases can be far too low for an adequate anesthetic depth; however, his results and the results of the Schneider group have major clinical importance. In a case of malfunction of the anesthetic equipment and subsequent changes in the anesthetic drug delivery, the Narcotrend monitor would have failed to assess the anesthetic adequately and without significant latency and patients could have been exposed to the danger of intraoperative awareness, although continuously monitored.

Entropy

The EEG presents more disorder and random patterns when patients are awake when compared to general anesthesia. The collection of these samples, the entropy makes use of this principal and the monitor system carries the same name: Entropy (GE Healthcare). The entropy is relatively new, non-linear statistical parameter, which describes the order of stochastical data, like the EEG. The principle of the Entropy monitor assumes that the EEG is not a sum of sinusoidal oscillations, but rather that the EEG presents a non-linear chaotic pattern. The approximate entropy and the Shannon entropy quantify the predictability of the EEG signal amplitudes [34], the spectral entropy describes the coincidence of the frequencies [lit].

Bruhn et al. investigated the approximate and the Shannon entropy during desflurane anesthesia. They found that both parameters are suitable to describe the anesthetic properties of a drug [35].

Beside the Narcotrend and the BIS monitors, 3 further monitors are in clinical use for the assessment of anesthetic depth: The patient state index (PSA; Hospira, Inc), SNAP 2 (Everest Biomedical) and the cerebral state index (CSM, Danmeter). The majority of randomized, controlled trials have been conducted in order to evaluate the clinical use of the BIS. The above mentioned monitor systems have merely been evaluated in small studies, but most of them have produced similar reductions in intraoperative anesthetic dosing in a smaller spectrum of anesthesia types, surgical procedures and patient profiles [36].

During the last decades, several monitor devices have been introduced to clinical practice in order to assess reliably the anesthetic depth. The BIS is the monitor system which has been most evaluated from all available systems. Although new algorithms and filters have developed by the manufacturers in order to minimize the interference of increased electromyographic activity and the quality of the BIS signal, this problem still remains unsolved and limits the reliability of this monitor. A monitor system, which has been actually developed in order to adjust individually the anesthetic depth and reduce the required amount of anesthetic drugs and neuromuscular blocking agents, fails to reproduce accurately the anesthetic depth in the absence of neuromuscular blockade and may mislead anesthesiologists, who are not familiar with this phenomenon to administer repetitive doses of neuromuscular blocking agents and/or increase the amount of anesthetic drugs, in order to "readjust" the anesthetic depth. Additionally, further investigation is required for the development of a Narcotrend algorithm that detects transition between consciousness and unconsciousness with a clinical relevant latency, which is also reproducible.

Summary

In conclusion, the impact of p-EEG monitoring appears to be a modest reduction in intraoperative primary anesthetic agent dosing of approximately 20-25%. This reduction in anesthetic dosing appears to be linked to the other benefits, e.g. decrease in the time for emergence or tracheal extubation, reduction in early recovery time or time to reach certain milestone recovery endpoints and a reduction in postoperative nausea and vomiting. In addition, p-EEG monitoring has been shown to have the potential to reduce the rate of awareness compared to traditional measures of anesthetic depth (clinical signs). Thus, p-EEG adjusted anesthesia may increase safety but neither improvement of clinical pathways nor cost effectiveness has yet been shown.

Anesthesiologists have the possibility to gain experience with monitors of anesthetic depth and increase patients′ safety, only when they know how to interpret the clinical signs and how to use anesthetic depth monitor systems and the possible pitfalls during their use.

REFERENCES

[1] Schwender D, Klasing S, Daunderer M, Madler C, Pöppel E, Peter K.Awareness during general anesthesia. Definition, incidence, clinical relevance, causes, avoidance and medicolegal aspects] *Anaesthesist.* 1995 Nov;44(11):743-54.

[2] Sandin RH, Enlund G, Samuelsson P, Lennmarken C. Awareness during anaesthesia: a prospective case study. *Lancet.* 2000 Feb 26;355(9205):707-11.

[3] Ostermann JE, van der Kolk BA. Awareness during anesthesia and posttraumatic stress disorder. *Gen Hosp Psychiatry* 1998; 20:274-281.

[4] Casati L, Fernández-Galinski S, Barrera E, Pol O, Puig MM. Isoflurane requirement during combined general/epidural anaesthesia for major abdominal surgery. *Anesthesia Analgesia* 2002; 94: 1331-7.

[5] Hodgson PS, Liu S. Epidural lidocaine decreases sevoflurane requirement for adequate depth of anaesthesia as measured by the Bispectral Index monitor. *Anesthesiology* 2001; 94: 799-803.

[6] Agarwal A, Pandey R, Dhiraaj S, Singh PK, Raza M, Pandey CK, Gupta D et al. The effect of epidural bupivacaine on induction and maintenance doses of propofol (evaluated by Bispectral Index) and maintenance doses of fentanyl and vecuronium. *Anesthesia Analgesia* 2004; 99: 1684-8.

[7] Mahla ME. Electroencephalogram in the OR. *Seminars in Anesthesia* 1997; 16:3-13.

[8] Snow J. *On the inhalation of the vapors of ether in surgical operations.* Containing a description of the various stages of etherization and a statement of the result of nearly eighty operations in which ether has been employed in St. Georges′s and University College Hospitals. John Churchill, London, 1947. Reproduced by Lea and Febiger, Philadelphia, 1959.

[9] Guedel AE. *Inhalational anesthesia. A fundamental guide.* Macmillan, New York, 1937.

[10] Loomis AL, Harvey EN, Hobart CA. Cerebral states during sleep as studied by human brain potentials. *Journal of Experimental Psychology* 1937; 21: 127-44.

[11] Woodbridge PD. Changing concepts concerning depth of anesthesia. *Anesthesiology* 1957; 18:536.

[12] Johansen Jw. Update on bispectral index monitoring. *Best Pract Res Clin Anaesthesiol.* 2006; 20:81-99.

[13] Rampil IJ. A primer for EEG signal processing in anesthesia. *Anesthesiology* 1998; 89: 980-1002.

[14] Gan TJ, Glass PS, Windsor A, Payne E, Rosow C, Sebel P. et al. Bispectral Index monitoring allows faster emergence and improved recovery from propofol, alfentanil and nitrous oxide anesthesia. BIS Utility Study Group. *Anesthesiology* 1997; 87:808-815.

[15] Johansen JW. Provider survey of bispectral index utility. *Anesthesia and Analgesia* 1998; 86:Suppl 212.

[16] Nelskyla KA, Yli-Hankala AM, Puro PH, Korttila KT. Sevoflurane titration using bispectral index decreases postoperative vomiting in phase II recovry after ambulatory surgery. *Anesthesia and Analgesia* 2001; 93:1165-1169.

[17] Song D, Joshi GP, White PF. Titration of volatile anesthetics using bispectral index facilitates recovery after ambulatory anesthesia. *Anesthesiology* 1997; 87:842-848.

[18] Song D, van Vlymen J, White PF. Is the bispectral index useful in predicting fast-track eligibility after ambulatory anesthesia with propofol and desflurane? *Anesthesia and Analgesia* 1998; 87:1245-1248.

[19] Masuda T, Yamada T, Takada K, Sagata Y, Yamaguchi M, Tomiyama Y et al. Bispectral index monitoring is useful to reduce total amount of propofol and to obtain immediate recovery after propofol anesthesia. *Masui* 2002; 51:394-399.

[20] Leslie K, Myles PS, Forbes A, Chan MT, Short TG, Swallow SK. Recovery from bispectral index-guided anesthesia in a large randomized controlled trial of patients at high risk of awareness. *Anaesthesia and Intensive Care* 2005; 33:443-451.

[21] Bruhn J, Bouillon TW, Shafer SL. Electromyographic activity falsely elevates the Bispectral Index. *Anesthesiology* 2000; 92: 1485-7.

[22] Hemmerling TM, Fortier JD. Falsely increased Bispectral Index values in a series of patients undergoing cardiac surgery using forced-air-warming therapy of the head. *Anesthesia Analgesia* 2002; 95: 322-3.

[23] Panousis P, Koch T, Heller AR. The effects of electromyographic activity on the Bispectral Index during combined anaesthesia. *Anesthesia Analgesia* 2006; 103: 1605.

[24] Ishiyama T, Oguchi T, Iijima T, Matsukawa T, Kashimoto S, Kumazawa T. Ephedrine, but not phenylephrine, increases Bispectral Index values during combined general and epidural anaesthesia. *Anesthesia Analgesia* 2003; 97: 780-4.

[25] Vivien B, Di Maria S, Ouattara A, Langeron O, Coriat P, Riou B. Overestimation of Bispectral Index in sedated intensive care unit patients revealed by administration of muscle relaxant. *Anesthesiology* 2003; 99: 9-17.

[26] Inoue S, Kawaguchi M, Sasaoka N, Hirai K, Furuya H. Effects of neuromuscular block on systemic and cerebral haemodynamics and Bispectral index during moderate or deep sedation in critically ill patients. *Intensive Care Medicine* 2006; 32: 391-7.

[27] Liu N, Chazot T, Huybrechts I, Law-Koune JD, Barvais L, Fischler M. The influence of a muscle relaxant bolus on Bispectral and Datex-Ohmeda entropy values during propofol-remifentanil induced loss of consciousness. *Anesthesia Analgesia* 2005; 101: 1713-18.

[28] Panousis P, Heller AR, Burghardt M, Bleyl JU, Koch T. The effects of electromyographic activity on the accuracy of the Narcotrend monitor compared with the Bispectral Index during combined anaesthesia. *Anaesthesia* 2007 Sep; 62:868-74.

[29] Kreuer S, Bruhn J, Larsen R, Bialas P, Wilhelm W. Comparability of Narcotrend index and bispectral index during propofol anaesthesia. *British Journal of Anaesthesia* 2004 Aug;93(2):235-40.

[30] Kraus G, Mogendorf F, Bartlog M et al. Propofoldosierungen und Aufwachzeiten bei Cartis-Operationen ohne und mit EEG-Monitoring (Narcotrend®). *Anästhesiologie Itensivmedizin* 2000; 41:390.

[31] Wilhelm W, Kreuer S, Larsen R. Narcotrend EEG monitoring during total intravenous anaesthesia in 4360 patients. *Anaesthesiat* 2002; 51: 980-988.

[32] Schneider G, Kochs EF, Horn B, Kreuzer M, Ningler M. Narcotrend® does not adequately detect the transition between awareness and unconsciousness in surgical patients. *Anesthesiology* 2004; 101: 1105-11.

[33] Russell IF. The Narcotrend "depth of anaesthesia" monitor cannot reliably detect consciousness during general anaesthesia: an investigation using the isolated forearm technique. *British Journal of Anaesthesia* 2006; 96: 346-52.

[34] Bruhn J, Roepcke H, Hoeft A. Approximate entropy as an electroencephalographic measure of anesthetic drug effect during desflurane anesthesia. *Anesthesiology* 2000; 92:715-726.

[35] Bruhn J, Lehmann LE, Roepcke H, Bouillon TW, Hoeft A. Shannon entropy applied to the measurement of the EEG effects of desflurane. *Anesthesiology* 2000, A265.

[36] Monk TG. Processed EEG and patient outcome. *Best Practice & Research Clinical Anesthesiology* 2006; 20:21-228.

In: Drugs: Approval and Evaluation, Delivery and Control ISBN: 978-1-60456-533-1
Editors: A.O. Hartmann, L.K. Neumann

Chapter 9

AMORPHOUS ENEMIES IN THE WAR ON DRUGS: HEROIN AS MEDIATED EXACERBATOR OF WORLD TURMOIL

Bryan E. Denham*

Department of Communication Studies, 412 Strode Tower, Clemson University, Clemson, SC 29634, USA

ABSTRACT

More than three decades have passed since Richard Nixon became the first U.S. president to declare "war" on drugs, and despite the investment of billions toward eradicating the abuse of substances such as cocaine and heroin, public officials continue to witness sustained use of the very drugs Nixon, followed by Ronald Reagan and George H. W. Bush, sought to curtail. To keep up the fight, as it were, and to keep at least part of the U.S. population in support of it, political actors who support the "war" on drugs have had to ensure that new threats continually emerge, thus allowing officials to call for intensified efforts and "new" approaches to the problem. Examining heroin reports in the *New York Times* and the *Los Angeles Times* from 1988 to 2003, this article identifies several enemies in the U.S. drug war, including the "Golden Triangle" (i.e., Laos, Thailand and Myanmar), the "Indian Connection," the "Nigerian Connection" and the "Notorious Bekaa Valley" in Lebanon. "Russian drug gangs" and "porous European borders" were also to blame for heroin problems during the last decade of the 20th century.

An amorphous enemy cannot be defined or defeated and exists largely on a symbolic level. Such an enemy poses an imminent threat to a way of life, stands to disrupt an established moral order and allows public officials to frame political issues in an over-simplified, dichotomous manner, with seemingly obvious choices to be made between good and evil, right and wrong. In the case of narcotic threats, the mass-communicated presence of

---

* Associate Professor. (864) 656-6392; bdenham@clemson.edu

an unidentifiable menace has combined with dominant conceptions of morality, or "symbolic moral universes" (Ben-Yehuda, 1990), and a series of abstract, unassailable rationales (e.g., the protection of at-risk populations) to perpetuate a losing "war" on drugs – one that costs the United States upward of $18 billion annually (MacCoun & Reuter, 2001; see also, Tierney, 2005).

"We set up our categories," Gould (2002) observed, "often by arbitrary division based on tiny differences; then, mistaking names for moral principles, and using banners and slogans as substitutes for reason, we vow to live and die for one or the other side of a false dichotomy" (p. 257). As an example of false dichotomization, after the terrorist attacks of September 11, 2001, U.S. President George W. Bush declared war on terror and called on world leaders to follow his "battle plans" unconditionally – to be "with us or against us." Consequently, discussions of policy approaches gave way to military actions almost immediately, and those who did not support invading Iraq, in particular, found themselves ostracized by the Bush administration. For their part, U.S. journalists who did not acquiesce to military plans were labeled unpatriotic (Zelizer & Allan, 2002) and their lack of reporting ultimately facilitated the attack of a country that may not have possessed weapons of mass destruction and may not have harbored or given safe passage to terrorists associated with 9/11.

Similar strategies have been applied to the war on drugs, with public officials demanding that individuals either join the "fight" or be considered an enemy of the struggle (see Mackey-Kallis & Hahn, 1994; Morales, 1989). The administrations of Ronald Reagan and George H.W. Bush, Morales (1989) suggested, grounded their respective campaigns against drugs in issues of national security, with Mackey-Kallis and Hahn (1994) adding that such representations shut down debate and critical inspections of policy proposals. Public officials constructed an external enemy and demanded nothing less than categorical support for plans to defeat it; pointing to the demand for narcotics instead of their supply, or questioning the amount of tax dollars allocated toward the entire war on drugs, amounted to aiding and abetting the enemy.

"War excuses everything," observed political commentator P. J. O'Rourke (2002). "You can drop an A-bomb on the Japanese. No sacrifice is too great, no expense too high to win a war. This is why politicians love the war thing. War is steroids and free weights for government. Budgets, bureaucracies, and the whole scope of legal and regulatory authority to get pumped and buff" (p. 192). Of course, "war" stands to alienate those who do not support it, which U.S. policymakers have learned since forces invaded Iraq in 2003.

Given "extensions" of the facts and the ease with which military metaphors enter political conversations, it perhaps should come as little surprise that the war on terror and the war on drugs have intersected. Monies from Afghan poppies have allegedly financed terrorist cells since 9/11, and thus one necessity for winning the war on terror, U.S. officials contend, is to continue allocating resources for combating the illicit use of narcotics, especially opiates such as heroin. As Lynch and Witte (2007) reported in the *Washington Post*, "The surge in opium production has frustrated U.S. and NATO military commanders, who believe that the trade plays a major role in funding a Taliban insurgency that has become increasingly deadly over the past two years. Commanders also believe that the involvement of public officials in the drug trade has undermined Afghans' confidence in their government" (p. A7).

Table 1. Select Heroin Headlines in the *Los Angeles Times* and the *New York Times*, 1988-2003

1988	
Violence feared as Asian heroin influx soars	*Los Angeles Times*, February 25
The Bombay connection: India is major player in world drug trade	*Los Angeles Times*, March 17
Afghan opium yield up as Pakistan curbs crop	*New York Times*, April 14
U.S. sees increase in Afghan opium	*New York Times*, September 6
1989	
Western officials look to Afghanistan and see a new problem – heroin	*Los Angeles Times*, January 1
Singapore hangs 2 as drug traffickers	*Los Angeles Times*, May 28
Malaysia hangs drug trafficker	*Los Angeles Times*, July 21
Iran hangs 8 accused heroin traffickers	*Los Angeles Times*, August 5
Guatemala seen slipping into a haven for drugs	*Los Angeles Times*, August 30
1990	
Southeast Asia is no. 1 source of U.S. heroin	*New York Times*, February 11
Dutch drug policy gains ground	*Los Angeles Times*, March 4
'Indian Connection' poppies throw a curve at U.S. drug policy	*Los Angeles Times*, March 19
Golden triangle's blooming threat	*Los Angeles Times*, July 24
1991	
Heroin spreads among young in China	*New York Times*, March 21
Kuwaiti Blueblood reportedly could face death penalty	*Los Angeles Times*, April 20
China pledges to help U.S. curb Asian heroin trade	*Los Angeles Times*, July 27
Colombian heroin may be increasing	*New York Times*, October 27
1992	
Colombia's drug lords add new product: Heroin for U.S.	*New York Times*, January 14
Syrians cash in on drug trade in Lebanon's Notorious Bekaa Valley	*Los Angeles Times*, January 26
Nigerian Connection floods U.S. airports with Asian heroin	*New York Times*, February 15
U.S. links trail of heroin to a 'Soviet connection'	*New York Times*, April 15
China executes 27 narcotics traffickers	*Los Angeles Times*, June 27
Surge in addiction linked to Russian drug gangs	*Los Angeles Times*, November 29
1993	
Heroin pouring through porous European borders	*New York Times*, February 9
Tracking the Russian Connection	*Los Angles Times*, June 6
1994	
Mexican police make record heroin seizure	*Los Angeles Times*, January 17
State Dept. labels Nigeria major trafficker of drugs to U.S.	*New York Times*, April 5
Frenchman's arrest cracks narcotics ring	*Los Angeles Times*, July 3
1995	
Vietnam makes its biggest drug bust	*Los Angeles Times*, February 4
Heroin from Burmese surges as U.S. debates strategy	*New York Times*, February 12

Table 1. Continued

1995 (Continued)	
Heroin scourges million Pakistanis	*New York Times*, April 5
Drug trade, militants thrive in Pakistan's rugged north	*Los Angeles Times*, April 9
Young addicts spur China to address its drug problem	*Los Angeles Times*, June 10
U.S. to help Myanmar fight drug production	*Los Angeles Times*, June 21
Colombia's heroin couriers: Swallowing and smuggling	*New York Times*, November 2
Heroin route via Africa a new worry	*New York Times*, December 26
1996	
Colombians enter the heroin market	*New York Times*, February 11
Dubliners outraged at sellers of heroin	*New York Times*, October 6
1997	
Colombians up quality, lower price of heroin	*Los Angeles Times*, February 24
Heroin is proving a growth industry for Colombia	*New York Times*, March 30
Movie underscores Scotland's heroin plague	*Los Angeles Times*, April 13
1998	
Colombian heroin dominates U.S. market, government says	*New York Times*, January 1
Today's silk road carries a different kind of import: Heroin	*Los Angeles Times*, January 11
1999	
On the case in China	*Los Angeles Times*, April 21
A drug pusher's life is rotten in Denmark	*New York Times*, May 7
2000	
Adding to Pakistan's misery, million-plus heroin addicts	*New York Times*, April 19
2001	
At heroin's source, Taliban do what 'Just say no' could not	*New York Times*, May 24
The opium trail has a new stop . . . Tajikistan	*Los Angeles Times*, July 25
Portugal takes away prison as a penalty for using drugs	*Los Angeles Times*, August 21
'Super' heroin was planned by bin Laden, reports say	*New York Times*, October 4
Most Afghan opium grown in rebel-controlled areas	*New York Times*, October 5
Taliban's drug war risks unraveling	*Los Angeles Times*, October 7
Afghan ban on growing of opium is unraveling	*New York Times*, October 22
Opium poppies take root once again in Afghanistan	*Los Angeles Times*, November 23
A war on terror meets a war on drugs	*New York Times*, November 25
2002	
U.S. fears a glut of heroin from a volatile Afghanistan	*New York Times*, April 1
China stepping up war against drugs	*Los Angeles Times*, August 4
Drug use, trafficking on the rise in Russia	*Los Angeles Times*, August 11
2003	
Old habit has China in its grip	*Los Angeles Times*, January 15
N. Korea's growing drug trade seen in botched heroin delivery	*Los Angeles Times*, May 21
N. Korea ship left more heroin, Australia says	*Los Angeles Times*, May 27
Latin American poppy fields undermine U.S. drug battle	*New York Times*, June 8
Myanmar tries to kick its habit	*Los Angeles Times*, August 10
U.N. aide says Afghan drug trade pays for terrorist attacks	*New York Times*, September 5

While drug monies may have been funneled to terrorist organizations operating in or near Afghanistan, the sheer number of "enemies" in the war on drugs, as identified in prominent media outlets since the mid-eighties, has created a boy-who-cried-wolf predicament for effective narcotics control. Table 1 lists headlines gathered from the *New York Times* and the *Los Angeles Times* for the period 1988 to 2003. Based on the table, the following nations struggled with the narcotics trade on some level: Afghanistan, China, Colombia, Denmark, France, Guatemala, India, Iran, Ireland, Kuwait, Malaysia, Mexico, Myanmar (Burma), Nigeria, North Korea, Pakistan, Portugal, Russia, Scotland, Singapore, Syria, Tajikistan, and Vietnam. In reviewing the headlines, one begins to question whether nations existed that did *not* struggle with heroin use and narcotics trafficking during those 16 years.

In the late eighties, Afghanistan and India emerged as "major players" in the heroin trade, with Iran, Malaysia and Singapore executing drug traffickers. An apparent "influx" of Asian heroin had created potential for violence, with the South American nation Guatemala "slipping into a haven for drugs." In the early nineties, countries in Asia and South America continued to struggle in controlling the heroin trade, with the "Golden Triangle" (i.e., Laos, Thailand and Myanmar) and the "Indian Connection" posing threats internationally. In 1992, China executed 27 drug traffickers, with the "Nigerian Connection," the "Soviet Connection" and the "Notorious Bekaa Valley" in Lebanon creating problems for law enforcement. "Russian drug gangs" and "porous European borders" were also to blame for heroin problems during the last decade of the 20th century.

As the nineties passed, Myanmar and Colombia continued as mediated drug threats, with the film *Trainspotting* focusing rare attention on a European nation, Scotland, for an alleged heroin problem. Headlines focusing on Columbia from 1995 to 1998 implied a new "growth industry" there each year, and also entering the pages of the *New York Times* and the *Los Angeles Times* were countries such as Vietnam, Pakistan and Denmark. Apart from the European nations and Scandinavia, many of the nations mentioned in Table 1 had contentious relationships with the United States independent of narcotics trafficking; becoming a drug threat only affirmed political tensions elsewhere and demonstrated for media audiences the need to continue funding, or "fighting," the war on drugs.

News Processes, in Brief

If the war on drugs owes much of its existence to the mass media, as scholars have asserted it does (Marez, 2004), then fundamental news processes become important to consider. In the United States, "official sources" in Washington, D.C. dominate the reporting of public affairs and political issues (see McLeod, Kosicki and McLeod, 1994), leading to a homogenous and ethnocentric news product that largely supports the status quo. In most instances reporters from major news outlets will not cover a political story without securing at least one quote from a public official; those who offer views in opposition to official definitions of news events often find themselves labeled radicals and extremists, when in fact they may be quite rational and measured in their perspectives.

For working journalists, government officials provide credibility and accessibility, and journalists in turn offer officials an opportunity to demonstrate initiative before constituents. The process is self-perpetuating, with officials building name recognition through mass communication and, as a result, becoming difficult to unseat. If a senior official tells reporters from the *New York Times* and/or the *Los Angeles Times* that Myanmar poses a heroin-trafficking threat to the United States (Greenhouse, 1995; Koss, 2003), or that methamphetamine is the new scourge in middle America (Zernike, 2005), the assertions become a mediated reality, reinforced each time they appear in print. Indeed, as Breen (1997) noted, "As well as setting the agenda for public issues, the news media can also set the agenda for themselves by their repetitious coverage of a single event and their collective definition of newsworthiness" (p. 348).

Media scholar Michael Schudson (2003) contends that content in major national newspapers is largely code-speak among political and economic elites – among official news sources. Consequently, news content often comes with an agenda, unbeknownst to media audiences. In the current war on terror, journalists initially did not question the link between Iraq and weapons of mass destruction, reporting on official definitions of the problem without moving deeper. Levenson (2004) lamented the resulting ambiguity:

> What, after all, is the war on terror? It's certainly the war against Al Qaeda. But is it the war in Iraq? Does the Israeli-Palestinian conflict qualify as a front? What about North Korea? For that matter, who are the terrorists? Osama bin Laden surely counts. But how about Moktada al-Sadr's army? Or ETA, the Basque separatists? Or the Armed Islamic Group in Algeria? For that matter, what about the IRA? Three years after the United States attacked Afghanistan, it is extremely difficult for the press to gauge where the United States stands in the war on terror because the term itself obscures distinction (p. 9).

Similarly, in the ongoing war on drugs, officials have kept journalists supplied with a steady list of amorphous enemies – nations, or combinations of nations, whose struggles with narcotics control would appear to pose a vague but salient threat to U.S. drug enforcement efforts. Countries enter the news periodically, and usually absent is contextual information regarding the scope of an alleged problem. Even more elusive are reports about problems ever being resolved; the more common practice is to simply introduce a new menace. In some cases, then, headlines and news reports simply remind news audiences that evil forces exist "out there," and consequently, monies must continue to fund interdiction efforts. One such effort continues in Afghanistan.

The Taliban: Eradicating and Cultivating Heroin in Afghanistan

Reporting from the Helmand Province in Afghanistan on May 24, 2001 – less than four months before the September 11 terrorist attacks on the United States – Barry Bearak of the *New York Times* discussed the successful eradication of opium there by the Taliban, a group of Fundamentalist Sunni Muslims who, by then, had protected Osama bin Laden and other Al Qaeda terrorists from being extradited to the United States following the 1998 bombings of U.S. embassies in Africa. In 2000, Bearak explained, Afghanistan had accounted for 75 percent of the world's entire opium crop, but in July of that year, Taliban leader Mullah Muhammed Omar had declared heroin cultivation a sin to the teachings of Islam, and as the headline accompanying the Bearak article indicated (see Table 1), Omar appeared to have accomplished what "Just Say No" could not. Bearak (2001) wrote:

> The world is unused to good news coming from Afghanistan, known these days as a womb for global jihad and an unsafe preservation site for Buddhist statues . . . But American narcotics officials who visited the country confirmed earlier United Nations reports that the Taliban had, in one growing season, managed a rare triumph in the long and losing war on drugs. And they did it without the usual multimillion-dollar aid packages that finance police raids, aerial surveillance and crop subsidies for farmers (p. A1).

Additionally, despite what Americans may have anticipated given representations of the Taliban, those caught growing poppies did not meet an unimaginable fate, as Bearak (2001) noted: "They whip women for exposing flesh at midcalf. They jail men for trimming their beards. They hold public executions in stadiums full of cheering people. But this spring's poppy crop seems to have died a relatively quiet death" (p. A1). One theory for the quiet demise of poppies involved the Taliban seeking legitimacy as a government and thus qualifying for financial aid toward controlling opiates. Although the possibility of poppies returning to the drug market certainly existed, Bearak explained, "the betting is that the ban will hold up" (p. A1).

As one might anticipate, after September 11, 2001, characterizations of Mullah Muhammed Omar and the Taliban changed dramatically. Instead of eradicating opium in Afghanistan, they allegedly had begun to cultivate it under the direction of Osama bin Laden and members Al Qaeda. On October 4, 2001, less than five months after the Bearak (2001) report, and less than one month after the terrorist attacks of 9/11, Barry Meier (2001) filed a report in the *New York Times* indicating that Osama bin Laden had been planning a "super" heroin to release among unsuspecting Americans and Western Europeans. In the sixth paragraph of his report, Meier wrote that "The announcements were made as United States officials, gearing up for a possible military action in Afghanistan, are seeking to portray the governing Taliban officials and Mr. bin Laden as critical cogs in the world drug trade. Although there is little dispute that the Taliban derived millions of dollars from opium production, the intelligence reports, if accurate, would provide a rare link between Mr. bin Laden's organization and drugs" (p. B3). It is difficult to argue the accuracy of that information, as linking drugs with terrorist threats is – on some level – relatively safe; the question is whether authorities ever make inroads on terror by attempting to make inroads on amorphous enemies who cultivate opium poppies.

On October 5, 2001, Meier reported in the *New York Times* that areas controlled by the Taliban did not contain as much opium as areas controlled by the Northern Alliance, a rebel group that U.S. officials hoped would destabilize the Taliban. Still, Meier explained, officials had warned "that the Taliban had large stockpiles of opium and heroin from record harvests in the years before the ban on cultivation" (p. B5).

By October 22, 2001, in an article headlined "Afghan ban on growing of opium is unraveling," Tim Golden offered the following lead in an article for the *New York Times*: "A highly successful ban on the growing of opium poppies in Afghanistan, which had been by far the biggest source of opium in the world, has begun to unravel as the United States presses its war against the ruling Taliban, American and United Nations officials say" (p. B1). With the United States assaulting Afghanistan in an attempt to remove the Taliban from power and destroy Al Qaeda networks, farmers had apparently been permitted to plant poppies; the crops could then be taxed, thus helping to fund the Taliban and, possibly, terrorist cells. On November 25, 2001, Golden wrote the following in a *New York Times* report:

> The problem that Afghanistan posed under the Taliban was not an isolated one. Over the last decade or so, as anti-drug campaigns have advanced in relatively coherent states like Pakistan, Iran, Thailand and Bolivia, more of the world's drug supply has begun to come from so-called rogue states, or from regions that government authority simply doesn't reach. After Afghanistan, the world's biggest opium producer these days is Burma. Most of the world's supply of coca, the raw material for cocaine, comes from regions of Colombia dominated by leftist rebels and right-wing paramilitary forces (p. D4).

Thus, to some extent, the production of opiates in Afghanistan appears to have correlated with the perceived severity of terrorist threats, and the *New York Times*, as a major national newspaper and agenda-setter for smaller news organizations, communicated the link between opium poppies and terror funding to media audiences. In addition, the *Times* kept readers aware of alleged threats from nations and territories elsewhere, implying a need to remain vigilant in the war on drugs.

Advancing to July 2007, Afghanistan continued to pose a threat, with *The New Yorker* publishing a lengthy report addressing difficulties encountered by American and international authorities charged with eradicating opium poppies. Jon Lee Anderson reported the following:

> Last year an estimated four hundred thousand acres of opium poppies were planted in Afghanistan, a fifty-nine percent increase over the previous year. Afghanistan now supplies more than ninety-two per cent of the world's opium, the raw ingredient of heroin. More than half the country's annual G.D.P., some $3.1 billion, is believed to come from the drug trade, and narcotics officials believe that part of the money is funding the Taliban insurgency (p. 62).

Consistent with the rhetoric of drug wars, Anderson posited that the Taliban had mounted a "concerted comeback" in the previous two years, tacitly indicating a need to continue spending millions of dollars in fighting Afghanistan opium production, given that Sunni Muslims would continue to fund terrorism with drug monies. Ultimately, press coverage of opiate threats from Afghanistan appears to have been consistent with coverage of other international drug threats and geo-political tensions.

SUMMARY

More than three decades have passed since Richard Nixon became the first U.S. president to declare "war" on drugs, and despite the investment of billions toward eradicating the abuse of substances such as cocaine and heroin, public officials continue to witness sustained use of the very drugs Nixon, followed by Ronald Reagan and George H. W. Bush, sought to curtail. To keep up the fight, as it were, and to keep at least part of the U.S. population in support of it, political actors who support the "war" on drugs have had to ensure that new threats continually emerge, thus allowing officials to call for intensified efforts and "new" approaches to the problem. As discussed, one approach used in rallying support for drug enforcement and interdiction has been to link narcotics with terror, the former being a funding source for the latter. Another approach has been to identify purported threats from nations and territories that existing intelligence has not identified.

As a common practice, news organizations rely on public officials to inform journalists and mass publics which nations do and do not pose a threat. The headlines in Table 1 revealed a variety of nations, and combinations of nations, whose involvement in the drug trade appeared to pose a threat on some level. In publishing these headlines, the *New York Times* and the *Los Angeles Times* implied a need to continue funding the "fight" against illegal narcotics. But, because mediated threats often receive little coverage beyond an initial alert (i.e., a headline in a prominent newspaper), a portion of the "breaking" news items amounted to little more than politically charged reminders – or exacerbators of world turmoil. In Table 1, with so many countries posing an alleged threat to the United States and to the world through heroin and narcotics trafficking, at least some of the news items stood to be dismissed given the sheer pervasiveness of alleged threats – or amorphous enemies.

REFERENCES

Anderson, J. L. (2007, July 9 & 16). Letter from Afghanistan: The Taliban's opium war. *The New Yorker*, pp. 60-71.

Associated Press (1989, July 21). Malaysia hangs drug trafficker. *Los Angeles Times*, p. A2.

Associated Press (1991, July 27). China pledges to help U.S. curb Asian heroin trade. *Los Angeles Times*, p. A4.

Associated Press (1995, February 4). Vietnam makes its biggest drug bust. *Los Angeles Times*, p. A12.

Barnetson, D. (1988, March 17). The Bombay connection: India is major player in world drug trade. *Los Angeles Times*, p. V20.

Bearak, B. (2000, April 19). Adding to Pakistan's misery, million-plus heroin addicts. *New York Times*, p. A1.

Bearak, B. (2001, May 24). At heroin's source, Taliban do what 'Just say no' could not. *New York Times*, p. A1.

Ben-Yehuda, N. (1990). *The politics and morality of deviance*. Albany, NY: State University of New York Press.

Bodeen, C. (2002, August 4). China stepping up war against drugs. *Los Angeles Times*, p. A3.

Breen, M. J. (1997). A cook, a cardinal, his priests, and the press: Deviance as a trigger for intermedia agenda setting. *Journalism & Mass Communication Quarterly, 74*(2), 348-356.

Burns, J. F. (1995, April 5). Heroin scourges million Pakistanis. *New York Times*, p. A12.

Carpenter, D. (1998, January 11). Today's silk road carries a different kind of import: Heroin. *Los Angeles Times*, p. A2.

Clarity, J. F. (1996, October 6). Dubliners outraged at sellers of heroin. *New York Times*, p. A4.

Colombian heroin may be increasing (1991, October 27). *New York Times*, p. A15.

Colombian heroin dominates U.S. market, government says (1998, January 1). *New York Times*, p. A19.
Cowell, A. (1993, February 9). Heroin pouring through porous European borders. *New York Times*, p. A3.
Dahlberg, J. T. (1993, June 6). Tracking the Russian Connection. *Los Angeles Times*, p. A1.
Dahlberg, J. T. (1995, April 9). Drug trade, militants thrive in Pakistan's rugged north. *Los Angeles Times*, p. A4.
Daniszewski, J. (2001, October 7). Taliban's drug war risks unraveling. *Los Angeles Times*, p. A1.
Darling, J. (1997, February 24). Colombians up quality, lower price of heroin. *Los Angeles Times*, p. A1.
Dixon, R. (2001, July 25). The opium trail has a new stop . . . Tajikistan. *Los Angeles Times*, p. A1.
Erlanger, S. (1990, February 11). Southeast Asia is no. 1 source of U.S. heroin. *New York Times*, p. A26.
Farley, M. (1995, June 10). Young addicts spur China to address its drug problem. *Los Angeles Times*, p. A1.
Forero, J. (2003, June 8). Latin American poppy fields undermine U.S. drug battle. *New York Times*, p. A1.
Freed, K. (1989, August 30). Guatemala seen slipping into a haven for drugs. *Los Angeles Times*, p. A1.
Gall, C. (2003, September 5). U.N. aide says Afghan drug trade pays for terrorist attacks. *New York Times*, p. A5.
Gates, A. (1999, May 7). A drug pusher's life is rotten in Denmark. *New York Times*, p. E23.
Girardet, E. (1989, January 1). Western officials look to Afghanistan and see a new problem —heroin. *Los Angeles Times*, p. A22.
Golden, T. (2001, October 22). Afghan ban on growing of opium is unraveling. *New York Times*, p. B1.
Golden, T. (2001, November 25). A war on terror meets a war on drugs. *New York Times*, p. D4.
Golden, T. (2002, April 1). U.S. fears a glut of heroin from a volatile Afghanistan. *New York Times*, p. A1.
Gould, S. J. (2002). The war on (some) drugs. In M. Gray (Ed.), *Busted: Stone cowboys, narco -lords and Washington's war on drugs* (pp. 257-259). New York: Nation Books.
Greenhouse, S. (1995, February 12). Heroin from Burmese surges as U.S. debates strategy. *New York Times*, p. A3.
Hahn, D. F. (1998). *Political communication: Rhetoric, government, and citizens*. State College, PA: Strata Publishing.
Hays, T. (1994, July 3). Frenchman's arrest cracks narcotics ring. *Los Angeles Times*, p. A2.
Holley, D. (2001, August 21). Portugal takes away prison as a penalty for using drugs. *Los Angeles Times*, p. A1.
Ingram, J. (2002, August 11). Drug use, trafficking on the rise in Russia. *Los Angeles Times*, p. A3.
Ivanko, A. (1992, November 29). Surge in addiction linked to Russian drug gangs. *Los Angeles Times*, p. A30.

Jehl, D. (1990, March 19). 'Indian Connection' poppies throw a curve at U.S. drug policy. *Los Angeles Times*, p. A17.

Kamm, H. (1988, April 14). Afghan opium yield up as Pakistan curbs crop. *New York Times*, p. A16.

Koss, M. (2003, August 10). Myanmar tries to kick its habit. *Los Angeles Times*, p. M2.

Kristof, N. B. (1991, March 21). Heroin spreads among young in China. *New York Times*, p. A1.

Levenson, J. (2004, November/December). The war on what, exactly? Why the press must be precise. *Columbia Journalism Review*, pp. 9-11.

Lynch, C., & Witte, G. (2007, August 28). Afghan opium trade hits new peak. *Washington Post*, p. A7.

MacCoun, R. J., & Reuter, P. (2001). *Drug war heresies: Learning from other vices, times, & places*. Cambridge: Cambridge University Press.

Mackey-Kallis, S., & Hahn, D. (1994). Who's to blame for America's drug problem? The search for scapegoats in the "War on Drugs." *Communication Quarterly, 42*(1), 1-20.

Mann, J., & Ostrow, R. J. (1995, June 21). U.S. to help Myanmar fight drug production. *Los Angeles Times*, p. A4.

Marez, C. (2004). *Drug wars: The political economy of narcotics*. Minneapolis: University of Minnesota Press.

McLeod, J. M., Kosicki, G. M., & McLeod, D. M. (1994). The expanding boundaries of political communication effects. In J. Bryant & D. Zillmann (Eds.), *Media effects: Advances in theory and research* (pp. 123-162). Hillsdale, NJ: Erlbaum.

Meier, B. (2001, October 4). 'Super' heroin was planned by bin Laden, reports say. *New York Times*, p. B3.

Meier, B. (2001, October 5). Most Afghan opium grown in rebel-controlled areas. *New York Times*, p. B5.

Morales, W. (1989). The war on drugs: A new U.S. national security doctrine? *Third World Quarterly, 11*, 147-169.

Navarro, M. (1995, November 2). Colombia's heroin couriers: Swallowing and smuggling. *New York Times*, p. A1.

Ni, C. C. (2003, January 15). Old habit has China in its grip. *Los Angeles Times*, p. A1.

O'Rourke, P. J. (2002). My problem with the war on drugs. In M. Gray (Ed.), *Busted: Stone cowboys, narco-lords and Washington's war on drugs* (pp. 187-195). New York: Nation Books.

Overend, W. (1988, February 25). Violence feared as Asian heroin influx soars. *Los Angeles Times*, p. A3.

Paddock, R. C., & Demick, B. (2003, May 21). N. Korea's growing drug trade seen in botched heroin delivery. *Los Angeles Times*, p. A1.

Pear, R. (1988, September 6). U.S. sees increase in Afghan opium. *New York Times*, p. A10.

Pogatchnik, S. (1997, April 13). Movie underscores Scotland's heroin plague. *Los Angeles Times*, p. A29.

Reuters (2003, May 27). N. Korea ship left more heroin, Australia says. *Los Angeles Times*, p. A11.

Rotella, S. (1994, January 17). Mexican police make record heroin seizure. *Los Angeles Times*, p. A3.

Schemo, D. J. (1997, March 30). Heroin is proving a growth industry for Colombia. *New York Times*, p. A3.

Schudson, M. (2003). *The sociology of news*. New York: W. W. Norton.

Sciolino, E. (1994, April 5). State Dept. labels Nigeria major trafficker of drugs to U.S. *New York Times*, p. A1.

Singapore hangs 2 as drug traffickers (1989, May 28). *Los Angeles Times*, p. A12.

Tempest, R. (2001, November 23). Opium poppies take root once again in Afghanistan. *Los Angeles Times*, p. A1.

Tierney, J. (2005, August 9). Debunking the drug war. *New York Times*, p. A19.

Treaster, J. B. (1992, January 14, 1992). Colombia's drug lords add new product: Heroin for U.S. *New York Times*, p. A1.

Treaster, J. B. (1992, February 15). Nigerian Connection floods U.S. airports with Asian heroin. *New York Times*, p. A1.

Treaster, J. B. (1992, April 15). U.S. links trail of heroin to a 'Soviet connection.' *New York Times*, p. B3.

United Press International (1989, August 5). Iran hangs 8 accused heroin traffickers. *Los Angeles Times*, p. A10.

United Press International (1991, April 20). Kuwaiti Blueblood reportedly could face death penalty. *Los Angeles Times*, p. A15.

United Press International (1992, June 27). China executes 27 narcotics traffickers. *Los Angeles Times*, p. A13.

Verschuur, P. (1990, March 4). Dutch drug policy gains ground. *Los Angeles Times*, p. A11.

Wallace, C. P. (1990, July 24). Golden triangle's blooming threat. *Los Angeles Times*, p. H1.

Welkos, R. W. (1999, April 21). On the case in China. *Los Angeles Times*, p. F1.

Williams, N. B. Jr. (1992, January 26). Syrians cash in on drug trade in Lebanon's Notorious Bekaa Valley. *Los Angeles Times*, p. A18.

Wren, C. S. (1995, December 26). Heroin route via Africa a new worry. *New York Times*, p. A13.

Wren, C. S. (1996, February 11). Colombians enter the heroin market. *New York Times*, p. A51.

Zelizer, B., & Allan, S. (2002). *Journalism after September 11*. London: Routledge.

Zernike, K. (2005, July 6). Officials across U.S. describe drug woes. *New York Times*, p. A12.

In: Drugs: Approval and Evaluation, Delivery and Control ISBN: 978-1-60456-533-1
Editors: A.O. Hartmann, L.K. Neumann

Chapter 10

STANDARDS AND NEW DEVELOPMENTS IN THE MEASUREMENT OF HEART RATE VARIABILITY

Matthias Burghardt
Technical University of Dresden, Germany

1. ABSTRACT

The existence of deterministic processes behind the beat-to-beat fluctuations of heart rate has been postulated since the 1970´s. As autonomic balance is believed to be one major driving force behind this phenomenon heart rate variability (HRV) and its measurement have attracted significant attention from several medical disciplines including neurology, cardiology, somnology, anaesthesiology and intensive care. The large number of methods that have been developed to analyse HRV not only reflects the wide range of information that can be gained from this parameter but also the fact, that there is no single algorithm that can be considered generally suitable for this task.

A short overview of the two basic classes of HRV algorithms (time domain and frequency domain methods) and their application will be given. The mathematical validity of Fourier Transform (FT), the most prevailing algorithm for frequency domain analysis, will be critically discussed. Wavelet Transform (WT) will be proposed as a possible alternative that does not share FT's theoretical limitations for this application.

2. INTRODUCTION

It is a well known fact that heart rate is not constant over time but rather reacts to physical and mental stress. Increased demand of oxygen and nutrient supply in brain, splanchnic organs or skeletal muscles is answered by an increase in heart rate. This physiological mechanism provides adaption of cardiac output to perfusion requirement.

Beside these large excursions there are small fluctuations of heart rate occurring ubiquitously throughout time. This so-called "Heart Rate Variability" (HRV) originates from a number of intrinsic pacemakers which have been shown to be under control of the sympathetic and parasympathetic branches of autonomic nervous system [1,]The prognostic value of HRV monitoring was first recognized in obstetrics for the diagnosis of fetal distress syndrome [2]. HRV analysis has since then received considerable interest from various medical disciplines dealing with autonomic disorders and has become a standard test of autonomic function in neurology.

As autonomic function is greatly influenced by anesthesia and critical illness measurement of HRV would be desirable for these situations. However, beside some scientific research there has been no widespread utilisation of HRV in anesthesiology and intensive care. Standard anesthesia monitors usually filter out the minor heart rate oscillations induced by HRV in order to enhance readability of numerically displayed heart rate. The main reason for this discrepancy is that existing applications of HRV measurement have been focusing on quantification of statical alteration of autonomic function. Broadening the scope of HRV monitoring to dynamical situations as they are commonplace in anesthesiology and intensive care imposes the need for new algorithms specifically tailored to the instantaneous detection of changes in autonomic function.

3. Principles of HRV Analysis

The widespread interest in HRV measurement has motivated the application of numerous statistical methods to HRV analysis. The traditional starting point for this analysis is a sequence of interval durations between two consecutive normal heart beats (so-called normal-to-normal intervals, NN intervals). Interbeat intervals adjacent to premature or compensatorily delayed heart beats are discarded prior to analysis. Alternatively, the reciprocal of interbeat duration is used to calculate so-called instantaneous heart rate (IHR). The graphical display of this sequence of interval durations or their respective IHRs as a function of time is known as tachogram.

It has become standard practice to treat the sequence of consecutive interbeat intervals or IHRs as a time series. The methods taken from the field of time series analysis, a branch of stochastics, basically fall into two classes [3]:

I. Time domain methods
II. Frequency domain methods

Analysis in time domain includes the calculation of various descriptive statistics from the series of intervals between two consecutive normal heart beats. The simplest of these parameters, standard deviation of NN intervals (*SDNN*) gives a measure of the whole oscillatory activity. Another parameter, *SDNN index* is obtained by calculating multiple SDNNs for subsequent short sections (about 5 min) and averaging over this series of SDNNs. SDNN index therefore represents only oscillations with shorter cycle lengths. Conversely, the standard deviation of short-time averages of NN intervals (*SDANN*) is used to restrict quantification to slower oscillations. While SDNN can be calculated from periods as short as 5 min SDANN and SDNN index require longer recording of heart rate. These parameters are usually calculated from 24h periods.

A slightly different approach is based on the series of differences between subsequent NN intervals instead of the absolute interval durations. This leads to parameters like *NN50*, the count of interval differences greater than 50 ms, and *pNN50*, the proportion of NN50 to the whole interval count. A more complex parameter from this class is *RMSSD*, the square root of the mean of squared interval differences. These measures emphasize beat-to-beat changes of heart rate and therefore express mostly high-frequency activity.

Beside the numerical description of the data there are also geometric methods which are used to extract certain variational properties from the NN interval series. Most of these methods are based on a plot of the distribution density of NN intervals. A common parameter of this type is *HRV triangular index*, the ratio of the whole number of NN intervals divided by the count of occurrence of the most prevalent interval duration. Triangular interpolation of NN intervals (*TINN*) is found by fitting a triangular shape to the density curve and measuring the base length of this triangle. These geometric measures of HRV quantify the diversity of NN intervals. They are more influenced by slow-oscillating activity, which is partly due to the need of a considerable number of NN intervals for reliable construction of the density plot.

Plotting the duration of each NN interval against the duration of its immediately subsequent interval yields the so-called *Lorenz plot*. The spread of dots in this plot is a geometric measure of total variation of NN intervals. It has been proposed to classify the pattern formed by the plot into categories like „comet“ or „torpedo“. This approach is limited by the lack of a clear definition of categories and is not suitable for results that can not be easily assigned to one of these classes [4].

4. Fourier Transform in HRV Analysis

As most of the time domain measures try to partition total oscillatory activity into slow-oscillating and fast-oscillating components it is an obvious choice to apply spectral methods to HRV analysis. This is achieved by transposing the tachogram, i.e. the time series of subsequent NN intervals or their respective IHRs from time domain into frequency domain. Fourier Transform (*FT*) is the most prevailing method for this transposition. This approach has become especially popular since the (re-)discovery of Fast Fourier Transform (*FFT*) in 1965, an efficient algorithm for the decomposition of the input sequence into a weighted sum of sinusoidal components, the so-called Fourier series. This method accomplishes discrimination between high-frequency and low-frequency portions and allows for simultaneous measurement of their magnitude. Plotting squared absolute magnitudes against frequency yields the power spectrum. From the multi-modal distribution of spectral power over the frequency axis three different frequency ranges have been defined and several physiological processes have been ascribed as intrinsic pacemakers to these frequency bands (Table 1). High-frequency (HF) variations of heart rate are attributable to respiratory sinus arrhythmia, a physiological mechanism that suppresses parasympathetic activity during inspiration thereby causing a periodic rise in heart rate synchronous to respiration. The magnitude of these HF oscillations is therefore a measure of basal parasympathetic activity. The low-frequency (LF) portion of HRV has been shown to represent a mixture of both sympathetic and parasympathetic activity [1]. The physiological meaning of very low and ultra-low frequency content is not yet clear [1].

Table 1. Frequency bands of HRV

Frequency band	Frequency range	Physiological relevance
High frequency (HF)	0.15..0.40 s^{-1}	parasympathetic
Low frequency (LF)	0.05..0.15 s^{-1}	sympathetic and parasympathetic
Very / ultra low frequency (VLF, ULF)	< 0.05 s^{-1}	undetermined

However, the application of Fourier transform to a series of NN intervals or IHRs is not unproblematic. FFT requires the points of the input series to be equidistantly sampled. This special case, however, would only be encountered if heart beat is controlled by an artificial pacemaker with fixed-frequency in which case HRV analysis would be senseless. In the general case variability of heart rate implies that heart beat arrivals and therefore sampling points are non-equidistant. There are two popular approaches to deal with this problem. A simplistic solution is to number all NN intervals and use interval numbers instead of time points to construct the input sequence for FT. The frequency axis of the spectrum obtained by this method has the unit [beat number]$^{-1}$ instead of the usual s^{-1} and therefore requires correction by mean heart rate during the time of recording. This is especially difficult for longer recordings where heart rate can not reasonably be assumed to be constant over the time of measurement.

A more complex workaround to the problem of non-equidistance is to interpolate the input sequence e.g. by spline methods and resample equidistant points from this curve. This method circumvents the problem of frequency axis scaling, but with added complexity and unpredictable distortion of the original information.

So far spectral HRV analysis has primarily been applied to situations where autonomic function was assumed to be in steady state. This assumption of constant frequency content is no longer valid when HRV measurement is extended to dynamical situations. Non-stationarity of oscillatory properties does not only violate the preconditions for FT but also requires the algorithm to allow for instantaneous detection and representation of changes in spectral content. This leads to methods that provide a time-frequency representation of the original time series. Similar to SDNN index where standard deviations are calculated for subsequent short epochs of the input time series some window function is shifted along the time axis to split the whole input sequence into short, optionally overlapping sections which are processed separately. This application of FT to windowed portions of the input time series is known as Short-Time Fourier Transform (*STFT*). Instead of one power spectrum for the whole recording time a series of spectra is obtained that forms a function of spectral content over discrete time thereby providing insight into the temporal dynamics of spectral power.

The time resolution of STFT depends on the width (technically speaking: support) of the window function, i.e. the narrower the window the more accurate the variation in time is depicted. However, narrowing the window also decreases the number of interbeat intervals that are considered for spectral analysis in each epoch. On the one hand, this renders the assumption of stationarity more valid, on the other hand frequency resolution decreases as time resolution increases. Basically this is due to the Heisenberg principle of uncertainty which, applied to the time-frequency information of a signal, states that exact time and frequency information of one spectral component cannot be known simultaneously. In fact, only the time interval and frequency band containing an amount of spectral power can be found. One extremum with respect to resolutional characteristics is formed by time domain where time resolution is maximal but no frequency information available. The other end of this continuum is its Fourier series where frequency resolution is perfect while time resolution is completely lost. The trade-off between time and frequency resolution in STFT is controlled by the support of the window function (Figure 1).

HRV consists of a mixture of high-frequency and low-frequency content. The HF portion is usually dominated by respiratory sinus arrhythmia which produces a single peak in this region of the spectrum. Changes in parasympathetic activity are rapidly reflected by the amplitude of this peak. Conversely, the LF region is populated by a number of spectral components with similar frequencies and slowly changing properties. This mixture would require higher time resolution for HF and higher frequency resolution for LF. The fact that time and frequency resolution are constant over the whole STFT spectrum implies that no optimal tuning of STFT's resolution properties for simultaneous analysis of LF and HF portions can be achieved.

Moreover, there is also fundamental criticism to the utilization of the tachogram as starting point for the application of FT (or any other frequency transform). The basis for this disagreement is the conception that HRV is only a surrogate parameter for the activity of autonomic nervous system that is actually to be assessed. Sympathetic-parasympathetic balance is a process that changes continuously over time. The time course of heart rate reflects these time-continuous changes of auonomic balance although it is no time-continuous parameter in itself, but rather a stochastic point process. The oscillations of heart rate are generated in correlation to autonomic balance through some kind of mapping. The optimal choice of techniques for HRV analysis depends on the characteristics of this connection. As autonomic balance can not be directly measured there is no straightforward way to analyse this mapping. However, there exist evidence that HRV is generated from sympathovagal balance by means of Integral Pulse Frequency Modulation (IPFM) [5].

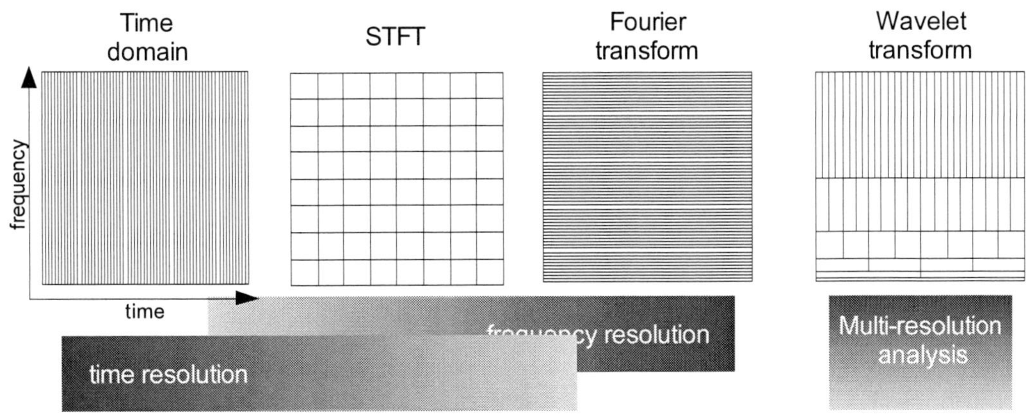

Figure 1. Resolutional characteristics of different representations of an oscillating time series.

Extraction of frequency information from a stochastic point process can be performed by two different ways (Figure 2). Applying frequency transform to the tachogram, i.e. to the sequence of interbeat interval durations, yields the so-called interval spectrum. On the other hand, by representing the arrival of every single heart beat by a delta function another time series is obtained that can be used as input to frequency transform. In practice, as beat arrival can only be detected with limited accuracy, the delta spikes are substituted by rectangles. The resulting time series is formed by values of [1 heart beat / sampling interval] = $f_{Sampling}$ for those sampling instants associated with beat arrival and values of zero elsewhere. Under the assumption that HRV is generated through IPFM low-pass filtering of this spike train yields an estimate of the underlying sympathetic-parasympathetic balance. Transformation of this spike train into frequency domain gives a so-called spectrum of counts as opposed to the interval spectrum resulting from frequency transform of the tachogram. Which of these two spectra is preferable to the other depends on the characteristics of the underlying process [6]. In the case of HRV analysis, where IFPM is assumed to generate the stochastic point process there is evidence to suggest that the spectrum of counts is a more valid estimator of the true frequency content.

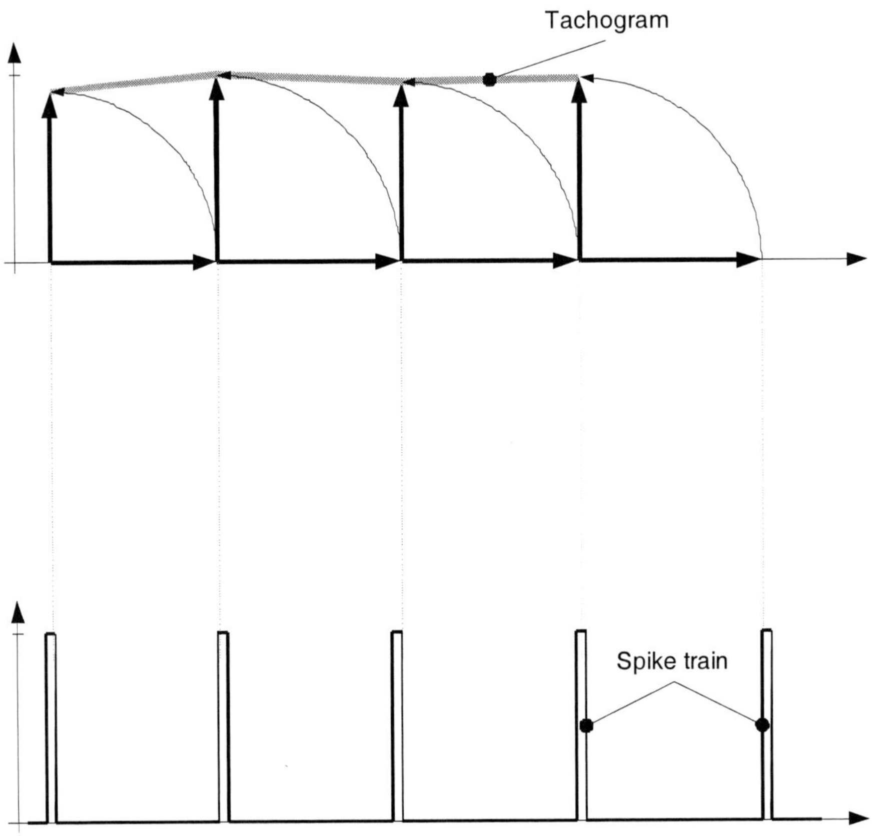

Figure 2. Preprocessing of raw ECG prior to frequency transform. Plotting interval duration against beat arrival time yields the tachogram (top), representing beat arrival by a rect function gives a spike train (bottom).

5. Multi-Resolution Analysis of HRV

On the basis of these theoretical limitations of Fourier Transform in HRV analysis we propose to employ Wavelet Transform (WT) as a possible alternative to Fourier methods. Wavelet Transform has been introduced to biomedical signal analysis in 1975 for the investigation of sound reception in the cochlea although its roots go back to the beginning of the 20th century [7]. The term wavelet describes a class of mathematical functions with fast-decaying oscillating waveform. Wavelets are therefore localized in both frequency (by their oscillating part) and time (by the decay of the envelope). By translating and scaling the mother wavelet along time axis a continuum of daughter wavelets is generated each being specific for one certain time point and frequency. Performing WT with various daughter wavelets yields one wavelet coefficient for each daughter wavelet describing the magnitude of oscillatory activity for the time-frequency pair of this daughter wavelet. Plotting squared wavelet coefficients against translation and scale of their respective wavelets gives a so-called translation-scale-plane (TSP). As scale is reciprocally related to frequency this TSP resembles a time-frequency representation of spectral power like the one obtained by STFT. WT is therefore applicable to input time series with non-stationary frequency content. However, unlike STFT, where time and frequency resolution are constant over the whole time-frequency grid, the support of the window function in WT changes (reciprocally proportional) with frequency. This allows for finer temporal resolution at high frequencies and better frequency resolution for low-frequency content. These particular resolution properties make WT especially well suited for simultaneous analysis of both high-frequency and low-frequency components of HRV. Moreover, the direct application of WT to the spike train formed by beat arrival times is not only a mathematically valid method to obtain the spectrum of counts avoiding the need for equidistant resampling but is also straightforward and computationally efficient.

A preliminary evaluation of this new method has been conducted in 12 (7 male, 5 female) subjects undergoing major visceral surgery [8]. In all subjects a thoracic epidural catheter was inserted and general anesthesia was maintained according to a standardized protocol with nitrous oxide and desflurane, supplemented with remifentanil as needed. Subjects were randomly allocated to receive local anesthetic or placebo via epidural catheter before skin incision and at regular intervals of 1 hour. WT was applied to the sequences of beat arrival times extracted from arterial blood pressure waveforms. We found a reduction of HRV in both LF and HF bands by the local anesthetic as compared to the placebo group. LF spectral power was negatively correlated with remifentanil dosage in placebo group. We concluded that the decrease of LF activity under thoracic epidural anesthesia can be attributed to cardiac sympathectomy induced by neuraxial blockade of sympathetic efference to the heart while the negative correlation between LF power and remifentanil dosage reflects general reduction of sympathetic activity due to the central blockade of nociception.

Our results indicate that WT is a viable method for the monitoring of autonomic function in an anesthesiologic setting. Whether this new method is preferable to traditional Fourier Transform in terms of scientific and clinical utility and especially in its applicability to dynamic situations has to be further determined.

6. References

[1] Akselrod S, Gordon D, Ubel FA, Shannon DC, Berger AC, Cohen RJ, Power spectrum analysis of heart rate fluctuation: a quantitative probe of beat-to-beat cardiovascular control., *Science,* 1981; 213: 220-2.

[2] Hon Eh, Lee ST, Electronic evaluation of the fetal heart rate. viii. patterns Preceding fetal death, further observations., *Am J Obstet Gynecol,* 1963; 87: 814-26.

[3] Task Force of the European Society of Cardiology the North American Society of Pacing Electrophysiology, Heart Rate Variability: Standards of Measurement, Physiological Interpretation, and Clinical Use, *Circulation,* 1996; 93: 1043-65.

[4] Malik M, Time-Domain Measurement of Heart Rate Variability, *Cardiac Electrophysiology Review,* 1997; 1: 329-34.

[5] Hyndman B, Mohn R, Model of the Cardiac Pacemaker and its Use in Decoding the Information Content of Cardiac Intervals, *Automedica,* 1975; 1: 239-52.

[6] DeBoer RW, Karemaker JM, Strackee J, Comparing spectra of a series of point events particularly for heart rate variability data., *IEEE Trans Biomed Eng,* 1984; 31: 384-7.

[7] Haar A, Zur Theorie der orthogonalen Funktionensysteme, *Math Ann,* 1910; 69: 331-71.

[8] Burghardt M, Heller AR, Complex Continuous Wavelet Transform for Quantification of Neuraxial Sympathetic Blockade by Thoracic Epidural Analgesia., *Biomedical Engineering,* 2005; 50 Suppl 1: 1503-4.

In: Drugs: Approval and Evaluation, Delivery and Control ISBN: 978-1-60456-533-1
Editors: A.O. Hartmann, L.K. Neumann

Chapter 11

DRUG CONTROL: INTERNATIONAL POLICY AND APPROACHES*

Raphael Perl

ABSTRACT

Efforts to significantly reduce the flow of illicit drugs from abroad into the United States have so far not succeeded. Moreover, over the past decade, worldwide production of illicit drugs has risen dramatically: opium and marijuana production has roughly doubled and coca production tripled. Street prices of cocaine and heroin have fallen significantly in the past 20 years, reflecting increased availability. The effectiveness of international narcotics control programs in reducing consumption is a matter of ongoing concern. Despite apparent national political resolve to deal with the drug problem, inherent contradictions regularly appear between U.S. anti-drug policy and other national policy goals and concerns. Pursuit of drug control policies can sometimes affect foreign policy interests and bring political instability and economic dislocation to countries where narcotics production has become entrenched economically and socially. Drug supply interdiction programs and U.S. systems to facilitate the international movement of goods, people, and wealth are often at odds. U.S. international narcotics policy requires cooperative efforts by many nations which may have domestic and foreign policy goals that compete with the requirements of drug control. The mix of competing domestic and international pressures and priorities has produced an ongoing series of disputes within and between the legislative and executive branches concerning U.S. international drug policy. One contentious issue has been the Congressionally-mandated certification process, an instrument designed to induce specified drug-exporting countries to prioritize or pay more attention to the fight against narcotics businesses. Current law requires the President, with certain exceptions, to designate and withhold assistance from countries that have failed demonstrably to meet their counternarcotics obligations. P.L. 106-246, "Plan Colombia," a $1.3 billion military assistance-focused initiative to provide emergency supplemental narcotics assistance to Colombia, was signed into law July 13,

* Excerpted from CRS Report IB88093, Updated February 2, 2006.

2000. Recently, U.S. policy toward Colombia has focused increasingly on containing the terror- ist threat to that country's security. The Bush Administration's FY2005 budget request continues a policy, begun in FY2002, to request authority for the State and Defense Departments to supply assistance to Colombia for counterterrorism purposes. For instance, U.S.-supplied helicopters and intelligence could be used to support military operations against guerrillas financed by drugs as well as against drug traffickers themselves. See CRS Report RL32337, *Andean Counterdrug Initia- tive (ACI) and Related Funding Programs: FY2005 Assistance.*

An issue likely to achieve increased attention in the 109th Congress is that of sky-rocketing opium poppy cultivation in Afghanistan and whether to press for aerial crop eradication against the wishes of the local Afghan leadership. See CRS Report RL32686, *Af- ghanistan: Narcotics and U.S. Policy.*

Drug control approaches addressed in this issue brief include:

- Expansion of efforts to reduce foreign production at the source.
- Expansion of interdiction and enforcement activities to disrupt supply lines.
- Expansion of efforts to reduce worldwide demand.
- Expansion of economic disincentives for international drug trafficking.

Most Recent Developments

On January 28, 2006, President Evo Morales of Bolivia appointed Felipe Caceres, a coca leaf grower, to head his government's fight against drug trafficking — escalating concern in U.S. policy circles that Morales will follow through on his pre-election pledge to roll back U.S. efforts to curb coca production in Bolivia. U.S. counternarcotics programs in Bolivia were funded at $79.2 million in FY2006 (alternative development and law enforcement). The Administration's FY2007 request is expected to be somewhat less.

A report released by the Government Accountability Office (GAO-06-200) argues for the development of better counter-drug performance measures by government agencies and warns that the diversion of military assets to Iraq and Afghanistan is likely to hamper the ability of U.S. law enforcement to intercept drug shipments in the future. Proponents of strong drug interdiction policies have long been concerned that the nation's focus on anti-terror objectives will detract from resources and political will needed to combat foreign source illicit drug production and trafficking.

Background and Analysis

Problem

More than 14 million Americans buy illicit drugs and use them at least once per month, spending by most conservative estimates over $60 billion annually in a diverse and fragmented criminal market. Such drugs are to varying degrees injurious to the health, judgment, productivity and general well-being of their users. The 2002 *National Drug Control Strategy* (hereafter *Strategy*) of the White House Office of National Drug Control

Policy (ONDCP) estimates the total costs of drug abuse to American society to be approximately $160 billion. The major components of this total are health care costs ($14.9 billion), workplace productivity losses ($110.5 billion) and losses related to crime, the criminal justice system, and social welfare ($35 billion). According to the *Strategy* more than 60% of the inmates in the federal prison system are drug law violators; moreover, the addictive nature and high price of most illegal drugs contribute significantly to the incidence of violent crime and property crime in the United States. Additionally, the U.S. illicit drug market generates billions of dollars in profits. Such profits provide international drug trafficking organizations with the resources to effectively evade and compete with law enforcement agencies, to penetrate legitimate economic structures, and, in some instances, to challenge the authority of national governments.

Calculated in dollar value terms, at least four-fifths of all the illicit drugs consumed in the United States are of foreign origin, including virtually all the cocaine and heroin and most of the marijuana, according to the ONDCP *Strategy* and the U.S. Drug Enforcement Administration (DEA) 2002 report, *Drug Trafficking in the United States*. According to DEA, the methamphetamine market is supplied predominantly from laboratories in both the United States and Mexico while most of the hallucinogens and illegally marketed psychotheraputic drugs and "designer" drugs are of domestic U.S. origin.

Drugs are a lucrative business and a mainspring of global criminal activity. According to a 2002 estimate by the State Department's Bureau of International Narcotics and Law Enforcement Affairs (INL), as much as 930 tons of cocaine could have been produced from coca leaf grown in South America in 2001. If sold internationally at an average U.S. street price per gram of $100, the drug would yield a gross value of $93 billion, a figure exceeding the Gross National Income of three-quarters of the world's nations. A November 2002 study by the United Nations Office on Drugs and Crime estimated the net regional earnings of the illicit drug industry in the Caribbean at $3.3 billion, or about half the Gross National Income of Jamaica or Trinidad. Little is known about the distribution of revenues from illicit drug sales, but foreign supply cartels exercise considerable control over wholesale distribution in the United States and illicit proceeds are often laundered and invested through foreign banks and financial institutions.

In December 2002, the Chief of Operations of the U.S. Drug Enforcement Administration (DEA) told a Congressional panel that the number of hard-core heroin users in the United States had increased to "almost a million" from an estimated 630,000 in 1992. The DEA Heroin Signature Program, which identifies the sources of that drug seized by U.S. federal authorities, found that 56% of the seized heroin was of Colombian origin.

The federal anti-drug initiative has two major elements: (1) reduction of demand and (2) reduction of supply. Reduction of demand is sought through education to prevent dependence, through treatment to cure addiction and through measures to increase prices and risk of apprehension at the consumer level. Reduction of supply (which currently accounts for about 53% of the federal anti-drug control budget, according to the *Strategy*) is sought by programs aimed at destabilizing the operations of illicit drug cartels at all levels and severing their links to political power, and by seizing their products, businesses, and financial assets. As most illicit drugs are imported, a major interdiction campaign is being conducted on the U.S. borders, at ports of entry, on the high seas, and along major foreign transshipment routes and at production sites. An international program of source crop eradication is also being pursued. As reported in the *Strategy*, approximately 18% of the requested federal drug control budget of $11.7 billion for FY2004 is for interdiction and 9.2% is for international assistance programs. These ratios continue to remain relatively constant. The major international components of federal policies for the reduction of illicit supply are discussed below.

On or about March 7, 2005, the State Department released its annual International Narcotics Control Strategy Report (INCSR), a comprehensive assessment of the efforts of foreign nations to combat the illicit drug trade and drug related money laundering.

Current International Narcotics Control Policy

The primary goal of U.S. international narcotics policy is to reduce the supply of illicit narcotics flowing into the United States. A second and supporting goal is to reduce the amount of illicit narcotics cultivated, processed, and consumed worldwide. U.S. international narcotics control policy is implemented by a multifaceted strategy that includes the following elements: (1) eradication of narcotic crops, (2) interdiction and law enforcement activities in drug-producing and drug-transiting countries, (3) international cooperation, (4) sanctions/economic assistance, and (5) institution development. The U.S. State Department's Bureau of International Narcotics and Law Enforcement (INL) has the lead role coordinating U.S. international drug intervention and suppression activities.

In April 2001, the President requested $882 million in economic and counternarcotics assistance for Colombia and regional neighbors as part of an Andean Regional Initiative (ARI). The ARI proposal differed from the Plan Colombia program in two key areas: (1) spending on economic and social programs would be roughly equal to the drug control and interdiction components that had been the primary focus of Plan Colombia; and (2) more than half of the assistance was targeted to neighboring countries experiencing spillover effects from Colombia's civil conflict and from narcotrafficking activities in that country. The enacted appropriations bill (P.L. 107-115) cleared by Congress on December 20, 2001, provided $783 million for the Initiative, a cut of $99 million from the President's request. Of the appropriation, not less than $215 million was to be apportioned directly to the Agency for International Development (AID) for economic and social programs. The enacted bill included conditions on the use of funds for purchase of chemicals for the aerial spraying program in Colombia, limited the number of U.S. civilian and military personnel involved in Colombia to 800, and blocked funding for restoration of flights in support of the Peruvian air interdiction program until a system of enhanced safeguards is in place. The State Department's request for its Andean Drug Counter Drug Initiative (ACI) for FY2003 and FY2004 totaled $731 million for each year respectively. The Administration requested $731 million for the Andean Counterdrug Initiative for FY2005, and $114 million for economic assistance programs. Congress also raised from 400 to 800 the level of U.S. military personnel and from 400 to 600 the level of civilian contractor personnel allowed to be deployed in Colombia, in response to an Administration request.

Eradication of Narcotic Crops

A long-standing U.S. policy regarding international narcotics control is to reduce cultivation and production of illicit narcotics through eradication. The United States supports programs to eradicate coca, opium, and marijuana in a number of countries. These efforts are conducted by a number of U.S. government agencies administering several types of programs. The United States supports eradication by providing producer countries with chemical herbicides, technical assistance and specialized equipment, and spray aircraft. The U.S. Agency for International Development (AID) funds programs designed to promote economic growth and to provide alternative sources of employment for the people currently growing, producing, or processing illicit drugs. AID also provides balance of payments support (especially to the Andean countries) to help offset the loss of foreign exchange (from diminished drug exports) occurring as a result of U.S.-supported anti-drug programs. U.S. eradication policy receives informational support from the State Department's Office of Public Diplomacy and Public Affairs (formerly the U.S. Information Agency (USIA)) which publicizes the dangers of drug abuse and trafficker violence. In addition, AID sponsors drug education and awareness programs in 33 Latin American, Asian, and East European countries.

The eradication program in the Andes resulted in the elimination of an estimated 110,000 hectares of coca in Peru and Bolivia between 1995 and 2001, or almost 70% of the combined cultivated area in those countries. Nevertheless, cultivation in Colombia increased by 119,000 hectares or 234% over the same period.[1] The shift in cultivation has had implications for Colombia's civil conflict, putting more "taxable" resources into the hands of Colombia's leftist guerrillas. The State Department's International Strategy report for 2001 notes that "The Colombian syndicates, witnessing the vulnerability of Peruvian and Bolivian coca supply to joint interdiction operations in the late 1990s, decided to move most of the cultivation to Colombia's southwest corner, an area controlled by the FARC, the country's oldest insurgent group." This trend continues in Colombia today.

On January 2, 2005, the *Los Angeles Times* reported that the Bush Administration is split over how to respond to Afghanistan's skyrocketing opium poppy production. The debate reportedly centers over whether to push for large scale aerial eradication, or to leave the issue to the discretion of local officials. Central to the debate is what some view as potentially competing U.S. policy objectives in the war-torn nation, i.e., counterterrorism, counter-narcotics, and political stability.

Interdiction and Law Enforcement

A second element of U.S. international narcotics control strategy is to help host governments seize illicit narcotics before they reach America's borders. A related imperative is to attack and disrupt large aggregates of criminal power, to immobilize their top leaders and

---

[1] Note, however, that in Congressional testimony on July 10, 2003, Acting State Department INL Assistant Secretary Paul E. Simons announced that coca cultivation in Colombia during the year 2002 had declined overall by more than 15%, a development he characterized as a "direct result of the robust U.S.-assisted aerial eradication program."

to sever drug traffickers' ties to the economy and to the political hierarchy. Training of foreign law enforcement personnel constitutes a major part of such endeavors. The Department of State funds anti-narcotics law enforcement training programs for foreign personnel from more than 70 countries. In addition, the Department of State provides host country anti-narcotics personnel with a wide range of equipment, and U.S. Drug Enforcement Administration (DEA) agents regularly assist foreign police forces in their efforts to destabilize trafficking networks. U.S. efforts to promote effective law enforcement against narcotics traffickers also include suggestions to nations on means to strengthen their legal and judicial systems. Finally, an important judicial tool against drug dealers is extradition. Since 1997, the U.S. government has successfully extradited at least 14 major traffickers from Colombia to face justice in the United States.

International Cooperation

Essentially all elements of U.S. international narcotics control strategy require international cooperation. By use of diplomatic initiatives, both bilateral and multilateral, the Department of State encourages and assists nations to reduce cultivation, production, and trafficking in illicit drugs. These bilateral agreements and international conventions have thus far been largely ineffective in reversing the growth of international narcotics trafficking, in part because they lack strong enforcement mechanisms and are not uniformly interpreted by member nations.

U.S. international narcotics control strategy also requires cooperation among governments to coordinate their border operations to interdict traffickers. To this end, the U.S. government has provided technical assistance for anti-drug programs in other countries. For FY2005, the State Department's international narcotics control budget request totaled $1.05 billion to assist programs globally, including $90.2 million for Bolivia, $115.4 million for Peru, $462.8 million for Colombia, and $25.8 million for Ecuador. Also requested was $69.4 million for interregional aviation support, to provide aircraft for anti-drug programs in other countries. The United States also participates in multilateral assistance programs through the U.N. International Drug Control Program and actively enlists the aid and support of other governments for narcotics control projects. The U.N. currently assists 67 developing countries through development, law enforcement, education, treatment, and rehabilitation programs. For FY2005, the Bush Administration requested $15 million for general anticrime/anticorruption programs and $5 million for narcotics control-related contributions to international organizations; the majority of the latter constituted the U.S. voluntary contribution to the U.N. drug control program.

Sanctions/Economic Assistance

A fourth element of U.S. international narcotics control strategy involves the threat of, or application of, sanctions against drug producer or trafficker nations. These range from suspension of U.S. foreign assistance to curtailment of air transportation. Current law on International Drug Control Certification Procedures (P.L.107-228, Section 706) requires the President to submit to Congress not later than September 15 of the preceding fiscal year a report identifying each country determined to be a major drug transit or drug producing country as defined in section 481(e) of the Foreign Assistance Act of 1961. In the report the President must designate each country that has "failed demonstrably" to meet its counternarcotics obligations. Designated countries would be ineligible for foreign assistance unless the President determined that that assistance was vital to the U.S. national interest or that the country had made "substantial efforts" to improve its counternarcotics performance. Previous certification requirements had established a 30- calendar day review process in which the Congress could override the President's determinations and stop U.S. foreign aid from going to specific countries, but this process is no longer extant.

A multilateral [drug performance] evaluation mechanism (MEM) has also been established under the auspices of the Organization of American States (OAS). This mechanism is seen by many as a vehicle to undermine and facilitate abolishment of the existing U.S. sanctions-oriented unilateral certification process which is often viewed as an irritant to major illicit drug-producing countries, and which, opponents argue, does little to promote anti-drug cooperation.

U.S. sanctions policy has been augmented with programs of economic assistance to major coca producing countries (see "Use of Sanctions or Positive Incentives" and "Bush Administration Anti-Drug Strategy," below). For FY2005 the State Department requested for drug related alternative development: approximately \$124.7 million for Colombia, \$53.9 million for Peru, \$41.7 million for Bolivia and \$14.9 million for Ecuador.

On June 2, 2003, President Bush submitted to Congress a list of foreign narcotics kingpins subject to U.S. legislative efforts to deny such individuals and entities access to U.S. financial systems and to prohibit U.S. individuals and companies from doing business with these kingpins. For the first time, foreign "entities" such as the Colombia's FARC and United Self-Defense Forces (AUC) are included in the list.

Institution Development

A fifth element of U.S. international narcotics control strategy increasingly involves institution development, such as strengthening judicial and law enforcement institutions, boosting governing capacity, and assisting in developing host nation administrative infrastructures conducive to combating the illicit drug trade. Institution development includes such programs as corruption prevention, training to support the administration of justice, and financial crimes enforcement assistance.

Policy Approaches

Overview

The primary goal of U.S. international narcotics control policy is to stem the flow of foreign drugs into the United States. A number of approaches have been proposed to reshape U.S. international narcotics control policy and implement it more effectively. Whatever ideas are ultimately selected will have to consider the scope of the drug problem. It is estimated that the illicit drug trade generates as much as half of the approximately $750 billion in illegal funds laundered internationally each year. Policymakers face the challenge of deciding the appropriate level of funding required for the nation's international narcotics control efforts within the context of competing budgetary priorities.

Another challenge facing the U.S. international narcotics control efforts concerns how to implement policy most effectively. Some observers argue that current U.S. policy is fragmented and overly bilateral in nature. These analysts suggest that to achieve success, policy options must be pursued within the context of a comprehensive plan with a multilateral emphasis on implementation. For example, they point out that some studies indicate that interdiction can actually increase the economic rewards to drug traffickers by raising prices for the products they sell. They agree, however, that interdiction as part of a coordinated plan can have a strong disrupting and destabilizing effect on trafficker operations. Some analysts suggest that bilateral or unilateral U.S. policies are ill-suited for solving what is in effect a multilateral problem. They cite the need for enhancing the United Nations' ability to deal effectively with the narcotics problem and for more international and regional cooperation and consultation on international narcotics issues. Proponents of bilateral policy do not necessarily reject a more multilateral approach. They point out, however, that such multinational endeavors are intrinsically difficult to arrange, coordinate, and implement effectively.

Between 1981 and 2001 The United States spent $8.57 billion on international narcotics control, mostly in Latin America. Yet estimated potential production of South American cocaine over the period increased from 140 to 170 tons to almost 870 tons, according to State Department and other U.S. government figures. According to ONDCP's *Strategy* the average price per pure gram of cocaine in 2000 was $212, approximately half what it was in 1981, and the average purity of a gram of street cocaine was 69% higher. For heroin the price and purity respectively were 77% lower and 147% higher in 2000 than in 1981. Some analysts believe, viewing such trends, that current efforts to reduce the flow of illicit drugs into the United States have essentially failed and that other objectives, policies, programs, and priorities are needed. Four major approaches which have been suggested, in various combinations as part of an overall effort, are set out below.

Expansion of Efforts to Reduce Production at the Source

This option involves expanding efforts to reduce the volume of narcotic plants and crops produced in foreign countries before the crops' conversion into processed drugs. Illicit crops may either be eradicated or purchased (and then destroyed). Eradication of illicit crops may be accomplished by physically uprooting the plants, or by chemical or biological control agents. Development of alternative sources of income to replace peasant income lost by nonproduction of narcotic crops may be an important element of this option.

Proponents of expanded efforts to stop the production of narcotic crops and substances at the source believe that reduction of the foreign supply of drugs available is an effective means to lower levels of drug use in the United States. They argue that reduction of the supply of cocaine — the nation's top narcotics control priority — is a realistically achievable option.

Proponents of vastly expanded supply reduction options, and specifically of herbicidal crop eradication, argue that this method is the most cost-effective and efficient means of eliminating narcotic crops. They maintain that, coupled with intensified law enforcement, such programs will succeed since it is easier to locate and destroy crops in the field than to locate subsequently processed drugs on smuggling routes or on the streets of U.S. cities. Put differently, a kilogram of cocaine hydrochloride is far more difficult to detect than the 300 to 500 kilograms of coca leaf that are required to make that same kilogram. Also, because crops constitute the cheapest link in the narcotics chain, producers will devote fewer economic resources to prevent their detection than to concealing more expensive and refined forms of the product.

In addition, eradication successes have been recorded in individual countries. According to INL's *International Narcotics Control Strategy Report* of 2002, for example, Pakistan has reduced opium cultivation by more than 95% since 1995 and Taliban-controlled Afghanistan accomplished a similar feat in a single year, eliminating more than 62,000 hectares or 97% of the opium crop between 2000 and 2001. However, INL reports that cultivation surged beginning in 2002 under the relatively weak Afghan political authority that succeeded the Taliban, suggesting that an effective central government presence in drug crop areas is critical to the success of eradication projects.

Opponents of expanded supply reduction policy generally question whether reduction of the foreign supply of narcotic drugs is achievable and whether it would have a meaningful impact on levels of illicit drug use in the United States. They argue that aerial spraying in Colombia has failed to contain the spread of coca cultivation and point to drug syndicates' moving into opium poppy cultivation in Colombia and (more recently) Peru. Total Andean cultivation, in fact, has remained relatively stable in the past decade despite U.S. efforts, and because farmers are finding ways to increase productivity per unit of land according to INL figures. Critics also suggest that even if the supply of foreign drugs destined for the U.S. market could be dramatically reduced, U.S. consumers would simply switch to consumption of domestically-grown or synthetic drug substitutes. Thus, they maintain, the ultimate solution to the U.S. drug problem is wiping out the domestic market for illicit drugs, not trying to eliminate the supply in source countries.

Some also fear that environmental damage will result from herbicides. As an alternative, they urge development, research, and funding of programs designed to develop and employ biological control agents such as coca-destroying insects and fungi that do not harm other plants. Others argue that intensified eradication will push the drug crop frontier and the attendant polluting affects of narcotics industries farther into ecologically sensitive jungle areas, with little or no decrease in net cultivation. In addition, reports have surfaced in Colombia of toxic effects of herbicides on legal crops and on the health of animals and humans, although the veracity of such accounts is debated.

Others question whether a global policy of simultaneous crop control is politically feasible since many areas in the world will always be beyond U.S. control and influence. Such critics refer to continuously shifting sources of supply, or the so-called "balloon syndrome": when squeezed in one place, it pops up in another. Nevertheless, many point out that the number of large suitable growth areas is finite, and by focusing simultaneously at major production areas, substantial reductions can be achieved if adequate funding is provided.

Some also question the value of supply reduction measures since world production and supply of illicit drugs vastly exceeds world demand, making it unlikely that the supply surplus could be reduced sufficiently to affect the ready availability of illicit narcotics in the

U.S. market. Such analysts also suggest that even if worldwide supply were reduced dramatically, the effects would be felt primarily in other nation's drug markets. The U.S. market, they argue, would be the last to experience supply shortfalls, because U.S. consumers pay higher prices and because U.S. dollars are a preferred narco-currency.

Political and Economic Tradeoffs

Some suggest that expanded and effective efforts to reduce production of illicit narcotics at the source will be met by active and violent opposition from a combination of trafficker, political, and economic groups. In some nations, such as Colombia, traffickers have achieved a status comparable to "a state within a state." In others, allegations of drug-related corruption have focused on high-level officials in the military and federal police, as well as heads of state; In Mexico, according to a *Washington Times* report, smugglers often are protected by heavily-armed Mexican military troops and police who "have been paid handsomely to escort the drug traffickers and their illicit shipments across the border and into the United States." In addition, some traffickers have aligned themselves with terrorist and insurgent groups, and have reportedly funded political candidates and parties, pro-narcotic peasant workers and trade union groups, and high visibility popular public works projects to cultivate public support through a "Robin Hood" image. Because some constituencies that benefit economically from coca are well armed, if the United States were successful in urging foreign governments to institute widespread use of chemical/biological control agents, cooperating host governments could well face strong domestic political challenge and violent opposition from affected groups. Heavy military protection, at a minimum, would be required for those spraying or otherwise eradicating drug crops.

Some critics have argued, with respect to Colombia, that eradication campaigns can have the unintended effect of aggravating the country's ongoing civil conflict. Since Colombia's guerrilla groups pose as advocates of growers, spraying may broaden support for such groups, thereby contradicting the objectives of the government's counterinsurgency efforts in the affected zones. Such observers believe that Colombia's enforcement priorities should shift to targeting critical nodes in transportation and refining and, to the extent possible, sealing off traffic routes to and from the main coca producing zones. The argument is made that interdiction can disrupt internal markets for coca derivatives and that, compared to eradication, it imposes fewer direct costs on peasant producers and generates less political unrest.

For some countries, production of illicit narcotics and the narcotics trade has become an economic way of life that provides a subsistence level of income to large numbers of people from whom those who rule draw their legitimacy. Crop reduction campaigns seek to displace such income and those workers engaged in its production. In this regard, these campaigns may threaten real economic and political dangers for the governments of nations with marginal economic growth. Consequently, some analysts argue that the governments of such low-income countries cannot be expected to launch major crop reduction programs without the substitute income to sustain those whose income depends on drug production.

Use of Sanctions or Positive Incentives

Those promoting expansion of efforts to reduce production at the source face the challenge of instituting programs that effectively reduce production of narcotic crops and production of refined narcotics without creating unmanageable economic and political crises for target countries. A major area of concern of such policymakers is to achieve an effective balance between the "carrot" and the "stick" approach in U.S. relations with major illicit narcotics-producing and transit countries.

Proponents of a sanctions policy linking foreign aid and trade benefits to U.S. international narcotics objectives argue against "business as usual" with countries that permit illicit drug trafficking, production, or laundering of drug profits. They assert that this policy includes a moral dimension and that drug production and trafficking is wrong, and that the United States should not associate with countries involved in it. Such analysts maintain that U.S. aid and trade sanctions can provide the needed leverage for nations to reduce production of illicit crops and their involvement in other drug related activities. They argue that both the moral stigma of being branded as uncooperative and the threat of economic sanctions prod many otherwise uncooperative nations into action. They further stress that trade sanctions would be likely to provide a highly effective lever as most developing countries depend on access to U.S. markets.

Opponents of a sanctions policy linking aid and trade to U.S. international narcotics objectives argue that sanctions may have an undesirable effect on the political and economic stability of target countries, making them all the more dependent on the drug trade for income; that sanctions have little impact because many countries are not dependant on U.S. aid; that sanctions historically have little effect unless they are multilaterally imposed; and that sanctions are arbitrary in nature, hurt national pride in the foreign country, and are seen in many countries as an ugly manifestation of "Yankee imperialism." Finally, an increasing number of analysts suggest that if sanctions are to be fully effective, they should be used in conjunction with additional positive incentives (subject perhaps to an expanded certification/approval process) to foster anti-drug cooperation.

Alternatively, some suggest positive incentives instead of sanctions. They believe that narcotics-producing countries must be motivated either to refrain from growing illicit crops, or to permit the purchase or destruction of these crops by government authorities. Many argue that since short term economic stability of nations supplying illegal drugs may depend upon the production and sale of illicit narcotics, it is unrealistic to expect such nations to limit their drug-related activities meaningfully without an alternative source of income. The House Appropriations Committee report on the 1993 foreign operations appropriations bill suggested that when it comes to narcotics related economic development "there is too little emphasis in either actual funding or policy."

It has been suggested by some analysts that a massive foreign aid effort — a so-called "mini-Marshall Plan" — is the only feasible method of persuading developing nations to curb their production of narcotic crops. Such a plan would involve a multilateral effort with the participation of the United States, Europe, Japan, Australia, other industrialized nations susceptible to the drug problem, and the rich oil producing nations. The thrust of such a plan would be to promote economic development, replacing illicit cash crops with other marketable alternatives. Within the framework of such a plan, crops could be purchased or else destroyed by herbicidal spraying or biological control agents while substitute crops and markets are developed and assured.

Any such program would be coupled with rigid domestic law enforcement and penalties for non-compliance. Thus, it could require a U.S. commitment of substantially increased enforcement assets to be used against both growers and traffickers, and some observers assert it might require direct U.S. military involvement at the request of the host country. Significant coercion might be required, since drug crops typically produce a better cash flow than licit crops grown in the same region. For example, in Afghanistan a hectare of opium earns 30 to 45 times as much as a hectare of wheat at prevailing prices ($13,000 compared to $300 to $400). Even if the international community bought up the entire Afghan opium crop, the temptation to plant new opium could prove irresistible to farmers.

Critics have concerns regarding positive incentive concepts. They warn of the precedent of appearing to pay "protection" compensation, that is, providing an incentive for economically disadvantaged countries to go into the drug export business. They also warn of the open-ended cost of agricultural development programs and of extraterritorial police intervention. Finding markets for viable alternative crops is yet another major constraint. Some experts argue that typical conditions of drug crop zones, such as geographical remoteness, marginal soils and, in certain countries, extreme insecurity, tend to limit prospects for legal commercial agriculture. According to one report, the soils in Colombia's Putumayo Department, an important center of coca cultivation, are simply too poor to support the number of people currently farming in the province if all converted to growing legal crops. Such observers believe that a more promising strategy is to foster development of the legal economy in other locales, including urban settings, in order to attract people away from areas that have a comparative advantage in coca or opium production. In the view of these analysts, the best "substitute crop" for coca or opium could well be an assembly plant producing electronic goods or automobiles for the international market.

Expansion of Interdiction and Enforcement Activities to Disrupt Supply Lines/Expanding the Role of the Military

Drug supply line interdiction is both a foreign and domestic issue. Many argue that the United States should intensify law enforcement activities designed to disrupt the transit of illicit narcotics as early in the production/transit chain as possible — well before the drugs reach the streets of the United States. This task is conceded to be very difficult because the United States is the world's greatest trading nation with vast volumes of imports daily flowing in through hundreds of sea, air, and land entry facilities, and its systems have been designed to facilitate human and materials exchange. This has led some analysts to suggest that the military should assume a more active role in anti-drug activities.

Some in Congress, in the late 1980s and prior to appropriations for FY1994, had urged an expanded role for the military in the "war on drugs." The idea of using the military is not novel. Outside the United States, U.S. military personnel have been involved in training and transporting foreign anti-narcotics personnel since 1983. Periodically, there have also been calls for multilateral military strikes against trafficking operations, as well as increased use of U.S. elite forces in preemptive strikes against drug fields and trafficker enclaves overseas.

The military's role in narcotics interdiction was expanded by the FY1990-1991 National Defense Authorization Act. The conference report (H.Rept. 100-989) concluded that the Department of Defense (DOD) can and should play a major role in narcotics interdiction. Congress, in FY1989 and FY1990-1991 authorization acts, required DOD to promptly provide civilian law enforcement agencies with relevant drug-related intelligence; charged the President to direct that command, control, communications, and intelligence networks dedicated to drug control be integrated by DOD into an effective network; restricted direct participation by military personnel in civilian law enforcement activities to those authorized by law; permitted the military to transport civilian law enforcement personnel outside the U.S. land area; expanded the National Guard's role in drug interdiction activities; and authorized additional $300 million for DOD and National Guard drug interdiction activities.

DOD's requested drug budget total for FY2005 was 852.7 million as compared to $908.6 million for FY2004 and as compared to $905.9 million for FY2003.

Despite the military's obvious ability to support drug law enforcement organizations, questions remain as to the overall effectiveness of a major military role in narcotics interdiction. Proponents of substantially increasing the military's role in supporting civilian law enforcement narcotics interdiction activity argue that narcotics trafficking poses a national security threat to the United States; that only the military is equipped and has the resources to counter powerful trafficking organizations; and that counter drug support provides the military with beneficial, realistic training.

In contrast, opponents argue that drug interdiction is a law enforcement mission, it is not a military mission; that drug enforcement is an unconventional war which the military is ill-equipped to fight; that a drug enforcement role detracts from readiness; that a drug enforcement role exposes the military to corruption; that it is unwise public policy to require the U.S. military to operate against U.S. citizens; and that the use of the military may have serious political and diplomatic repercussions overseas. Moreover, some in the military remain concerned about an expanded role, seeing themselves as possible scapegoats for policies that have failed, or are likely to fail.

Expansion of Efforts to Reduce Worldwide Demand

Another commonly proposed option is to increase policy emphasis on development and implementation of programs worldwide that aim at increasing public intolerance for illicit drug use. Such programs, through information, technical assistance, and training in prevention and treatment, would emphasize the health dangers of drug use, as well as the danger to regional and national stability. The State Department's Office of Public Diplomacy and Public Affairs and AID currently support modest efforts in this area. Some believe these programs should be increased and call for a more active role for the United Nations and other international agencies in development and implementation of such demand reduction programs.

Expansion of Economic Disincentives for Illicit Drug Trafficking

Proponents of this approach say that the major factor in the international drug market is not the product, but the profit. Thus, they stress, international efforts to reduce the flow of drugs into the United States must identify means to seize and otherwise reduce assets and profits generated by the drug trade. Some critics point out the challenges of tracking, separating out and confiscating criminal assets. These include the huge volume of all international electronic transfers — more than $2 trillion each day — and the movement of much illegal money outside of formal banking channels (through hawala-type chains of money brokers).

Policymakers pursuing this option must decide whether laws in countries where they exert influence are too lenient on financial institutions, such as banks and brokerage houses, which knowingly facilitate financial transactions of traffickers. If the answer is "yes," national leaders might then take concerted action to promote harsher criminal sanctions penalizing the movement of money generated by drug sales, including revocation of licenses of institutions regularly engaging in such practices. Finally, those supporting this option favor increased efforts to secure greater international cooperation on financial investigations related to money laundering of narcotics profits, including negotiation of mutual legal assistance treaties (MLATs).

THE GEORGE W. BUSH ADMINISTRATION'S ANTI-DRUG STRATEGY

The direction of drug policy under President George W. Bush does not appear to be an immediate top foreign policy priority for the Administration. To date, issues of international terrorism and homeland security appear to command more attention. However, Bush administration officials are beginning to portray Colombia's counter-insurgency campaign as part of the broader worldwide campaign against terrorism. While Congress has stipulated that U.S. military aid to Colombia be dedicated to fighting drugs, support is reportedly growing in Congress and the Administration for providing direct support to Colombia's efforts to rein in the rebel groups. The extent of any such support — and whether it might involve the use of American combat forces — remains to be determined.

On or about February 23, 2005, the White House released its annual National Drug Control Strategy, [http://www.whitehousedrugpolicy.gov/publications/policy/ndcs05/]. Central to the international component of the strategy is disrupting the operations of drug traffickers "including destroying the economic basis of the cocaine production business in South America by fumigating the coca crop, seizing enormous and unsustainable amounts of cocaine from transporters, and selectively targeting major [drug] organization heads for law enforcement action and, ultimately, extradition and prosecution in the United States."

Possible issues of concern to Congress relating to international drug control policy include the following:

(1) Can the Plan Colombia and the Andean Regional Initiative as currently envisioned have a meaningful impact on reducing drug shipments to the U.S. or in reducing the current level of violence and instability in Colombia? To what degree can a counter-drug plan which does not aim to deal a decisive blow to insurgent operations in Colombia be expected to meaningfully curb drug production and violence there?

(2) To what degree might a more regional approach to the drug problem in Colombia prove more effective and how might such an expanded initiative be funded?

(3) How does U.S. involvement in anti-drug efforts in the Andean nations affect other aspects of American foreign policy in the region, and in Latin America generally? Does a concentration on drug-related issues obscure more fundamental issues of stability, governance, poverty , and democracy (i.e., to what degree are drugs a major cause, or result, of the internal problems of certain Latin American countries)? Might U.S. pursuit of drug control objectives conflict in certain ways with efforts to resolve

Colombia's ongoing civil conflict, for instance by alienating large rural constituencies in contested regions of the country?

(4) In the case of Colombia and other nations where insurgents are heavily involved in the drug trade, how can the United States ensure that U.S. military aid and equipment is in fact used to combat drug traffickers and cartels, rather than diverted for use against domestic political opposition or used as an instrument of human rights violations? How great is the risk that such diversions could take place, and is the degree of risk worth the possible gains to be made against drug production and trafficking?

(5) How extensive is drug-related corruption in the armed forces and police of the Andean nations? What impact might such corruption have on the effectiveness of U.S. training and assistance to these forces?

(6) Will an active role for the military in counter-narcotics support to foreign nations (i.e. Colombia) result in U.S. casualties? If so, is there an exit strategy and at what point, if at all, might presidential actions fall within the scope of the War Powers Resolution; that is, does the dispatch of military advisers to help other governments combat drug traffickers constitute the introduction of armed forces "into hostilities or into situations where imminent involvement in hostilities is clearly indicated by the circumstances"? (The War Powers Resolution requires the President to report such an introduction to Congress, and to withdraw the forces within 60 to 90 days unless authorized to remain by Congress.)

(7) Will the evolving strategy under the Bush Administration produce better results than previous strategies in reducing illicit drug use in the United States and in supporting U.S. narcotics and other foreign policy goals overseas? Is a proper balance of resources being devoted to domestic (the demand side) vs. foreign (the supply side) components of an overall national anti-drug strategy? Are efforts to reduce the foreign supply level futile while domestic U.S. demand remains high? Are efforts to reduce domestic demand fruitless as long as foreign supplies can enter the country with relative impunity?

(8) To what extent will the Administration's current priority in fighting terrorism affect implementation of antidrug policy? Has repositioning of equipment and resources to improve U.S. defenses against acts of terrorism, for example the shift of Coast Guard vessels from the eastern Pacific and the Caribbean to perform coastal patrols and port security functions, lowered defenses with respect to curbing drug flows? On the flip side of the issue, to what degree has committing anti-drug resources to support anti-terrorism objectives significantly enhanced the effectiveness of counterterrorism efforts?

(9) To what extent should U.S. military assistance programs in Colombia target groups that use narcotics operations to finance terrorist activities (including leftist guerrillas and paramilitaries), as opposed to the narcotics trafficking infrastructure itself?

Certification Status

In December 2001, legislation on "Modifications to the Annual Drug Certification Procedures" in the Foreign Operations, Export Financing and Related Programs Appropriations Act (P.L. 107-115, Section 591) was enacted that effectively waived the drug certification requirements for FY2002. It required the President to withhold assistance from the countries most remiss in meeting their international drug-fighting obligations, but permitted the President to determine what countries to put in the "worst offending" category and (under specified conditions) to provide U.S. foreign assistance to a designated country. Legislation on "International Drug Control Certification Procedures" in the Foreign Relations Authorization Act of September 2002 (P.L. 107-228) extended the waiver to FY2003, and subsequently provided for a *de facto* ongoing waiver. Such changes may reflect the fact that spokesmen from many countries have complained for years about the unilateral and noncooperative nature of the drug certification requirements, and have urged the United States to end the process or at least to replace it with multilateral evaluation mechanisms. Acting under this legislation, President Bush made designations on a transitional basis for FY2002 and FY2003, and then made designations on the designated date for FY2004 and FY2005.

On February 23, 2002, the President designated Afghanistan, Burma and Haiti as having "failed demonstrably" in counter-narcotics efforts, but granted national interest waivers to Haiti and Afghanistan under the new government.

On January 31, 2003, he designated Burma, Guatemala, and Haiti, but granted national interest waivers to Guatemala and Haiti.

On September 15, 2003, he designated Burma and Haiti, but granted a national interest waiver to Haiti.

On September 15, 2004, he removed Thailand from the list of major illicit drug transit or producing countries, and designated Burma as having "failed demonstrably" in counter-narcotics efforts.

On September 15, 2005, President Bush issued the annual determination that lists major illicit drug producing or drug transit countries. The President identified 20 countries to be included on the so-called "majors list": Afghanistan, The Bahamas, Bolivia, Brazil, Burma, Colombia, Dominican Republic, Ecuador, Guatemala, Haiti, India, Jamaica, Laos, Mexico, Nigeria, Pakistan, Panama, Paraguay, Peru, and Venezuela. Burma was again singled out a county which had "failed demonstrably" to adhere to its obligations under international counternarcotics agreements. Venezuela was singled out as well as having failed demonstrably, but was granted a national interests waiver exempting it from U.S. aid and trade sanctions and possible access to loans from international financial institutions. China and Vietnam were removed from the list.

Plan Colombia

On July 13, 2000, U.S. support for Plan Colombia was signed into law (P.L. 106-246). Included was $1.3 billion in emergency supplemental appropriations in equipment, supplies, and other counter narcotics aid primarily for the Colombian military. The plan aimed to curb trafficking activity and reduce coca cultivation in Colombia by 50% over five years. Though focused on military and law enforcement initiatives, Plan components included helping the Colombian Government control its territory; strengthening democratic institutions; promoting economic development; protecting human rights; and providing humanitarian assistance. Included as well was $148 million for Andean regional drug interdiction and alternative development programs. Supporters of the Plan argued that without enhanced U.S. aid, Colombia risks disintegration into smaller autonomous political units — some controlled by leftist or rightist guerrilla groups that are heavily involved in drug trafficking and violent crime -for- profit activity. Other observers cautioned that narcotics-related assistance to Colombia can, at best, produce serious reductions in illicit drug production only within a multi-year timeframe. They warn against enhanced U.S. involvement in a conflict where clear- cut victory is elusive and to a large degree dependent on reduction of the so far intractable U.S. domestic appetite for illicit drugs. Still others warned of the so-called "spillover" effect of Plan Colombia on neighboring nations such as Ecuador where narco-linked insurgents and paramilitaries increasingly operate. For additional data on issues relating to Plan Colombia see CRS Report RL32774, *Plan Colombia, a Progress Report*, CRS Report RL30541, *Colombia: Plan Colombia Legislation and Assistance (FY2000-FY2001)*, and CRS Report RS20494, *Ecuador: International Narcotics Control Issues.*

Andean Regional Initiative

In April 2001, the Bush Administration unveiled an Andean Regional Initiative (ARI) as a successor to Plan Colombia, requesting $882 million for the program. Of these funds approximately 45% percent were intended for Colombia and the remainder for six regional neighbors of Colombia (Bolivia, Brazil, Ecuador, Panama, Peru, and Venezuela) affected by drug trafficking and drug- related violence. By contrast, Colombia received two-thirds of the funds allocated under Plan Colombia. In December 2001, Congress passed the Foreign Operations Appropriations bill for FY2002, allocating $783 million to the ARI. Of the $783 million, 49% were provided to Colombia and the rest to the other six countries. Of the Colombia funds, 36% were earmarked for economic and social and governance purposes and 64% for counternarcotics and security, a ratio largely reflecting the enforcement orientation of Plan Colombia. In the case of Peru and Bolivia, the economic and social share was significantly higher — 61% in both countries. For FY2003, the Bush Administration requested $980 million in ARI funding, of which 55% was for Colombia. The ARI request for FY2004 totaled $990.7 million of which $463 million was for State Department Andean Counterdrug Initiative (ACI) programs for Colombia. For FY2005, Congress appropriated $731 million for the ACI (of which $466.5 was for Colombia) and an additional $106.5 million for Foreign Military Financing (FMF) funding.

INDEX

A

B

D

E

F

I

J

N

O

P

T

U

V

W

X

Y

Z